1992

BIOMEDICAL POLITICS

Kathi E. Hanna, *Editor*

Division of Health Sciences Policy
Committee to Study Biomedical Decision Making

INSTITUTE OF MEDICINE

NATIONAL ACADEMY PRESS
Washington, D.C. 1991

NATIONAL ACADEMY PRESS · 2101 Constitution Avenue, N.W.· Washington, D.C. 20418

NOTICE: The project that is the subject of this report was approved by the Governing Board of the National Research Council, whose members are drawn from the councils of the National Academy of Sciences, the National Academy of Engineering, and the Institute of Medicine. The members of the committee responsible for the report were chosen for their special competences and with regard for appropriate balance.

This report has been reviewed by a group other than the authors according to procedures approved by a Report Review Committee consisting of members of the National Academy of Sciences, the National Academy of Engineering, and the Institute of Medicine.

The National Academy of Sciences is a private, nonprofit, self-perpetuating society of distinguished scholars engaged in scientific and engineering research, dedicated to the furtherance of science and technology and to their use for the general welfare. Upon the authority of the charter granted to it by the Congress in 1863, the Academy has a mandate that requires it to advise the federal government on scientific and technical matters. Dr. Frank Press is president of the National Academy of Sciences.

The Institute of Medicine was established in 1970 by the National Academy of Sciences to secure the services of eminent members of appropriate professions in the examination of policy matters pertaining to the health of the public. The Institute acts under the responsibility given to the National Academy of Sciences by its congressional charter to be an adviser to the federal government and, upon its own initiative, to identify issues of medical care, research, and education. Dr. Samuel O. Thier is president of the Institute of Medicine.

Support for this activity was provided by the Howard Hughes Medical Institute. The opinions and conclusions expressed here are those of the authors and do not necessarily represent the views of the Howard Hughes Medical Institute, the National Academy of Sciences, or any of their constituent parts.

Library of Congress Cataloging-in-Publication Data
Biomedical politics / Kathi E. Hanna, editor ; Division of Health
    Sciences Policy, Committee to Study Biomedical Decision Making,
    Institute of Medicine.
          p.   cm.
      Includes bibliographical references and index.
      ISBN 0-309-04486-3
      1. Medical policy–Case studies. 2. Health planning–Case
    studies. I. Hanna, Kathi E. II. Institute of Medicine (U.S.).
    Committee to Study Biomedical Decision Making.
      [DNLM: 1. Decision Making. 2. Health Policy–United States.
    3. Politics–United States. WA 540 AA1 B52]
    RA393.B48 1991
    362. 1–dc20
    DNLM/DLC
    for Library of Congress   91-18394
                                    CIP

Printed in the United States of America

The serpent has been a symbol of long life, healing, and knowledge among almost all cultures and religions since the beginning of recorded history. The image adopted as a logotype by the Institute of Medicine is based on a relief carving from ancient Greece, now held by the Staatlichemuseen in Berlin.

COMMITTEE TO STUDY BIOMEDICAL DECISION MAKING

CARL W. GOTTSCHALK (*Chair*), Kenan Professor of Medicine and Physiology, Department of Medicine, University of North Carolina, Chapel Hill, North Carolina

PAUL BERG, Director, Beckman Center for Molecular and Genetic Medicine and Willson Professor of Biochemistry, Stanford University, Stanford, California

PETER F. CARPENTER, Visiting Scholar, Center for Biomedical Ethics, Stanford University, Stanford, California

LEON EISENBERG, Presley Professor and Chairman, Department of Social Medicine, Harvard Medical School, Boston, Massachusetts

WALTER HARRELSON, Distinguished Professor of Hebrew Bible, emeritus, The Divinity School, Vanderbilt University, Nashville, Tennessee

WILLIAM HUBBARD, Jr., Retired President, The Upjohn Company

WILLIAM R. KENNEDY, Professor of Neurology, University of Minnesota Health Center, Minneapolis, Minnesota

PATRICIA A. KING, Professor of Law, Georgetown University Law Center, Washington, D.C.

ERNEST R. MAY, Charles Warren Professor of History, Kennedy School of Government, Harvard University, Cambridge, Massachusetts

DOROTHY NELKIN, Professor, Department of Sociology and Affiliated Professor, School of Law, New York University, New York, New York

STANLEY JOEL REISER, Griff T. Ross Professor of Humanities and Technology in Health Care, University of Texas Health Science Center, Houston, Texas

PAUL SLOVIC, President, Decision Research and Professor of Psychology, University of Oregon, Eugene, Oregon

STAFF

RUTH ELLEN BULGER, Division Director, Division of Health Sciences Policy

KATHI E. HANNA, Study Director

CATHARINE CHETNEY, Senior Secretary

LOUISE GILLIS, Senior Secretary

LEAH MAZADE, Staff Editor

SHELLEY MEYERS, Senior Secretary

APRIL POWERS, Senior Secretary

Preface

Scientists like to believe that they operate in a rational world, one in which interpretations and predictions are based on objective data and evaluated through a systematic process. While some question whether these suppositions hold true for science, they certainly fall apart when science becomes a public issue, as it so often does in biomedicine. Decisions about how to proceed with the funding, ordering, and use of biomedical research are made in the public arena. The interests of scientists, regulators, politicians, patients, practitioners, and interest groups converge and often clash. These clashes may slow the progression of science and medicine while simultaneously advancing moral, ethical, or democratic causes. Sometimes, the interests of all groups can be advanced. In other cases, rigid deadlock occurs with little movement in any direction. Is there a better way by which to deal with controversial biomedical issues confronting us today? Can we better anticipate the forces that will emerge on the various sides of an issue, or are we destined to muddle through and make policy incrementally and contentiously?

These were some of the questions posed in the summer of 1989 to our committee, a group of individuals with diverse backgrounds and experiences. We were given the task of using case studies as a first step toward answering some of these questions. This document is the result of our efforts. As we chose the topics for case study we were mindful of the fact that we were exploring possibilities, not necessarily testing hypotheses. We knew we needed to understand in great detail how several decisions were made before we could attempt to postulate guidelines or prescriptions for better decision making. What we found was both illuminating and complex. The politics of decision making are easily described but difficult to predict. Each decision or set of decisions faces different paths, publics, and constraints, as the cases in this book so beautifully demonstrate.

In our deliberations, we stopped short of recommending a normative approach to decision making. Case study methodology militates against such an approach. What we chose to do was define areas of research to be examined that would move the study of decision making to a more analytical level. Our greatest contribution may well be providing six individuals the opportunity to tell compelling stories about how we arrive at public biomedical decisions.

ACKNOWLEDGMENTS

The committee thanks all who contributed to its work. We greatly appreciate the opportunity provided by the Howard Hughes Medical Institute to investigate the process of biomedical decision making. The committee is grateful to the six individuals who prepared and presented the case studies. These studies were the information base for the committee's deliberations.

We wish especially to thank and to acknowledge the contributions of Kathi E. Hanna, the study director and editor. With the able assistance and advice of Ruth E. Bulger, division director, she planned and organized the meetings, analyzed the data, edited drafts, and prepared the Introduction and Conclusions sections. The project was also assisted by the excellent support work of Catharine Chetney, Shelley Meyers, Louise Gillis, and April Powers, and the thorough copyediting of Leah Mazade.

Carl W. Gottschalk, *Chair*
Committee to Study Biomedical Decision Making

Contents

Introduction

Should scientists be allowed to pursue research on treatment of Parkinson's disease using fetal tissue from induced abortions?

Should American women be denied access to a nonsurgical abortifacient because some groups in the society feel its use is immoral?

Should the U.S. Congress make decisions about large-scale biomedical research projects that might affect the availability of funds for research in other areas?

Should scientists be the first to police and regulate their own work for potential safety risks?

Should federal reimbursement for and access to treatment be provided for victims of end-stage renal disease when other terminally ill patients are denied this entitlement?

Should patients terminally ill with acquired immune deficiency syndrome (AIDS) be allowed to take experimental drugs before their safety and effectiveness have been thoroughly assessed?

1

At one time it was accepted that the answers to these questions lay in the domains of science and medicine, and they would have been largely debated in those arenas. Today, biological and medical research have become a focus of public scrutiny. For each of the above questions, any public opinion poll would probably show a multitude of responses, including a healthy degree of uncertainty. Even among those questions for which a majority in the U.S. society can agree on the proper, moral response, organized vocal minorities can have considerable influence on how the debate is resolved.

There are many "publics" in any debate. In biomedical research decisions, the public can take the form of voters, taxpayers, special interest groups, community organizations, and patients. In the context of this report, the public refers to any group typically outside the process of biomedical research and its medical applications—that is, laypersons. When these groups have a say in what should and should not be allowed in biomedical research and practice, deciding what should be done involves listening, negotiating, advocating, judging, and implementing. This process of weighing alternatives is the process of decision making. When it is done in public, in the light of the competing values and interests of American pluralism, it is called policymaking. How the policy process is conducted has an effect on the outcome.

It is easy, with hindsight, to identify successful versus failed decisions. In the absence of outcomes, and when there is no precedent, as is often the case in biomedicine, predicting what is a correct decision becomes exceedingly difficult. Therefore, a useful strategy for examining decision making is to separate outcome from the quality of the decision process.

In recent years, numerous mechanisms have been established at the federal, state, and institutional levels to define, review, and regulate the application of biomedical advances and the content of biomedical research. In addition, various quantitative methods (e.g., use of indicators, cost-benefit and cost-effectiveness analyses, surveys of need, evaluation research, policy analysis, social experimentation) have been developed to help decision makers make better decisions. Some of these analytical methods and mechanisms have worked as intended; others have failed to produce desired results, and still others require more time before their adequacy can be judged.

The decision-making process is the focus of this report. Examining the way discourse proceeds among all affected parties in a policy debate may shed light on how the decision was made and could provide clues as to how similar decisions might best be debated in the future. It is not the purpose of this effort to judge whether the decisions described in the following cases were proper or improper. Rather, the goal is better understanding so that appropriate questions may be asked in the future when difficult decisions must be made.

This exercise does not presume to be scientific in that it produces specific results that are reproducible or even testable. The cases in this text were chosen because they so precisely reflect the social and political mechanisms used in democracy to decide and set policy. The complexities of the decisions described bear the message of democracy: it is a difficult and sometimes uneasy way to conduct a nation's business.

In 1987 the Howard Hughes Medical Institute (HHMI) awarded the Institute of Medicine (IOM) an endowment grant to develop a program of studies that would (1) identify fields of biomedical research that are candidates for accelerated development; (2) identify mechanisms that could facilitate the translation of basic biological discoveries into new health care technologies; and (3) anticipate the legal, ethical, and social issues that attend new technologies. This report is one of several IOM responses to the HHMI charge that focuses specifically on the processes by which decisions are made regarding advances in biomedical science. Early in 1989 the IOM formed the Committee to Study Biomedical Decision Making. Its membership is comprised of clinicians, researchers, industrialists, a theologian, an attorney, a historian, a sociologist, and a behavioral scientist.

The historical case study was chosen as the methodology for this effort, with the cases serving as prototypes for appropriate or inappropriate strategies for decision making. Case study methodology provides a mechanism for using hindsight to identify ways to improve future performance rather than to render a verdict on any individual or group (Neustadt and May, 1986). On issues as contentious as abortion, debates over principles, morality, and rights are argued on the level of high theory, much to the confusion of practical and possible outcomes (Jonsen and Toulmin, 1988). The zealots on each side of the debate, as in other issues, tend to concentrate on universal and invariable principles, as if these principles were exhaustive and authoritative. Rules and maxims are not necessarily helpful for making decisions when the action to be taken is marginal or even ambiguous. One finds that they might apply to certain situations quite directly but to others only marginally, making decisions difficult and full of conflict. Particularly controversial actions must be considered in their context and not judged against an arbitrary set of rules.

Cases, therefore, permit us to set problems in context and deal with them individually and on their own terms. Ideally, the cases sug-

TABLE 1 Criteria for Case Selection

Category	Criteria
Factors of contention	Ethical/religious concerns
	Equity and allocation
	Risk or perceived risk
	Fear of social control
	Conflicting world view
Decision maker	Public or citizen groups
	Legislators
	Regulators
	Scientists/universities
	Third party payers
	Clinicians
	Industry
	Funding agency
	Commission
	Courts
	Church
Stage of diffusion	Research and development
	Trial and approval
	Dissemination
	Use and acceptance
	Reimbursement
	Evaluation
Dualities	Consults and tribunes
	Expertise and ignorance
Outcome	Successful
	Uncertain
	Failure
	Yet to come

gest, at the margin, how the public's biomedical business might be better done in the future. Case study excuses us from addressing issues on the level of high theory and general principles by injecting a large measure of pragmatism. Indeed, democracy in America seems to preclude the development of fixed universal laws and immutable principles, and attempts to set policy on such assumptions tend to create irresoluble debate. The tales told in the following pages demonstrate that, as much as some would like to believe it so, there is little in modern life that is eternal and invariable.

The IOM committee was immediately faced with the logistics of conducting this project and with two tasks in particular: first, to develop a taxonomy for case selection that would meet the needs of the project's mission; and second, to develop a morphology for case construction. The cases were selected based on a set of criteria (Table 1) that constitute characteristic facets of a biomedical policy problem. The committee spent considerable time developing a framework from which to choose the cases to ensure that the complexities of decision making were comprehensively illustrated. The committee agreed that the cases should be considered in the aggregate and that no case, standing alone, could possibly fulfill all of the criteria. Thus, the reader is encouraged to read all of the cases because as a set they illustrate the texture of decision making in the field of health sciences research. To ensure that the six cases collectively encompassed the selection criteria, a matrix was developed to score candidate cases, and the six that best filled the cells of the matrix were chosen for the project. Many additional cases were considered and might have served equally well. They included the use of animals in biomedical research, deinstitutionalization of the mentally ill, vaccine development, and the use of maternal serum alpha-fetoprotein test kits. There are, and have been, numerous contentious issues in biomedical research. The cases described in this text are by no means exhaustively inclusive of the many issues raised by advancing technology.

The committee organized the criteria in five categories.

1. The basis of the disagreement, or factors of contention. Was the problem a problem because of ethical or religious differences, inequities or misallocations, risk or perceived risk, fear of social control, or conflicting philosophical or world views? Decisions might be made differently and by different mechanisms depending on the nature of the contention. None of these factors are mutually exclusive—just convenient ways of dissecting the problem.

2. The decision maker. Presumably the process and outcome of decision making will differ depending on the stature, authority, and power of the person or persons making the decision.

3. The point in the diffusion process at which the innovation entered the policy arena. For example, innovations in the research and development stage are subject to different sets of decisions and decision makers than innovations that have entered the realm of treatment, reimbursement, and evaluation. Is the type of advance predictive of public involvement? For instance, is the public more likely to get involved if the advance is a therapeutic drug (because there is greater potential for immediate benefit) than if the advance is a medical procedure (because the medical model entrusts those decisions to the practitioner)? At what point in the process of diffusion were critical decisions made? Banta's (1984) diffusion-adoption

continuum indicates that the factors influencing adoption of a new practice may be different at each stage.

4. Dualities in terms of expertise and ignorance. Who was consulted, who provided advice, and how was that advice received and used by those with the authority to act?

5. The perceptions of the decision or decisions after the fact. Was the decision considered to be an effective one in that intentions were met? Were goals not met? Is the outcome uncertain? Is it too early to tell?

The group of case writers chosen to prepare the stories of these decisions counted among their ranks an ethicist, an attorney, a policy analyst, an activist, a scientist/public official, and a political scientist (biographies can be found in Appendix B). Each author provided a unique viewpoint, coming to his or her specific issue with different working knowledge and experiences. The task set by the committee for the case writers, however, was the same: to identify and expose the underlying values held by all those described in their decisions and to determine if and how the moral response to the problem or issues changed under pressure. (Pressure could be created by time, special interest groups, perceived risk, administrative duties or obligations, economics, or the law.) The writers were also asked to describe the process by which decisions were made and identify all known constituencies and the extent to which they were involved in the decision. The writers were to consider whether the implications of the decision were well thought out or discussed during deliberations. In a sense, the writers were asked to serve as reporters, documenting what happened and what led up to the decision that was made.

In the first case, activist Jeffrey Levi reports on the activities that led to the 1989 Food and Drug Administration decision to approve the use of dideoxyinosine (ddI), an as yet unproven AIDS therapy, in a parallel track protocol. The case illustrates an extraordinary confluence of action on the part of diverse groups—scientists, regulators, and activists—directed toward the possibility of providing relief and saving lives.

In the second case, attorney R. Alta Charo provides an overview of action and inaction in the heated debate over the inavailability of RU-486 (the "French abortion pill") in the United States. The case highlights the sometimes paralyzing influence of special interest groups on a decision that involves not only moral but economic values. Thus, it is really a case about delayed or postponed decision making, only the first chapter from an ongoing and as yet unresolved debate.

In the third case, Robert Cook-Deegan, a physician-turned-policy analyst, chronicles the events of 1986-1990 leading to congressional action on the human genome project. The case describes the events surrounding decisions made by executive agencies, scientific constituencies, science spokespersons, and Congress to fund a large-scale project to map and sequence the entire human genetic complement. It spotlights science policy formation and implementation and will surprise readers who believe that the process is rational.

The fourth case, prepared by Richard Rettig, a political scientist, analyzes the events leading to the passage of Section 299I of the Social Security Amendments of 1972, which produced an entitlement program for victims of end-stage renal disease. This entitlement remains the only one of its kind, and the decision remains controversial today. The case exemplifies the way law making about life-threatening illness is affected by politics, chance, spending assumptions, and human foibles or capabilities. It also provides a realistic view of how the U.S. Congress operates.

In case five, bioethicist James Childress describes the deliberations of the Human Fetal Tissue Transplantation Research panel in its efforts to provide advice to the Department of Health and Human Services on the morality of using fetal tissue obtained from induced abortions for therapeutic transplantation. The case offers insight on how experts can disagree, as well as agree to disagree, and yet arrive at a consensus on whether a particular research effort should continue.

In the last case, former National Institutes of Health Director Donald Fredrickson takes us back to the 1970s and describes the events that led to and included the Asilomar conference on recombinant deoxyribonucleic acid (DNA). In this case we are treated to an inside look at how the scientific community came to terms with their own uncertainty about the safety of a new biotechnique and how they negotiated a moratorium.

Some of the decisions described in the cases have been well documented; for example, numerous articles have been written about the events at Asilomar that led to the moratorium on certain types of recombinant DNA research, and audio transcripts of the meetings are available. Written transcripts are on record for the Human Fetal Tissue Transplantation Research panel meetings. Hearing records exist that document the congressional debate on entitlement for end-stage renal disease and funding for the human genome project. In other cases a variety of communications, both public and personal, provide the bases for the author's documentation. In some cases, such as the ones on ddI and the human genome project, the author was a participant in the process and can rely on the authority of experience as well as secondary references. The case of RU-486 has not yet been played out, and the primary documents available to the author were those provided to the press by the actors involved and media accounts of the events as they unfolded. Because the case study approach is inherently a subjective process, the writers were urged to use all available sources of reference for their work and describe the process by which they investigated the case study. Endnotes and references can be found at the conclusion of each case.

Also following each case are two commentaries, written and signed by individual members of the IOM committee, all of whom have their own rich experiences on which to draw. They present different aspects and viewpoints on the decisions—their unique perspectives as opposed to the conclusions of the full committee. The last chapter summarizes the committee conclusions and suggests areas for continued research. In Appendix A, committee member Stanley Reiser provides a historical perspective on the public and the expert in biomedical policy controversies.

These cases illustrate the complexity and evolution of decision making related to the diffusion and adoption of advances in biomedicine. The committee did not judge whether the cases were resolved adequately; in fact, in many of these cases the debate is still in process. What makes this collection different from other "technology transfer" reports is the deliberate intent to include the impact of values and the role of the public in the discussion. The cases do not merely present a historical, descriptive documentation of the diffusion process. Integral to the final analyses is a discussion of the myriad moral, religious, political, legal, psychological, and economic forces that influence how and when certain decisions are made.

REFERENCES

Banta, H. D. 1984. Embracing or rejecting innovations: Clinical diffusion of health care technology. In The Machine at the Bedside, S. T. Reiser and M. Anbar, eds. Cambridge: Cambridge University Press.

Jonsen, A. R., and S. Toulmin. 1988. The Abuse of Casuistry: A History of Moral Reasoning. Berkeley, California: University of California Press.

Neustadt, R. E., and E. R. May. 1986. Thinking in Time: The Uses of History for Decision Makers. New York: The Free Press.

Unproven AIDS Therapies:
The Food and Drug Administration and ddI

Jeffrey Levi

The scientific decision-making process in the case of the acquired immune deficiency syndrome (AIDS) has been characterized by un- precedented involvement of the persons affected by the disease. Initially, the AIDS crisis involved one group of people who were already political- ly organized—in this instance, gay men. Most other diseases affect a far more heterogeneous population from the start. By the time the first AIDS case was diagnosed in 1981, gay men, together with lesbians, had become a growing political presence in U.S. society and were already psychologically and strategically primed to challenge the system.

Indeed, gay men came to the AIDS crisis with a predisposition to question and distrust the health and scientific establishments. In many of the larger cities across the nation, gay men had formed gay health clinics some 10 to 15 years before the advent of AIDS because of their distrust of the medical establishment in treating gays for sexually transmitted diseases. Past actions by health agencies fueled the dis- trust. For example, the Public Health Service (PHS), of which all the federal agencies responding to AIDS are a part, including the Food and Drug Administration (FDA), was, until late 1990, responsible for en- forcement of a ban on immigration by homosexuals based on the deter- mination that gays and lesbians are mentally ill—even though the

Jeffrey Levi is a Washington-based health policy consultant working with several groups on AIDS issues, including the National Gay and Lesbian Task Force, the Gay Men's Health Crisis, and the Institute of Medicine.

American Psychiatric Association removed homosexuality from its list of illnesses in 1976. It is from this past experience that AIDS activists of all stripes—from mainstream lobbying organizations to street groups using direct action (demonstrations and civil disobedience)—came to challenge some of the fundamental assumptions of the public health community's response to AIDS: from traditional public health control measures to how research ought to be conducted to determining who should make decisions about access to experimental therapies.[1]

Decision making regarding early release of dideoxyinosine (ddI), a promising antiretroviral drug that has been seen as a potential replacement for the often highly toxic drug zidovudine (AZT) in the treatment of human immunodeficiency virus (HIV) infection, occurred in a context of more general discussions within the AIDS scientific and activist communities about early access to experimental treatments for persons with AIDS that were to be offered on a "parallel track" with ongoing clinical trials. In effect, ddI became a prototype for early access before a model for implementing the broader parallel track program was developed or approved by the relevant government agencies. The success of the parallel track concept will be closely linked to the improvised approach developed for ddI.

The support for early release of ddI and the general notion of parallel track represented a remarkable shift in attitudes among government researchers and regulators, a change inspired by discussions with and pressure from the AIDS activist community. The endorsement of parallel track by top PHS officials occurred in a context of agency jockeying for support from the AIDS activist community. Parallel track and early release of ddI have also resulted in an unusual confluence of interests among AIDS activists, regulators, drug companies, and some key scientific researchers. Government officials saw early release as a means of showing compassion and responsiveness at a time when existing research and regulatory structures seemed rigid and uncaring. Drug companies and top government regulators saw early access as another step toward the reduced regulation of the pharmaceutical industry that was a hallmark of Frank Young's tenure as FDA commissioner. Finally, activists saw parallel track as providing greater autonomy in decision making for persons with HIV infection.

This paper reviews and describes the decision-making process that led to the early release of ddI. It is not an attempt to judge the merits of early release of ddI or the entire parallel track concept. Rather, it is meant to paint a picture of how and why decisions were made, with the hope that it might provide a basis for better, more rational decision making in the future.

To lay the groundwork for the discussion of early release of ddI, the paper first reviews the history of increased drug regulation in the United States. It then discusses the trend toward deregulation during the Reagan administration that coincided with the AIDS crisis, the initial discussions and pressures for creation of a parallel track, and, finally, the process leading to early release of ddI. The paper also assesses some of the motivations of the actors involved.

The sources for the paper are primarily interviews of participants in the process conducted by the author. The outcome is necessarily the author's synthesis—but one that, it is hoped, reflects what actually happened when the analysis of the individual participants and the public record are pieced together.[2]

THE DRUG REGULATION PROCESS

Federal regulation of the drug industry in the United States[3] is a product of twentieth-century legislation that, until the 1980s, produced increasingly tight restrictions on pharmaceutical companies. Prior to this century, regulation of the food and drug industries was left to state and local governments, but as the federal role increased, the state role in this area began to disappear.[4] Each significant federal initiative for closer regulation of the drug industry coincided with a major catastrophe with a drug, which brought political pressure for greater premarketing protection of consumers.

The first major federal legislation designed to protect consumers was the Food and Drugs Act of 1906. No premarketing approval was proposed; the law merely required that drugs meet official standards of strength and purity. The next major legislation was the Federal Food, Drug, and Cosmetic Act of 1938, prompted by the elixir sulfanilamide scandal in 1937. In this case the drug was marketed without any safety testing and caused the death of 107 persons because it contained a chemical commonly used in antifreeze. The 1938 law required that a manufacturer prove the safety of a drug before it was marketed. Thus, from 1938 until 1962, regulation was focused on safety and involved minimal review by the FDA. A manufacturer simply sent a new drug application to the agency, and if there was no response within 60 days, the drug was deemed to be approved. The FDA had authority to veto an application, and it also had the option of using informal authority to try to convince a company not to market a product.

In 1962, in reaction to the thalidomide scandal overseas, the Kefauver amendments to the Food, Drug, and Cosmetics Act resulted in a requirement that manufacturers demonstrate not only the safety of a drug but also its efficacy.[5] This requirement led to far more complex clinical trials and the regulatory system that is the basis for today's drug approval process.

The Drug Approval Process Today

A pharmaceutical company wishing to begin human clinical trials of a new drug must first submit an investigational new drug (IND) application to the FDA. The IND must contain laboratory data on the drug, the results of any animal studies or foreign trials, and the proposed research protocols for trials in humans. Trials may begin within 30 days of submission of an IND if the FDA does not order a hold on clinical trials.

Although not required by regulation, there are generally three stages to the clinical trials process. During Phase I, initial safety studies are conducted, usually among a small number of healthy patients, with gradual increases in dosage to determine safe levels. These trials average between six months and one year. Because they normally take place among healthy research subjects, usually no data are collected regarding efficacy. If a drug is considered toxic, however, as is the case for many cancer and AIDS drugs, Phase I trials are conducted among those who are already sick. As a result, some information regarding efficacy may be obtained, which is the basis for some of the pressure for early release of experimental drugs. These trials were not designed to test for efficacy, however, and as a result it is risky to draw any firm conclusions about the potential usefulness of a drug from Phase I trials. About 29 percent of drugs do not continue in trials past the Phase I stage.

Phase II trials test the effectiveness of the drug and provide further evidence on safety. These studies, which usually take up to two years and involve several hundred patients with the disease for which the therapy is intended, are designed to assess the value of the drug as a treatment. Another 39 percent of drugs under development fail at this stage.

Phase III trials are long-term safety and efficacy studies, involving thousands of patients at numerous research centers, that are designed to assess the risk-benefit value of the drug. They take between one and three years. Very few drugs (3 to 5 percent) fail at this stage. Indeed, there are some in the scientific community who believe that the distinction between Phase II and Phase III trials is often artificial and that, in fact, the two phases run into one another at a certain point in the research process.

At the end of Phase III, the FDA begins its formal review of the data. A new drug application (NDA) is the basis for the agency's final approval of a drug for marketing. The NDA summarizes the findings of all the research, and the FDA has 180 days to approve the application. After the drug is placed on the market, the FDA and the pharmaceutical company monitor it for unexpected toxicities, which could cause the FDA to revoke the marketing approval. In some instances, the FDA may even require what are called Phase IV, or postmarketing, studies to learn more about the drug.

Speeding Up the Process: The "Bush Initiative"

The length of the drug approval process has been a source of frustration to the drug industry for many years and a source of anger to many advocates for patients with life-threatening diseases. Partially in response to this pressure, and with the urging of the President's Task Force on Regulatory Relief, chaired by then Vice President George Bush, the FDA announced in the fall of 1988 new regulations to expedite availability of promising therapies for patients with life-threatening and serious diseases. In a sense, the purpose of the regulations was to short-circuit the three clinical trials phases and, in the words of then FDA Commissioner Frank Young, "be able to reach a scientifically defensible decision to approve or disapprove marketing of drugs intended to improve the outcome in such diseases, based on the results of well-designed Phase II controlled trials" (Young, 1989).

Essentially, the new approach assumes that patients and physicians will use a different risk-benefit analysis for drugs to treat life-threatening illnesses and will be willing to use those drugs with less complete data than are usually available for approved drugs. The FDA's new regulations called for early consultation between the FDA and drug sponsors in the preclinical stage to ensure a clear understanding between regulators and industry as to the data required for approval. The regulations also permitted submission of an NDA after Phase II. If the drug were approved, the FDA might still require postmarketing studies (referred to as Phase IV above).

As mentioned earlier, the distinctions among the clinical trials phases are considered artificial by some, and so it is difficult to assess how dramatic this change will be. On the other hand, the more active involvement of the FDA in the design of trials is also dependent on the willingness of the sponsoring company to work actively with the FDA early in the process and on the availability of FDA personnel, who are already stretched thin owing to agency understaffing. It is too early to know what effect the new procedures are having on drug approval times.

Prelicensing Availability

Under ordinary circumstances, access to a drug that is still in the investigational (IND) stage is limited to those patients participating in the clinical trials. The FDA, however, has a number of regulatory options to make the drug more widely available under certain circumstances. The primary vehicle is the treatment IND, which allows distribution of a promising therapy to limited populations before completion of an NDA.

Prior to 1987, the uses and criteria for a treatment IND were relatively vague, which left tremendous discretion to the FDA regulators. The FDA issued new regulations in 1987 that attempted to clarify procedures and standards. According to these regulations, a treatment IND can be issued at any time between the end of Phase I trials and the submission of an NDA for promising therapies to treat the desperately ill—those with immediately life-threatening illnesses—provided there is no comparable or satisfactory alternative therapy that has already been licensed.

The FDA also has a special mechanism for early access to promising cancer treatments. Known as Group C drugs, these agents are investigational drugs under development at the National Cancer Institute that are shown to have a certain level of efficacy but are some time away from full NDA approval.

The primary criticism of the treatment IND process offered by patient advocates, particularly in the AIDS community, was that the standard of proof for treatment INDs was almost as high as that for an NDA and that in practice the treatment IND was functioning simply as a bridge between Phase III and the NDA while the FDA reviewed the data. Some in the FDA and in the research community were concerned that if treatment INDs were granted any earlier, the ability to collect good research data might be compromised and would delay even further the final NDA for a drug. This concern was based on the assumption that if a drug were available outside of clinical trials, few people would enroll in randomized trials because there was no guarantee of actually receiving the drug in question.[6]

It is in this context—with frustration over the length of time it took new drugs to move through the entire drug approval process and a feeling that existing mechanisms for early release of promising drugs were not being sufficiently employed—that AIDS activists began to call for a new mechanism for earlier release of AIDS drugs in the drug development process. This new mechanism is what became known as parallel track.

PARALLEL TRACK

The concept of parallel track—a system for expanded access to experimental therapies—originated in the AIDS activist community and posed some fundamental challenges to assumptions within the scientific community about how clinical research should be conducted and how access to drugs should be regulated. The most formal iteration of the parallel track concept came from the Treatment and Data Committee of the New York-based AIDS activist organization ACT UP (AIDS Coalition to Unleash Power), a direct action group more often seen protesting government policies than developing them. But the Treatment and Data Committee had also acquired a reputation for substantive understanding of AIDS drug development issues, and, more often than not, this arm of ACT UP could be found at the conference table at the National Institutes of Health (NIH), the FDA, or the PHS, particularly during the course of the discussions around parallel track and early access to ddI.

Jim Eigo, a leader of the Treatment and Data Committee, defined parallel track as follows: "At the beginning of phase two (efficacy) trials, this parallel track would make investigational AIDS drugs available to people with HIV disease who are ineligible for the drugs' clinical trials and have no reasonable treatment alternatives" (Eigo, 1989). As Eigo explains it, the parallel track concept grew out of the failure of existing mechanisms to "deliver drugs to people with serious or life-threatening conditions who have no treatment alternative before full FDA marketing approval" (Eigo, 1989). It was first presented in April 1988 to principal investigators and officials of the National Institute of Allergy and Infectious Diseases (NIAID), the lead NIH agency working on AIDS. This presentation was the start of a long series of discussions and an education process directed at the NIH leadership, in particular NIAID's director Anthony Fauci, primarily through conversations with ACT UP and Project Inform's Martin Delaney. (Delaney, who heads the San Francisco-based group, is one of the leading voices for greater patient access and autonomy in decision making regarding the use of experimental therapies.)

Fauci was probably the most critical player in the transformation of parallel track from an idea advocated by outsiders to one embraced by the federal public health establishment. He initially held the standard scientific community view on these proposals—that scientific controlled trials were the only way to establish the effectiveness of a drug and that expanded access could not be allowed to compete with these trials. Fauci believed the success of those trials was paramount as well as the most compassionate route in the long term, and would ultimately help more people than would be helped through early access.

Through his conversations with the activists, however, Fauci became convinced that expanded access would not have to compromise the integrity of the trials if the parallel track was limited to those who could not otherwise participate in a clinical trial. There was also, at this time, growing concern within the NIH-funded AIDS clinical trials program that patients were not complying with the trial protocols. If patients did not see the clinical trials as their only means of obtaining a drug, it might be possible to conduct more efficient trials and have better patient compliance.

Although there were hints from NIH officials at the Fifth International AIDS Conference in Montreal in early June 1989 that there might be more flexibility in NIH's position regarding earlier access, the formal declaration of a change of heart occurred in a speech given by Fauci in San Francisco later that month. "My commitment to carefully designed, controlled clinical trials for AIDS has not changed," said Fauci. "Such trials are absolutely essential if we are going to get the answers needed by physicians who are treating patients." But, he declared, "[a]t the same time, we have to be creative and flexible so we can provide increased access to promising drugs to patients who cannot participate in clinical trials" (Zonana and Cimons, 1989).

Once Fauci broke the ice, there was almost a bandwagon effect on the rest of the PHS leadership. Fauci had given no warning to his colleagues in the FDA or to Dr. James Mason, the assistant secretary for health. Mason, who was Fauci's boss, reportedly was angry at receiving no advance notice that such a major initiative was going to be announced without prior consultation or approval. FDA Commissioner Young, eager to maintain his leadership position as an early advocate of quick access to experimental drugs, was quoted as saying, "I've been pushing it [parallel track] as much as Tony has" (Kolata, 1989a).

Fauci presented his endorsement of the concept in principle without detailing how the program would actually work. Essentially, he announced that early release would not interfere with NIH's conduct of scientifically sound clinical trials and that personally he felt there was a moral obligation to make such therapies available earlier. He then tossed the ball into the FDA's court, correctly saying that, from a legal standpoint, all decisions regarding early release had to come from the regulatory agency, not the research arm. This maneuver was a source of considerable annoyance on the part of the other branches of the PHS, which were now handed a hot political potato with no prior warning or discussion. Overnight, Fauci became the hero of the activist community and, from the perspective of the FDA at least, made the regulators into the stumbling block to reform.

It was not just the regulators and his political superiors in the assistant secretary's office whom Fauci took by surprise. Little if any groundwork had been laid within the research community or within the NIH AIDS program. This lack of preparation left considerable room for open opposition (or covert backbiting) to the proposal from the traditional research community. Indeed, some principal investigators in the AIDS Clinical Trials Group (ACTG) of NIAID suggested that Fauci was undercutting good science. Fauci did not have direct discussions on this topic with the principal investigators until the regular meeting of the ACTG the following month.[7]

There has been some suggestion that Fauci, in announcing the parallel track initiative, was trying to abate the rather harsh personal criticism he had been receiving from the activist community. In a sense the activists were the squeaky wheel that got the attention. Little was done to address the consequences of a parallel track endorsement to the rest of Fauci's political base—or the impact on internal agency morale of such a surprise announcement. It fell to the assistant secretary's office, through its National AIDS Program Office (NAPO), to try to produce a bureaucratic consensus on parallel track and ensure that the PHS was speaking with one voice. Essentially, Fauci was told that, although NIH should participate in discussions on parallel track, FDA and NAPO would be taking the lead roles.

The need for a PHS-wide consensus was heightened by the pressures of a congressional hearing, a common mechanism to force decisions within in the bureaucracy. Congressman Henry Waxman called a hearing on parallel track for July 19, 1989. As chair of the House health subcommittee, Waxman was the key AIDS legislator in the House and was concerned about the momentum Fauci's idea had gained. He was also wary of how such a policy was to be implemented and how the broader research community would react.

At the hearing, Mason presented an administration position on parallel track that was astonishingly similar in its broad outlines to that of the AIDS activist community. Said Mason, "As contemplated, the availability of investigational therapeutic agents through this mechanism would be limited to those persons for whom there are no satisfactory alternative drugs or therapies available to treat that stage of disease and who, for some reason, are not eligible for or not able to participate in a clinical trial" (Mason, 1989).

Although initially parallel track seemed like a simple proposal, NAPO and the FDA soon realized that its formulation was going to be quite complex, and that nailing down the details of the policy was going to take some time. At the hearing on July 19, Mason announced that the many unresolved questions around parallel track—which ranged from safety monitoring of released drugs, informed consent, and specific patient eligibility criteria to liability and reimbursement issues—would be presented to an expanded meeting of the FDA's Anti-Infective Drugs Advisory Committee on August 17. In preparatory meetings with PHS, activist, and research community representatives, however, it became clear to NAPO officials that a much lengthier process would be needed. The August 17 meeting became, instead, a public forum for the discussion of the various options and positions, pro and con, on the parallel track concept. At that meeting, NAPO Director James Allen announced that a smaller working group would be established to develop guidelines for parallel track that included the PHS agencies as well as researchers, activists, care providers, and pharmaceutical company representatives.

The concepts of parallel track and ddI were first linked publicly after Fauci's San Francisco speech. When asked what would be a likely first candidate for parallel track, Fauci suggested ddI, although at the time only very preliminary discussions were taking place at FDA and with the drug's manufacturer, Bristol-Myers, regarding some form of early release. While ddI was always closely linked with the concept of parallel track, once it became clear that it would take time to develop the concept into a working system, ddI and parallel track decoupled, at least in terms of a bureaucratic response. As early as the July 19 congressional hearing, Assistant Secretary Mason stated that efforts to release ddI would not be constrained by any delays in the parallel track discussions. In a sense, ddI and parallel track were on parallel tracks of their own. As discussions were held at the NAPO level regarding guidelines for the parallel track policy, the FDA, NIH, Bristol-Myers, and AIDS activists were negotiating protocols for the early release of ddI. In these talks everyone took pains to make it clear that the ddI package was not meant to be the prototype for parallel track. Nevertheless, everyone also was very conscious that the success or failure of early release of ddI would greatly influence the outcome of the overall parallel track policy development.

PARALLEL TRACK: PROS AND CONS

Because attitudes toward parallel track are so closely tied to attitudes about early release of ddI, it is important to consider how the various players perceived parallel track before looking at some of the specifics of the decision making regarding ddI.

The Food and Drug Administration

The push for support of parallel track as a separate, new mechanism came from the commissioner's office. Frank Young's tenure at FDA had been marked by efforts to speed up the drug review process and reduce the level of regulation without compromising the safety and efficacy standards required by law. His 1987 effort to create greater flexibility in the use of treatment INDs, as discussed earlier, was met with skepticism by some patient groups who felt that FDA was merely repackaging old ineffective concepts and with criticism by some members of Congress and consumer advocates who believed FDA was allowing questionable reductions in safety and efficacy.

Young clearly communicated to career officials in charge of the drug review process that he wanted them to act expeditiously on parallel track and early release of ddI. At this juncture, Young was increasingly an embattled commissioner, with his administration of the FDA under close scrutiny by congressional oversight committees. He perceived the AIDS activist community as a source of strong support, perhaps the last stronghold, and was eager, if not anxious, to be seen moving the bureaucracy along on this issue.[8]

Alone, however, Young could only do so much. Considerable power in the federal bureaucracy is held by career officials, who make most of the regulatory decisions. In the minds of many activists, as well as some at NIH, one of the stumbling blocks to quicker approval or access to promising drugs was Ellen Cooper, then head of the Anti-Viral Drug Products Division. Cooper was perceived by some to be rigid in her adherence to traditional standards and inflexible in adapting to the new pressures associated with the AIDS epidemic. This perception changed somewhat during the course of the negotiations around release of ddI. Activists sensed a change of heart, and Cooper felt the activists were finally listening to what she had been saying all along.

Certainly, career officials at the FDA were angry with Fauci at his refusal to consult with them before his speech on parallel track. They had heard of the proposal and had actually sought out discussions with Fauci but were ignored. Yet despite some lingering frustration and anger, the bureaucrats were pushed forward by deadlines on both the parallel track and ddI fronts set by the political appointees, including their own commissioner. This haste was a source of annoyance, as some felt that their responsibility to ensure that all decisions were based on sound data or policy was being undermined.

To some career FDA officials, parallel track was simply the articulation of what had been their intent all along. In their view, the mechanisms for early release were there but had not been formalized, a condition that in some ways made the system potentially more flexible. In fact, they traced some of the difficulties in early access to Young's formalization of the treatment IND rules. This policy, they said, created false expectations among the AIDS activists and resulted in pressures to totally overhaul the system.

These officials were concerned that parallel track might be hard to contain; that in implementing policies that showed sympathy for the dying, the FDA still needed to maintain an orderly system of access to experimental agents. Some officials felt that activists, in their frustration with some of the kinks in the established system, wanted to throw it out entirely rather than devise ways to make it work better.

Career officials were also concerned about a "drug of the month" mentality on the part of activists. Because activists had been correct in arguing that AZT and aerosolized pentamidine were effective therapies, many believed they should be able to obtain early access for any drug they considered promising. Scientists, on the other hand, pointed to the many instances, even in the context of the AIDS crisis, in which the popular perception that a drug worked simply was not borne out in clinical trials.

In the end, the bureaucracy has supported, at least on its face, the parallel track concept. It is less willing to concede that parallel track and the early release of ddI are at all different. The experience of working ddI through the system, however, as discussed below, has reassured them to some degree.

The Research Community

As leader of the AIDS research community, Fauci committed the research agency with the largest research program and the greatest level of AIDS research funding to the parallel track concept. However, as noted earlier, his was a solitary decision within NIAID that did not involve much prior consultation—especially not with the principal investigators of the ACTG, the primary vehicle for academic AIDS drug trials. Although dependent on NIH for their funding, these investigators were known for their independence, a source of some frustration to Fauci on this and other matters.

Prior consultation may well have bogged down the process and resulted in a proposal so watered down as to be meaningless—as well as insufficient to meet the demands of the activist community. On the other hand, the lack of prior consultation also resulted in an initially tentative and later mixed reaction from the research community, which resigned itself to the inevitability of parallel track but over time became more vocal about its doubts.

Some in the medical community also raised objections to parallel track because drugs were being made available on the basis of very little data and might later prove to be unsafe. As Robert T. Schooley of Massachusetts General Hospital explained, potential toxicity "might be missed" in Phase I studies, a situation he said had occurred "with several AIDS drugs" (Zonana and Cimons, 1989).

The first full discussion of Fauci's proposal with principal investigators took place at a regularly scheduled meeting of the ACTG executive committee in July 1989. The principal investigators, who believed that people enrolled in clinical trials mainly to gain access to experimental drugs, challenged Fauci's assumption that clinical trials could maintain participant levels even with parallel track. The investigators argued that an alternative source for experimental drugs would mean fewer enrollees in randomized trials, the backbone of the ACTG approach to research. Already under attack for low levels of enrollment in ACTG clinical trials, the researchers were concerned that parallel track would further exacerbate their problems.

The chairman of the ACTG executive committee, University of Washington researcher Larry Corey, gave a lukewarm, often rambling endorsement of parallel track at the FDA's Anti-Infectives Advisory Committee hearing. The bulk of his statement focused on the greater value of good clinical trials in improving access in the long run: "I believe in expanded access in selected areas. I guess as a researcher I believe more passionately that the goal of clinical research is to define if a drug is effective and how to use it for the practicing physician and that truly is increasing access. To turn off the clinical research program in any way, shape or form, I think, will end up being a detriment to the overall good rather than benefit. But I am a true believer that if designed correctly, that these programs could actually enhance each other" (FDA, 1989). In addition to such statements within the scientific community, researchers also began expressing their concerns about recruitment to the press. Newton E. Hyslop, Jr., a principal investigator for the Tulane-Louisiana State University AIDS Clinical Trials Unit, told the *Los Angeles Times* that he was "concerned that the establishment of a parallel track process would affect the selection process for formal trials in a way that could bias the outcome because participants would no longer represent a statistically valid sample group" (Cimons, 1989).

Although much has been said about concerns within the research community regarding recruitment for ddI trials, others have suggested that the real problems may occur in recruiting participants for trials of different drugs. Clear distinctions are possible between parallel track and research eligibility for ddI alone; what happens, however, when trials for another drug seek participants and discover that many individuals in their potential recruitment pool are receiving a drug under the parallel track mechanism? Should or can they be forced to leave parallel track participation when a new clinical trial of a different drug, for which they meet the eligibility requirements, begins? Another concern among researchers and regulators—as well as among activists—is that there is no impartial monitoring mechanism within the context of parallel track or early release of ddI. Without such a component, proponents and opponents of parallel track may seek to fit the data to their arguments if there are any questions at all about its interfering with ongoing research.

The AIDS Activists

The parallel track issue brought an unusual level of unanimity to the AIDS constituency. Although all elements in the community were supportive of expanded access to clinical trials, early release of drugs outside the research setting was an issue pushed initially by the ACT UP and Project Inform sector, which then brought along, in growing numbers, more of the mainstream groups. Indeed, parallel track was considered to be of such importance to the AIDS constituency that a wide range of organizations signed a consensus statement presented to the August FDA Anti-Infectives Advisory Committee meeting that became the basis for much of the debate at the meeting. The document defined parallel track as follows:

Parallel Track should encompass post-Phase I open-label treatment protocols for people unable to participate in controlled clinical trials for AIDS and HIV-related conditions. Drugs should be eligible for Parallel Track as soon as a tolerably safe dose range has been defined and preliminary evidence of efficacy has been obtained.[9]

The document went on to offer the following eligibility criteria for early access:

• People with a condition for which there is no standard treatment.
• People who cannot tolerate the standard treatment for their condition.
• People who are failing on standard treatment.
• People who must stay on concomitant medications forbidden, but not expressly contraindicated, in trials of new experimental treatments.
• People who live too far from the site of an appropriate controlled trial.
• People who are too sick to participate in an appropriate controlled trial.[10]

Yet despite the apparent solidarity this consensus statement seemed to symbolize, disagreements continue to surface from time to time within the activist community. Some groups have adopted an essentially libertarian approach: that individuals have the right to make decisions about what drugs to take, even before clinical trials have been completed. They argue that even if people are eligible for trials, they should not be prevented from taking advantage of the parallel track.

Others are more cautious. Representative of that viewpoint is Neil Schram, chairman of the AIDS Task Force of the American Association of Physicians for Human Rights, the gay/lesbian physicians' group. Schram, in a *Los Angeles Times* op-ed piece asked: "Why shouldn't people who want the drug be allowed to have it? Shouldn't people with a life threatening illness be given any hope they want?" He responded to his own question by saying, "There is no doubt that people who are sick and cannot tolerate AZT, or are getting sick in spite of AZT, need ddI as their only current hope. But for others, a proven alternative is available." In more general terms, Schram made the argument common to more mainstream AIDS groups: "To completely do away with regulations that protect people from unproven drugs would lead to chaos and many unnecessary deaths. Even if the right to choose were granted, people would not have sufficient information to make an intelligent choice among untested drugs. So research and appropriate regulations must be protected" (Schram, 1989).

Other Consumer Interests

To a large degree, the discussion around parallel track took place in a vacuum. Other consumer or patient interests were not well represented in the discussion, and it was assumed that the guidelines being developed for parallel track would be limited to AIDS drugs. But William Schultz, then with the Public Citizen Health Litigation Project, told the FDA's Anti-Infectives Advisory Committee, "I do not see how this can be formulated without talking about the impact on drugs for other diseases. Whatever program the FDA adopts, it is going to be argued that it ought to be applied to other diseases" (FDA, 1989).

Schultz, while supporting the parallel track concept, urged greater attention to both safety and efficacy issues. He warned that "not every drug . . . is going to turn out to be sufficiently safe to be available at the beginning of Phase II or right after Phase I testing. . . . I do not think it should be advertised as a program where all AIDS drugs are going to be available at the beginning of Phase II" (FDA, 1989). Schultz also said, "I do not think it can be emphasized enough that there has to be some evidence of efficacy before such drugs can be made available. . . . One sort of test to apply to any program adopted would be to ask the question, would this program allow the drug laetrile to be made available during an investigational test? Laetrile, presumably, could pass the safety test. There is no evidence of efficacy and if the program would make laetrile available, then I would argue that there is a serious problem with it." Schultz did not claim that the parallel track program as outlined would, indeed, have such a result (FDA, 1989).

Earlier, Schultz's boss, Sidney Wolfe, had also urged caution and warned the presidentially appointed National Committee to Review Current Procedures for Approval of New Drugs for Cancer and AIDS that parallel track could create "an extraordinary conflict between researchers and patients." He expressed concern that parallel track could place clinical trials at risk. "Nothing will happen if science isn't applied," Wolfe said. "The parallel track is fraught with that possibility" (Science, 1989).

EARLY RELEASE OF ddI

Although many of the players, particularly the activists, insist that the early release of ddI was not carried out through the parallel track mechanism, the two were closely linked in the minds of the regulators, the public, and the press. It is hard to believe that, in formulating the structure for early release of ddI, the arguments regarding parallel track were not part of the thinking of the responsible actors in the process and that there was not some awareness that the success or failure of the ddI early release would directly affect support for parallel track. The stakes were clearly higher than simple negotiation of a treatment IND for one drug.

After several years of experience with AZT as the only approved antiretroviral drug in the arsenal against AIDS, it was clear that something better was needed. ddI was the first new antiretroviral to clear Phase I studies successfully, and thus, in the spring of 1989, it was finally possible to talk of another potential therapy besides AZT. Once that was clear, according to the FDA, some form of early access or compassionate use proposal was immediately put on the table—and supported by the FDA and the drug's sponsor, Bristol-Myers.

The activist community seized on ddI after the June 1989 Fifth International AIDS Conference in Montreal, at which promising early data were presented. It appeared, as several people observed later, that ddI would be AZT "without tears," that is, without some of the severe toxicities experienced by people on AZT. (It took lengthier trials for some of the toxicities associated with ddI to be revealed.) ddI's image was certainly enhanced by what some perceived as a ringing endorsement of the drug from National Cancer Institute Director Samuel Broder during a plenary speech in Montreal.

The activist community quickly began a push to gain early access to the drug on a broad scale, and in June, ACT UP/New York initiated discussions with Bristol-Myers and the FDA. As the sponsor of the drug, Bristol-Myers had no legal obligation to release it before the entire licensing process was completed (especially since it might not be able to charge for the treatment). The company's participation in these conversations and its commitment to negotiate early release of the drug with FDA and the activists was a remarkable breakthrough.

Although some form of compassionate availability might have occurred in any event, Fauci's speech on parallel track and his immediate suggestion that ddI might be the first candidate for this new initiative increased public attention and bureaucratic pressure on both the FDA regulators and the drug company. From mid-July on, there were regular meetings of all the involved parties to discuss what form early release would take. The fundamental disagreement was on the extent to which early release would be offered. Initially, both Bristol-Myers and FDA advocated a fairly narrow release, whereas the activists argued for full individual choice: anyone who wanted to take an informed risk should have access to ddI. By the end of the negotiations, the parties had agreed on a middle ground. A meeting held in New York in late July was a major turning point, in large part because it was the first time all the players had been in one room together (rather than participating in two-way conversations that often became scrambled when related to third parties). FDA, Bristol-Myers, and NIH officials sat down with activists and community physicians to determine just what level of access should be permitted. They finally agreed that ddI should be made available to those with no other options. From then until the September release of the drug, the discussions focused on the definition of "no other options" and on the research protocols associated with early release.

This meeting was a dramatic departure from standard operating procedure for the FDA. Normally, such discussions were limited to the FDA and the drug's sponsor, and researchers were only occasionally involved. Time pressures were also very different in that normally the drug company set the pace for negotiations. In this instance, the players were under pressure from both Commissioner Young and the NIH. ACT UP also claimed it had a commitment from Bristol-Myers that the drug would be available by the end of August.

Above all, the meeting represented an unusual level of involvement by activists and nonscientist patient representatives in issues normally reserved to the scientific community. Many activists felt the New York meeting marked a breakthrough in relations with Ellen Cooper, who led the FDA team in the ddI negotiations. They had arranged for community physicians to attend to introduce a real-world perspective, and the activists felt that this contact with the dilemmas facing physicians contributed to Cooper's more flexible approach. Cooper, on the other hand, argues that the meeting was not as critical a juncture in her attitude as the activists think. She said she had always been open to input but that this meeting, in contrast to more confrontational approaches in the past from the activists, was a very constructive one. When she asked to be invited to the New York meeting, she said she felt the activists were shocked to find that a bureaucrat was willing to leave Washington.

The end result was early release of ddI a little later than the activists had hoped for but a little sooner than some of the regulators felt was wise. Data cannot be rushed, they argued, and a little more time would have avoided some of the protocol changes that had to be made after they were announced.

Commissioner Young does not agree with those who worked under him. He blames NIH for the delays. He says that the FDA's part—the treatment IND—was held up because it was hoped that the patient access and research arms could be announced simultaneously. By having the treatment IND ready, Young felt the FDA placed needed pressure on the NIH to resolve its end of the discussions sooner.

Throughout the early release process, the assistant secretary for health's office had minimal involvement regarding ddI and was only involved through NAPO in the parallel track discussion. Toward the end, however, the office did ensure that all relevant pieces of the release were coordinated and in place.

On September 28, 1989, the secretary of health and human services announced a three-part program for early release of ddI.

- First, research would continue on the longer-term safety and efficacy of ddI through three Phase II clinical trials in the NIH's ACTG units among 2,600 patients: (1) comparing AZT and ddI among those with little or no exposure to AZT; (2) comparing AZT and ddI among those with more than a year's experience with AZT; and (3) comparing various doses of ddI among those who were intolerant of AZT.
- Second, the Phase I studies were used as the basis for issuing a treatment IND for ddI, allowing those who were intolerant of AZT to receive ddI.
- Third, an open safety protocol was permitted for those who had shown evidence of failing to respond to AZT.

The criterion for access to both the treatment IND and the open safety protocol was the inaccessibility of clinical trials: either because the individual did not meet the entry criteria or because there was no geographically accessible trial for the individual to join.

The details of these protocols had been the subject of substantial negotiation. Often, individual activists brought their personal experiences to the table—and were surprised to find them accommodated in the discussion. For many activists this was the first time they had been on the "inside," negotiating with the decision makers, and the shift in roles sometimes made them uncomfortable. In addition, those activists who remained on the outside soon questioned some of the protocols, as well as the activists who had participated in their design.

Questions also arose in short order from some in the traditional academic community. As mentioned above, it was a deliberate policy decision to issue all three parts of the early release program simultaneously because of the commitment to continuing the research process. Everyone involved in the early release decision was painfully aware of the criticisms of parallel track—that it had the potential for undermining clinical trials, thus preventing clear answers as to the usefulness of a therapy. But what had not been considered was that enrollment in the treatment IND and the open safety protocol—a relatively simple process of physicians contacting Bristol-Myers—would move much faster than enrollment of patients in the ACTG trials. The ACTG system was already under heavy criticism for its sluggishness in enrolling patients. By late November, when enrollment in ddI clinical trials seemed to be foundering while enrollment in the Bristol-Myers open safety program was booming, some scientists began to criticize the early release program openly. For example, Jerome Groopman of Boston's New England Deaconess Hospital told the *New York Times*, "People talked about and tried to reassure the academic community that, yes, parallel track will not dismantle our ability to do organized studies. But we have to face this head on. There really are conflicting issues here. If the philosophy is that anyone can decide at any point what drugs he or she wants to take, then you will not be able to do a clinical trial." Donald Abrams of San Francisco General Hospital said in the same article, "Nobody ever said it was logical. It was a matter of acquiescing to political pressure. In our effort to get things to go a little faster, we can only hope that we are not slowed down" (Kolata, 1989b).

NIH officials were significantly less concerned: they felt it was too early to know the impact of early release. The activist community suggested that parallel track might become the whipping boy for larger recruitment problems within the ACTG system. Bristol-Myers, for its part, also was not concerned. They were keeping close tabs on applications, and their data showed that those receiving the drug through early access were following the established criterion; that is, they were not able to join trials for one reason or another.

At this writing, it is too soon to determine the impact of early release on clinical trials and on the trials' ultimate goal of learning whether ddI does, indeed, work. One thing, however, is clear: despite the claims of many of the players, including Young, Fauci, and the activists, that early release of ddI is not necessarily parallel track in its pure form, the success or failure of the ddI early release program will determine the willingness of the FDA, the NIH, and drug companies to go down this path again.

Indeed, Ellen Cooper argues that if the ddI early release is not parallel track, she does not know what would be. The draft guidelines for parallel track now making their way through final bureaucratic review do not in any way create a new regulatory setup but instead use systems quite similar to those used for ddI. What makes the guidelines different— and perhaps therefore necessary from a policy standpoint—is that they bring together in a philosophical construct a commitment by the government to early release of promising AIDS therapies and make clear to all what methods will be available for accomplishing that end. Cooper admits that the FDA's commitment to early release, which she believes has always been present, has never before been clearly articulated, and these guidelines might solve that problem. But ultimately, she is correct. Because each drug will pose different issues, the exact nature of parallel track in the future will vary from drug to drug—and the ddI example will probably fit as closely as any successor drug might to a strict development structure.

One of the missing components of the ddI experiment with early access is a systematic review mechanism. With so much riding on the success of this experiment, it is unfortunate that no objective system of evaluation has been established. Ex post facto review is possible, but the fact remains that the need for ongoing evaluation should have been recognized by those responsible for developing the early release program, if only to prevent evaluation by press comment. In fact, there is very little in the way of hard data to support either side's claim regarding the impact of early release on clinical trial enrollment. The significance of parallel track or early release as a break with traditional practice and its potential importance to those with life-threatening illnesses call for systematic review and evaluation to supply the answer to this question.

MOTIVATIONS

The story for the moment must necessarily stop here, but it might be useful at this point to step back and assess some of the motivations and views of the key actors in this process. In a sense, all were thrust into new or dramatically altered roles. A consensus was reached through a confluence of self-interest, but some of that self-interest, while supportive of the immediate outcome, could well lead to future discord.

Bristol-Myers

Bristol-Myers' support and role in early release of ddI is perhaps the most interesting because in many respects company officials had the greatest capacity to insulate themselves from the political pressures being placed on them by the activist community. Instead, they embraced the efforts of the activists, even if they were not always in total agreement. In a process that depends heavily on the support of the drug sponsor, Bristol-Myers actively moved the discussions forward. In fact, all of the players in and observers of the ddI early release negotiations agree that Bristol-Myers believed in their drug, had actually sought out expedited processes within the FDA for review of AIDS drugs, and was willing, even before some of the publicity, to consider expedited release. Bristol-Myers was known as a cautious company; this history reassured some, especially in Congress, who might otherwise have been suspicious of a drug company's desire to expedite release of one of its products.

The activists perceived the company as acting sincerely during the negotiations. According to one company official, the firm understood the activists' message that people would be dying while waiting for approval of ddI. But seeking early release after only Phase I trials was a "quantum leap" from the past experience of the company (Paul Worrell, Bristol-Myers, personal communication, 1989). In addition, the scope of the early release undertaking may also have been beyond what Bristol-Myers initially anticipated. There is, apparently, some concern within the company about the costs associated with such a large program of distribution. The ability and willingness to set into motion the manufacture and distribution, at no cost, of an unapproved drug is a risk that probably only a larger company would be willing to take. A smaller company often waits until approval to gear up for manufacture and distribution—or to align itself with a larger company for this purpose. A small company would not have had the resources to undertake what the activist community wanted in terms of the scope of early access.

But the early release of ddI also served some of the corporate interests of the company. It certainly generated good will and positive media coverage for Bristol-Myers, a stark contrast to the feelings among AIDS activists toward Burroughs Wellcome, the manufacturer of AZT. Burroughs is under almost constant attack from the very same activists for its pricing structure. (Interestingly, no one who participated in the discussions with Bristol-Myers seems to have raised the issue of pricing postlicensure—and whether the cost of the early release program would be factored into that market price.)

There was also an important opportunity, through this program, for Bristol-Myers to educate the overwhelming majority of physicians treating the nation's AIDS patients about their drug, something normally forbidden before a drug is licensed. Early release resulted in a great deal of free advertising and marketing, all with the FDA's blessing and encouragement. From the regulatory perspective there was also the belief, probably not unfounded, that if Bristol-Myers went along with a process that seemed important to the FDA, it would be hard for the FDA to turn down the firm's new drug application for ddI unless the data proved to be very negative. Judgment calls are always made at critical points in the licensing process; had Bristol-Myers not gone along with the FDA on early release, some of those calls might not have been favorable.

The Food and Drug Administration

There were two levels of participants at the FDA. Commissioner Young, who was described by one activist as "tired of being out-Fauci-ed" in terms of favorable publicity among AIDS activists, wanted to use ddI as an example of how the FDA could make things work. He also saw the ddI case as an opportunity to vindicate his advocacy for the changes in the treatment IND regulations that allowed earlier release of drugs for life-threatening illnesses. Young believes that the ddI experience is a demonstration of the success of those changes, even though they were attacked by some activists and congressional leaders when they were announced, many of whom later supported early release of ddI. Under the regulations, the commissioner personally approves issuance of the treatment IND—the only FDA regulatory decision made in the commissioner's office. At a time when he was under increasing attack for his stewardship at the FDA, Young felt that his support of such early release mechanisms gave him a chance to exercise power that would generate good press.

Yet much greater regulatory power rests with Ellen Cooper as head of the antiviral division. She, too, saw the ddI experience as a vindication of her role and the positions she had taken—but in a very different way from Commissioner Young. She saw no need for the codification of the treatment IND regulations; she strongly believed that early release had always been an option for the agency and that codification created false expectations when no drugs were ready for treatment INDs. She saw parallel track in a similar vein. Accomplishing early release of ddI within existing constructs proved the flexibility of the system, and there was no need to codify the process. She felt strongly that there had been too little experience with early access after only one drug to try to write firm guidelines and that each drug would pose very different issues. Indeed, she felt the ddI experience was parallel track as it was meant to be structured.

The National Institutes of Health

Technically, the NIH role in the early release process was somewhat limited. NIH was responsible for negotiating and initiating the protocols for Phase II trials, which would have occurred even without early access to ddI.[11] In fact, however, the whole process was set in motion by Fauci's proposal for parallel track and his immediate linking of it to ddI. In his effort to gain support within the AIDS activist community, as well as out of sincere support for the concept, Fauci began something of which the ultimate outcome was not at all clear to him—and whose far-reaching implications were probably not considered and thrashed out within NIH before the concept was introduced. This kind of process can be effective if one has faith that the events will play out as one would like them to. Given the number of competing players, however—and the fact that much of the ultimate authority for the success of parallel track rested with his competitors at the FDA—if Fauci's initiation of the process was deliberate, it was an unusual display of trust because the entire exercise ran the risk of turning out very differently from what Fauci and the original proponents intended.

One of the most important roles the NIH could play in this process was to gain the support of the academic research community for early access, whether as parallel track or for ddI specifically. One of the recurrent criticisms from the other players in the early release effort was that they assumed that Fauci, as head of the NIH's AIDS research effort, had consulted with or would in some way limit criticism from the academic community. In fact, most NIH officials and the NIH principal AIDS investigators were in the dark about his proposal until it was made public. This lack of consultation and briefing raised the specter, which is still present, that the academic researchers would actively oppose early access or otherwise try to undermine its success.

The Activists

The philosophical imperative behind the work of the activists was simple: to the extent possible, patient autonomy in the drug availability process should be respected. Government interference should be limited in these decisions, and the sooner the opportunity for informed choice was permitted, the better.

The push for early access to ddI was motivated by the belief that ddI was, indeed, going to prove successful as an antiretroviral therapy and also by a more personal imperative: many of the activists and their friends needed an alternative to AZT. The activists knew that the process that had been agreed to for ddI release was going to be a prototype against which the ultimate parallel track initiative would be measured. It may not have been the systematic structure they envisioned for parallel track—and they felt very strongly that a systematic structure was needed—but it at least provided an opportunity to pilot-test some of the structure's components.

In a certain sense, the activists helped create something new by their participation in the early release negotiations. The system may always have been open to this kind of input or may always have had this level of flexibility, as government and company officials often claimed; but in the case of ddI the activists achieved an unprecedented level of involvement by consumer and patient advocates in the drug regulation process, normally a very tightly held series of negotiations, and forced real-world considerations into the decision making of the regulators and the sponsor.

Several fortunate political circumstances enhanced the activists' influence. There was a bidding war for community support between Young and Fauci that gave the activists an advantage, even if they were not conscious manipulators of that competition. In addition, ddI had gotten good press, which created public and media interest in how negotiations were faring. And above all, Bristol-Myers was a relatively open company.

From a policymaking perspective, some questions can certainly be raised. The personal imperative that motivated many of the activists involved in the process added urgency to the discussions. But some activists also recognized that there may have been a fuzzy line between good policy and what they as individuals needed; for example, were accommodations being made, one activist asked himself, because they met his personal medical needs or because they also represented appropriate modifications in the protocols?

Major precedent-setting changes were occurring in drug access policy. Both the ddI and parallel track decisions were made as though there was no carryover to diseases other than AIDS. The limited experience of the activists in broader health advocacy issues may have closed off opportunities for broader reform—or created problems for other disease groups. Even within the context of AIDS, decisions were made based on the immediate urgency of finding an alternative to AZT, while at the same time precedents were being set for future AIDS-related decisions.

It is not entirely clear whether the activists were aware of the situational nature of the alliances they were making. Bristol-Myers may appear to be aligned with their concerns at this stage of the drug development process, but the company's decision was based on sound business imperatives and not on moral factors alone. It is not inconceivable that those same imperatives may drive a wedge between Bristol-Myers and the activists later in the process.

Similarly, the activists seemed dependent on the support of FDA Commissioner Frank Young, particularly to push the career officials to accept earlier access. Young's sudden departure from the scene startled them—and taught them what many advocacy groups and career bureaucrats with longer experience have known for some time: political appointees come and go, and their value is of limited duration. Educating and building alliances with career officials may be more painstaking and less public, but they can, over the long term, provide lasting support. Given the substantial discretion that career officials have at a regulatory agency such as the FDA, it is not at all clear what impact Young's departure and a long transition period at the agency will have on the influence of the activists on future drug policy decisions.

There is also a question of accountability with regard to the activists who participated in the early release negotiations. Although nominally affiliated with specific organizations, they were very much a part of the negotiating process as individuals who were respected for their expertise on the issues and for their ties to certain parts of the AIDS constituency. Through force of intelligence and personality they won their way into the decision-making process—a measure of their capabilities. But it left them open to second-guessing from other activists and to questions from players on the other side of the negotiating table as to how much political strength they were bringing to the process. In a sense, whatever naivete the activists brought to the negotiations regarding the drug industry and bureaucratic politics was matched by the other participants' assumption that the activists were responsible to an organizational structure similar to that of their own employers.

CONCLUSIONS

All of the key players in the decision-making process publicly express support for the final outcome—early access to ddI. The process by which this decision was constructed lends itself to several general observations.

Competition and closely controlled decision making may move an agenda in the short term, but they may undermine long-term support. The competition between Fauci and Young caused Fauci to seek relatively little counsel beyond his inner circle regarding parallel track for fear Young would jump ahead of him. Young, for his part, pushed the FDA bureaucracy to move as quickly as possible on the ddI treatment IND so he could prove that he could make parallel track work before there was even a parallel track structure. In a sense, the strength of support from these two top health officials prevented the process from becoming bogged down in haggling over details. But that support also had its negative side: the lack of stability that accompanies dependence on a political appointee (Young) and the result of Fauci's lack of consultation with the academic community, whose long-term backing of parallel track remains very much in doubt. A process that allowed the academic community in particular to buy into the concept early on—to allow them, perhaps, the opportunity to be educated by the activists, as Fauci was— might have caused some frustration among the activists over delays, but it might also have assured a longer-term commitment, once the media and the politicians were no longer focusing on the subject.

A broader definition of decision makers produces better policy outcomes. The level of involvement in the ddI process by community physicians and advocates was unprecedented in FDA history, and all those who were part of the process agreed that the final outcome was the better for it. In particular, the New York meeting in late July that brought the FDA together with community physicians has been cited as introducing a critical and welcome real-world element to the discussion. FDA officials needed to hear from peers and fellow physicians, not just activists, to be convinced finally of the need for this level of expanded access. Yet no permanent mechanism currently exists to assure this level of involvement for future AIDS drugs or for drugs for any other disease.

Ellen Cooper, who has often been perceived by many as an obstacle to just this kind of involvement, is one who believes that there is a need for all relevant participants to meet on a more formal basis. By participants, she means the drug's sponsor, researchers, and patient advocates. At some point, the legally empowered decision makers need to make their choices, but those choices will be better if they are informed by the input of all interested parties. Logically, she feels, the FDA should call this group together. Yet because, at least in the context of AIDS, FDA is often perceived as part of the problem, an independent group may need to facilitate the process.

Even if the proposed parallel track guidelines are adopted, they would institutionalize advocacy involvement in only part of the drug access process. Broader solutions need to be proposed and debated, outside the context of a specific decision on one drug. The advocacy and activist groups, in facing the immediacy of the AIDS crisis, often neglect the longer-term value of institutionalizing their gains. Pressure for change needs to come from the outside, because even though regulators have been supportive of much that has happened in this individual case, the tendency is to fall back on familiar patterns that seem safer, even if not always better.

Evaluation of new initiatives is too often an afterthought. In this case, a fairly far-reaching change in standard procedures has been implemented without setting up evaluation mechanisms. The success or failure of the ddI experiment will affect the future of early access, but there is currently no independent means of assessing and auditing what is occurring. Advocates for the various points of view within the research, regulatory, pharmaceutical, and activist constituencies will be left to argue over whether problems arising during this experiment (such as difficulties in recruiting patients) are the result of the early access program or other causes. This new early access process is too critical a change to be left to this kind of debate. It may be too soon to draw conclusions, but it is not too soon to identify the data that should be collected and how they ought to be evaluated.

EDITOR'S NOTE: As of January 1991 clinical trial results suggest that ddI has promising retroviral activity and is generally well-tolerated.

NOTES

1. Not all AIDS activists come from the gay community, just as AIDS is not a gay disease. But within the AIDS constituency, much of the pressure around early access to experimental drugs has, indeed, come from the gay community. More fundamental issues of access—to primary care and to clinical trials—are also part of the AIDS constituency's agenda and have been pushed by the needs and advocacy of those minority and poverty community representatives active in the AIDS effort. These are antecedents, in a sense, to access to the experimental drugs that are the subject of this paper.

2. Among the individuals interviewed for this paper were James Allen, director of the National AIDS Program Office, and his deputy, Bruce Artem; Ellen Cooper, director of the Anti-Viral Drug Products Division of the FDA; Margaret Hamburg, then special assistant to Anthony Fauci, director of the National Institute of Allergy and Infectious Diseases, and now with the New York City Health Commission; Jay Lipner, a New York activist attorney; Tim Westmoreland, counsel to the House Subcommittee on Health and the Environment; Paul Worrell, of Bristol-Myers; and Frank Young, former commissioner of the FDA. The author, as an AIDS consultant working with several groups, including the National Gay and Lesbian Task Force and Gay Men's Health Crisis, also attended a number of the key meetings in question and had numerous conversations with participants in the ddI early release and parallel track process over the period under discussion in this paper.

3. The history of federal drug regulation and description of the regulatory process in this section draw heavily on an issue brief by the National Health Policy Forum (NHPF), "The Pharmaceutical Industry," and a talk by Peter Barton Hutt, at an NHPF panel on January 11, 1990 in Washington, D.C.

4. The AIDS crisis, however, brought a shift in thinking about the state role in drug regulation in this regard. Reflecting frustration with the slow pace

of federal drug approval for AIDS treatments, in 1987 the California legislature created its own version of the FDA in the hope that California-based pharmaceutical companies might move their drugs through an expedited state process.

5. The FDA had not permitted distribution of thalidomide in the United States, even without the additional authority and requirements granted with the Kefauver amendments.

6. Randomized trials are considered the "gold standard" for drug research. They involve assignment of patients to different parts of a study, to compare a new drug with a placebo (i.e., no treatment) or to compare the new drug with standard or current therapy. Patients are randomly assigned to a particular group, and researchers are not supposed to know to which study a patient is assigned.

7. This is not to say, however, that Fauci was caught by surprise at the attention his speech drew from the media. On the contrary, he personally called key AIDS reporters to make sure they would be covering the speech.

8. There was certainly some division within the AIDS activist community about Frank Young. New activists—such as those from ACT UP—had only relatively recent experience working with Young and saw him as trying sincerely to support their efforts and as responsive to the public demonstrations they undertook. Those with a longer history of AIDS lobbying were a bit more skeptical. They perceived Young as being supportive only as long as the interests of the AIDS community coincided with those of the pharmaceutical industry. And they had had some difficult experiences with Young in the early days of the AIDS epidemic around the licensing of the original antibody test for HIV.

9. "Guidelines for the Parallel Track Program for AIDS and HIV-Related Treatments," memo to James Mason, M.D., Assistant Secretary for Health, August 17, 1989, from the AIDS Action Council, ACT UP/New York, ACT UP/San Francisco, AIDS Project Los Angeles, American Association of Physicians for Human Rights, American Civil Liberties Union AIDS Project, American Foundation for AIDS Research, Community Research Alliance, Gay Men's Health Crisis, Human Rights Campaign Fund, Lambda Legal Defense and Education Fund, Mobilization Against AIDS, National Association of People with AIDS, National Gay and Lesbian Task Force, National Gay Rights Advocates, Project Inform, and San Francisco AIDS Foundation.

10. Ibid.

11. The NIH had a role in research protocol design only because ddI Phase II trials are being done through the NIH's ACTG system. Had Bristol-Myers decided to do the trials privately, there might have been no NIH role.

REFERENCES

Cimons, M. 1989. Coalition proposes criteria for AIDS drug trials. Los Angeles Times, August 17, 1989.

Eigo, J. 1989. Testimony before the Energy and Commerce Committee, Subcommittee on Health and the Environment, U.S. House of Representatives, July 19, 1989.

Food and Drug Administration Anti-Infectives Advisory Committee. 1989. Transcript of August 17, 1989 meeting.

Kolata, G. 1989a. AIDS studies head seeks wide access to drugs in tests. New York Times, June 26, 1989.

Kolata, G. 1989b. Innovative AIDS drug plan may be undermining testing. New York Times, November 21, 1989.

Mason, J. O. 1989. Testimony before the Energy and Commerce Committee, Subcommittee on Health and the Environment, U.S. House of Representatives, July 19, 1989.

Schram, N. R. 1989. Lives, research hinge on limiting new AIDS drug. Los Angeles Times, September 27, 1989.

Science. July 28, 1989. Quick release of AIDS drugs. Page 347.

Young, F. 1989. Testimony before the National Committee to Review Current Procedures for Approval of New Drugs for Cancer and AIDS, January 4, 1989.

Zonana, V. F., and M. Cimons. 1989. Ease AIDS drug rules, health chief urges. Los Angeles Times, June 24, 1989.

Commentary

Leon Eisenberg

The decision by the FDA to make ddI available early in the drug evaluation process is unique in that the "user" community (patients and potential patients) played a decisive role in the outcome. For this discussion, the bureaucratic dispute about whether the decision was implemented by an existing mechanism that permitted release for "compassionate use" or whether it represented the de novo creation of a parallel clinical trial is irrelevant. The important point is that the FDA responded to patient-generated pressure for release of ddI with only meager safety data and before randomized controlled trials (RCTs) had been completed. The FDA action was strongly opposed by those committed to RCTs as the only scientific way to evaluate efficacy and safety in a chronic disease with a highly variable course and duration. Moreover, even many of those who had been reluctantly persuaded by the case for compassionate use because of the dire prognosis of AIDS were concerned about the precedent-setting consequences of this action would this step mean that the FDA would subsequently release other drugs before thorough testing and thereby expose patients to unwarranted risk?

The epidemiology of AIDS and the historical moment of its appearance combined to create a singular set of circumstances. The first cases were exclusively male homosexuals; thereafter the syndrome was successively recognized in other population groups (transfusion recipients, hemophiliacs, intravenous (IV) drug users and their heterosexual partners, children born to infected mothers). The most recent case data (January 1990) show that gays

Leon Eisenberg chairs the Department of Social Medicine at Harvard University.

are still overrepresented in the caseload; the Centers for Disease Control attributes 60 percent of the 121,000 U.S. AIDS cases to male homosexual or bisexual behavior.

What gave this situation particular relevance was that white middle-class gays had organized an effective political movement *before* the disease was first recognized. Consequently, they were in a position to speak out—and they had powerful reasons for doing so because the federal response to the epidemic was grossly inadequate. In contrast to self-declared, politically active gays, many of the other AIDS patient constituencies (e.g., IV drug addicts, bisexuals, and men who engage in homosexual behavior but do not identify themselves as gay) were not and are not represented in health care decisions. Almost all diseases are differentially distributed in populations. But there is no other instance in recent memory of an epidemic of an infectious disease that has been so narrowly focused on a self-conscious, politically experienced patient group, one that has spoken out forcefully in its own interests.

It is not that concern for patients has been absent from prior FDA deliberations. Indeed, concern for health is the raison d'être of the FDA. Nor have patients lacked advocates. To the contrary, physician specialists have spoken up on behalf of their patients. What is different in the case of ddI is that for the first time patients spoke for themselves in the decision-making process.

Traditionally in FDA deliberations the dialogue has been confined to civil servants, pharmacologists, clinicians, and pharmaceutical representatives. With ddI, patient spokespersons in effect forced their way to the negotiating table, where the authenticity of their experience gave them a special expertise. Permitting laypersons to participate in a technical decision, even when they are highly educated, raised questions in the regulatory community. Can dialogue be meaningful when the premises from which each group starts are not shared, and often not understood, by the others? Furthermore, the gay spokespersons had no mandate to represent other AIDS patients—for example, drug users and closet gays in the minority communities, whose lives are also at risk but who are largely excluded from access to standard treatments no less than to experimental ones.

If the decision to proceed with the parallel track can be hailed in one sense as a victory for a more democratic process, what are its potential costs? Three risks can be foreseen: (1) the parallel track may impede or even block completion of the RCT; (2) early access to ddI may expose more patients to the risk of severe toxicity; and (3) the precedent may return to haunt us if it is applied unwisely. Let us consider each in turn.

Although gay advocates do not speak with a single voice, many agree that RCTs are necessary to evaluate drug efficacy and safety. They share the concern of clinical investigators that the ability to obtain ddI outside of trials may markedly decrease enrollment in clinical trials. Why should a patient agree to a 50-50 chance of getting the highly touted new drug in the RCT when he or she can be sure of receiving it through the parallel track? If enough RCT volunteers were to default, that would be a misfortune for all HIV-positive patients. Will that happen? Is it happening? As of the fall of 1990, there is no answer. Recruitment of participants for the ddI RCT has been slow; the same has been true, however, of earlier trials of other drugs.

What about undue toxicity? Recent reports indicate that the death rate among those in the parallel track is some 10 times higher than among those in the RCT. The explanation, however, is anything but certain. Criteria for admission into the RCT rule out patients with advanced disease, but such patients are allowed to receive the drug through the parallel track. The observed higher death rate in the parallel track may thus represent nothing more than the worse initial prognosis of the enrollees. The example of suramin, however, should remind policymakers that an RCT was necessary to discover that drug's unacceptably high toxicity.

The death rate from pancreatitis has also been much higher among those in the parallel track and probably does represent ddI poisoning. Again, this may be a dose-related phenomenon or interaction with stage of disease. Even if ddI use has caused pancreatitis and subsequent deaths, the fundamental question remains: does the chance to reverse a fatal disease justify the risk? Some patient advocates contend that life with advanced AIDS has such little value that hastening death is no tragedy. Unfortunately, during the FDA discussions, there was no agreement to spell out in advance (1) what data would justify abandoning the parallel track and (2) what evidence from the parallel track could properly be admitted into the evaluation process. Lack of such agreement led to predictable responses to the first mortality data. Those who had been against the parallel track from the first contended that the high mortality warranted its discontinuation; gay activists argue that the hope for benefit justified the risk.

At present, whether ddI will prove to be a safe, effective drug is not clear. What is more important for public health in the long run is the way we evaluate the parallel track as a response to clamor for access to new drugs. Surely this mechanism should be neither adopted nor abandoned without a close reading of the ddI story. Did it allow very sick patients to obtain a useful agent months before its official release? Did it lead to avoidable deaths because toxicity exceeded utility? Could either outcome have been predicted from the data on hand when the decision was made?

Whether ddI leads to early salvage or undue toxicity, should patients be given access to an agent they want to use when the risk is considerable and efficacy is uncertain? The recent example of laetrile raises serious questions about the wisdom of such a strategy. The danger is less the confraternity of charlatans ready to peddle expensive nostrums to credulous patients than the risk that even nontoxic nostrums, through their illusory promise of ready cure at no discomfort, can lead to great harm by diverting patients from appropriate (but unpleasant) treatment protocols.

Commentary

Peter F. Carpenter

This case study is a well-researched, balanced, unbiased review of the decision-making process that allowed release of the AIDS drug ddI for use prior to approval of the new drug application. The case is an excellent example of the difficulties involved in attempting to achieve an appropriate balance between the needs of individuals (people with AIDS), who desire access to an unproven therapy, and the needs of society, which must ensure proper testing of pharmaceutical products before they are made available for use outside of controlled clinical trials. There is no "right answer" to this dilemma: rather, the decision will reflect both the specific circumstances of the disease and of the unproven therapy. In the case of ddI, the expected outcome for patients who did not use the unproven therapy was sufficiently severe that none of the therapy's anticipated side effects would have been more serious than the outcome without therapy. In addition, more active involvement (than might have occurred even a few years ago) of patients in the decision-making process was a factor in shifting the balance toward making the drug available.

The case study also illustrates the importance of finding solutions within established rules, rather than forcing a change. Such an approach is not only face saving but, more importantly, avoids the often unexpected or unintended consequences of what was thought to be a simple change. However, the case

Peter F. Carpenter, a former pharmaceutical company (ALZA) and federal government (Office of Management and Budget) executive, is a visiting scholar at the Center for Biomedical Ethics at Stanford University.

does not carefully analyze the historical precedent of the availability of un-approved cancer drugs. These so-called Class C drugs and the controversy surrounding their use are, in many ways, quite similar to the ddl dilemma. It is unfortunate that we have failed to apply directly both the process and the substance of the lessons learned in developing the Class C system to ddl and other AIDS drugs.

Some key elements in the process examined by Jeffrey Levi were the identi-fication of concerned constituencies, clarity regarding the issue, and the role of certain key players in making things happen. A previously weak constituency, the gay community, consolidated recent increases in its political strength and was highly motivated by the impact of AIDS on its members to represent itself forcefully. The general public and the general scientific community, however, have not been represented in the process to date, which may have important long-term implications. The willingness of individuals in positions of formal power to engage in dialogue with the advocates of change was a procedural step that was critical in this decision-making process. In addition, the recog-nition that existing rules could be interpreted to accommodate the desired outcome was essential in reaching a timely decision. These procedural steps can and should be generalized to other decisions involving biomedical in-novations.

The two most important shortcomings of the ddl decision-making process were its failure to include representatives from all constituencies and to make provisions for evaluation. For example, the broader scientific community was not formally involved in the ddl decision and it is now beginning to question the apparent decision to move away from the "gold standard" of randomized controlled clinical trials, particularly in light of reports of adverse reactions among individuals receiving the drug outside of clinical trials. The FDA has published a formal proposal to revise its rules to permit the general applica-tion of the procedure used in the ddl case. The review process that the proposal will undergo could bring to light important constituencies that did not parti-cipate in the original ddl decision. Second, it is necessary and important to have a prospective evaluation mechanism to assess the soundness of the decision based on the actual results versus the expected results.

The following potential process guidelines emerge from this case:

1. Participants in the decision-making process should clearly identify the issue being addressed or, if they are starting from substantially different definitions, develop a convergent definition.

2. It is necessary to separate the specific from the general—realizing that the solution will later need to be generalized.

3. It is important to encourage dialogue among the broadest range of constituencies.

4. There is value in finding ways to use interpretations of existing policy as the solution rather than developing totally new policies.

A Political History of RU-486

R. Alta Charo

RU-486, a drug that interferes with uterine implantation of fertilized eggs, is a safe and effective alternative for early abortions. But it is not available in the United States. In fact, it is unavailable everywhere except France. The reason is not its cost, its side effects, or lack of consumer interest.

In fact, RU-486 is a captive of the abortion debate that has recently engulfed a number of tangentially related issues, such as appointment of the new director for the National Institutes of Health, the reconstitution of an Ethics Advisory Board to oversee federal funding of in vitro fertilization research, and the federal funding of fetal tissue transplant research for relief of Parkinson's disease symptoms. RU-486 is but the latest addition to this list.

Like the birth control pill, RU-486 has encountered strong resistance from moralists who fear it will trivialize sex, life, and human relations by "bolster[ing] the comparison between taking the drug and swallowing an aspirin" (Glasow, 1990i). These objections often contain statements of concern over women's health or the potential for contraceptive genocide in developing countries. But it is the moral opposition of a minority of Americans that underlies the so far effective campaign to keep this drug from coming to market. "When pro-lifers have the opportu-

---

R. Alta Charo holds a joint appointment at the University of Wisconsin Law and Medical Schools.

nity," wrote Richard Glasow, education director for the National Right to Life Committee (NRLC), "they should emphasize how RU-486 both cheapens the value of human life even more than surgical abortion and contributes to a general decline in moral standards" (Glasow, 1986).

RU-486 is available in France during the first 49 days of amenorrhea for the purpose of terminating a pregnancy, provided that (1) it is taken under a physician's supervision and in conjunction with a follow-up dose of prostaglandin derivative; (2) there is no contraindication to mifepristone (adrenal insufficiency, long-term administration of glucocorticoids, clotting disorders) or to prostaglandins (asthma, severe hypertension); and (3) it is taken in accordance with French abortion law, which requires a one-week waiting period between the request for an abortion and the procedure.

Anecdotal reports of only 90 percent effectiveness and some side effects (including two cardiac complications) were made by Meredeth Turshen of Rutgers University at an October 1990 meeting of the American Public Health Association (Contraceptive Technology, 1990). Turshen reported on conversations with French government researchers unaffiliated with Roussel whose preliminary data had not yet been peer-reviewed or published (Contraceptive Technology, 1990; Voelker, 1990). This was consistent with comments by an inquiry commission chaired by French researcher de Vernejoul that concluded that the prostaglandin follow-up to RU-486 administration posed potentially life threatening complications (Le Quotidien du Médecin, 1990).

Peer-reviewed studies, however, show that RU-486 is safer than suction techniques for early abortion. According to a 1990 study by researchers affiliated with the drug's manufacturer and published in the *New England Journal of Medicine*, pregnancy terminations reach 98.7 percent effectiveness when 600 milligrams (mg) of mifepristone is followed three days later with a 0.5-mg intramuscular injection of the prostaglandin analogue sulprostone. Side effects were minimal.

Of 2,115 French women using the drug in 1988, in various dosages of prostaglandin analogues, failures included persisting pregnancies (1.0 percent), incomplete expulsions (2.1 percent), and the need for hemostatic procedure (0.9 percent). The average time to expulsion ranged from 4.5 hours to 22.7 hours depending upon the dose of prostaglandin, and on average uterine bleeding continued for 8.9 days (range, 1 to 35 days). Use of the drug was characterized by transient abdominal bleeding after receiving prostaglandin, but few other side effects. One woman of the 2,115 received a blood transfusion. Incomplete abortions were completed by suction technique (Silvestre et al., 1990).

Besides being safer than suction abortions and causing few side effects, RU-486 is relatively inexpensive. An abortion performed by a pri-

vate physician in the United States costs $500 to $1,000. Clinics usually charge $200 to $300 (Abrams, 1988). In France, the cost of an abortion using RU-486 is approximately $233. This includes the RU-486, the
prostaglandin, and three medical visits. Roussel receives $44 for the RU-
486. French social security covers 75 percent of the cost, so the client
pays $58 (Aubény et al., 1990).

In France, more than 100 women a day (accounting for a third of all
abortions) take RU-486 (Herman, 1989). More than 40,000 women in
France (Herman, 1989) and 4,000 women in Britain, China, the United
States, and elsewhere have also tried it on an experimental basis
(Greenhouse, 1989a). China currently allows women to use RU-486.
The drug will probably not, however, play a leading role in the country's
contraception and abortion services. Other countries use the drug only
on an experimental basis, although it is hoped that it will become widely
available in Britain and Scandinavia by mid-1992. It may also become
available in other European countries. Although the drug is effective
only within the first seven weeks following conception, experts estimate
that it could replace one-half to two-thirds of the 30 to 40 million surgical abortions performed annually worldwide (Stein, 1988).

The prospects for RU-486 in the United States are dim. At best, it
could be available by 1997, but that would require several actions that
do not seem very likely to occur. A U.S. pharmaceutical company would
have to open negotiations almost immediately to obtain the rights to
produce and market the drug in this country. Soon thereafter, the firm
would have to begin the process of obtaining Food and Drug Administration (FDA) approval. No U.S. company has yet been willing to take
on the expense, an estimated $50 million, and difficulty of obtaining
FDA approval, especially in light of concerns about FDA's ability to
withstand pressure from the Bush administration and to review the
drug dispassionately. Another obstacle is the drug's 5 percent failure
rate, which is perceived as a significant potential liability. Finally, and
most importantly, marketing this drug in the United States would undoubtedly be a public relations nightmare. Boycott threats at the retail
and investment level are real—and so far, effective.

It seems that only a small, single-product company could withstand
these pressures. Family planning and feminist health groups have
discussed starting a company devoted to bringing RU-486 to the market,
but no concrete progress has been made. Ironically, the biggest stumbling
block is the drug's French manufacturer, Groupe Roussel Uclaf, which
has refused to license it in the United States. At least six groups of
financiers have expressed serious interest in forming a company for
U.S. development and distribution, and a coalition of interested feminists, lawyers, and researchers have combined under the name "Repro-

ductive Health Technologies Project" to develop wider public support for the drug. Roussel and its German parent company, Hoechst, however, fear an organized retail and investment boycott in the United States, and not only will not license the drug in the United States but even hesitate to supply it for research on nonabortion applications.

The company's fears are not groundless. The lives of Roussel executives and their families have reportedly been threatened. Organized campaigns to boycott Roussel products, to block investment in Hoechst, and to seek out potential product liability claims against both have dogged the companies ever since Roussel announced it had developed an "abortion pill."

Reassurance from the U.S. government may be a precondition to persuading Roussel to license the drug here. The company refused to market the drug in France without a direct order from the French Ministry of Health. Roussel has announced it will license RU-486 only to companies in countries whose governments have specifically requested the drug. In the United States, such a request is unlikely, despite the drug's other possible applications in the treatment of Cushing's syndrome, breast cancer, menangioma, endometriosis, and even obesity (Carey, 1990; Ullman et al., 1990). "It would be a tragedy to deny cures to Americans with life threatening diseases because of an ideological agenda," says Congressman Ron Wyden (D-Ore.) (Carey, 1990). But that is just what may happen unless there is a surge of support in the United States for the drug's abortion applications. "[Roussel] wants a groundswell of doctors who will run interference for them," says one researcher. "Then the company, with a Gallic shrug, can tell antiabortion protestors that it was forced to distribute the drug" (Carey, 1990).

For the moment, limited clinical trials have been completed in the United States; for example, small-scale trials were conducted at the University of Southern California (USC) under the auspices of the New York-based Population Council. Progress toward FDA approval will be slow, however, because the prostaglandins used in the United States in conjunction with RU-486 are different from those used in the European protocols. Even with new trials, once the studies are completed the patent on RU-486 will be close to expiring. Once that happens, the question of licensing (although not FDA approval) becomes moot.

In the end, it appears that American women are going to be denied this safe, effective form of early abortion for at least the next decade. As shown by the early history of the controversial birth control pill, it appears that in the United States there is a need for much patience.

The purpose of this case study is to trace the network of political, economic, and historic forces that have converged to slow the introduction of RU-486 into the U.S. market. It is a study of the absence of a decision, that is, the absence of FDA consideration of the drug, the absence of a U.S. license issuance, and the near absence of any government hearings. It is also a story of perceptions: the perception that RU-486 will trivialize abortion, that the abortion controversy makes any new contraceptive or abortifacient commercially risky, and that contraceptive development proceeds without full regard for women's health and safety.

One persistent theme in this story is that members of the women's health and family planning communities, the pharmaceutical industry, or the antiabortion movement have publicly questioned the sincerity of the public statements made by each other. The NRLC, for example, has consistently complained of distortions in press coverage and scientific journals (Andrusko, 1991). As a result, there is no single authoritative source of information on the motivations of those who have worked to promote or to discourage the development of the so-called abortion pill. It is therefore difficult to present the "truth" about why RU-486 is not likely to be on the U.S. market in the near future.

This article is based largely on the published statements of official representatives of these various groups and published rebuttals by their opponents. Most of the research is based on a full-text review of over 500 articles in leading newspapers and news services, as reproduced in the Mead Data electronic NEXIS service. Additional sources include the *National Right to Life News* (which itself relies heavily on popular press articles), leading medical journals, and recent congressional hearings. Those hearings have not yet been published by Congress and are described in this article on the basis of *New York Times* coverage. Because leaders of the various interest groups have often reacted to one another on the basis of these news articles, newspaper coverage has become not only a source of news reporting but a news event in itself.

INTRODUCING CONTRACEPTIVES TO THE UNITED STATES

Family planning is now an accepted part of American life. Planned Parenthood, for example, is supported by 250,000 donors and has 24,000 volunteers and staff, "by any measure . . . a mainstream organization" (Steinbrook, 1988). Supreme Court Justice Sandra Day O'Connor's husband was the emcee for two of its events in Phoenix, and her sister has sat on its board in Tucson. Dwight D. Eisenhower and Lyndon Johnson were once members of its honorary national board (Steinbrook, 1988). Today it is one of several organizations supporting access to RU-486.

Yet only a relatively short while ago in this country, contraceptives were considered obscene. They were also illegal, and there were several vigorous campaigns in the 1950s and 1960s to keep them that way.

look up cases

The battle in the United States was lost, however, when the Supreme Court ruled—first in *Griswold* v. *Connecticut* in 1965 and then in *Eisenstadt* v. *Baird* in 1972—that there is a constitutionally protected zone of privacy that extends to the purchase and use of contraceptives.

It would be a mistake, however, to view that battle as simply one centered on contraception or even on sexual morality. Rather, it was part of a larger debate about the power of women to control their reproductive capabilities and their lives. It began with nineteenth-century "voluntary motherhood" organizations fighting for contraception. This movement did not reject the idealization of motherhood; it fought merely to make the timing one of discretion rather than chance. The twentieth-century family planning movement went further, supporting a broader effort to ensure equal opportunity and independence for women. Personal control of reproduction was a crucial first step toward women's rights (Gordon, 1976).

This mix of concerns over immediate reproductive freedom and long-term creation of equality for women has affected past development of contraceptive options for women, and today its impact is being felt in the development of RU-486. The early birth control pill trials in Puerto Rico, for example, were heatedly attacked by feminists who accused the trial sponsors of paying inadequate attention to the safety of the study participants. Although directed toward a worthy goal—contraceptive choice—the trials appeared to violate the health and autonomy of the subject women (Seaman and Seaman, 1977).

Feminist health organizations often assert that supporters of "population control" put slowing global population growth ahead of protecting women's health and choice, and that commercial interests in contraceptives sales exacerbate this problem (Gordon, 1976). There is little question that A. H. Robins resistance to complaints about its Dalkon shield hardened skepticism of contraceptive development within the feminist community, which resulted in pitched battles over Depo-Provera (see the later discussion) and even a less than enthusiastic initial response to RU-486. "As women, we have learned that we cannot trust assurances given to us by doctors," activist and Harvard biology professor Ruth Hubbard has been reported to say (Glasow, 1988a).

But the autonomy offered by RU-486 overcame feminist skepticism of contraceptive innovations. The drug offers the prospect of performing abortions in any physician's office and even at home. The prospect of eliminating abortion clinics, which are easy targets for picketing and bombing by the radical antiabortion movement, has made feminists enthusiastic supporters of the drug. This alarmed abortion opponents, who characterized RU-486 as ushering in an era of "guilt-free, responsibility-free, carefree living—better killing through chemistry, so to speak" *good church quote*

(Andrusko, 1991). "Let's have the courage to say so openly," stated the Vatican, "a way of killing with no risk for the assassin has finally been found" (Reuters, 1989c).

THE EARLY DEVELOPMENT OF RU-486

The central actors in the RU-486 history are Etienne-Emile Baulieu, a 62-year old endocrinologist with a "breezy, almost brash manner and hyperkinetic nature [that] give him the air more of a populist politician than of a meticulous medical researcher" (Greenhouse, 1989a), and Edouard Sakiz, chairman of Groupe Roussel Uclaf, a $1.7 billion French pharmaceutical group. A native of Turkey who arrived in Paris at age 20 to pursue his studies, Sakiz is described as reserved and cautious (Greenhouse, 1989a). Although much attention has been paid to Baulieu's involvement in developing RU-486, it was Sakiz who played the instrumental role in determining the future of the so-called abortion pill in France.

Baulieu started investigating fertility control in 1961 as a postgraduate researcher at Columbia University in the United States. While at Columbia, Baulieu developed a relationship with Gregory G. Pincus, who had worked during the 1950s to develop a birth control pill. Pincus helped Baulieu obtain a sizable grant from the Ford Foundation for his basic research on hormones—even though Baulieu did not want to work on refining the birth control pill (Rosenfeld, 1986). Back in France, however, Baulieu became a member of the government committee appointed during the administration of Charles de Gaulle that was instrumental in getting birth control legalized in 1966. The tremendous social implications of hormonal control research were not lost on Baulieu (Greenhouse, 1989a).

In 1966, Baulieu recommended Sakiz for the position of director of biological research at Roussel. Just returning from a teaching position at Baylor Medical School, Sakiz took up the post and worked with the company during the turbulent 1960s. During that time Roussel decided not to pursue production of the contraceptive pill because it did not want to risk offending the Catholic Church. "We lost the market for contraceptives even though we were the most important steroid company in the world," Sakiz said regretfully in a 1989 *New York Times* interview. "And now contraceptives are considered natural; they aren't controversial at all" (Greenhouse, 1989a).

In 1970, Baulieu and his team at the University of Paris were the first to identify receptors within the uterine cells that receive messages from progesterone. They realized that it might be possible to use this knowledge to create a method for blocking or terminating pregnancy.

"The receptors are like a keyhole," explained Baulieu, "and we were trying to produce a false key" (Greenhouse, 1989a). Baulieu in turn gave the idea to Roussel, which had the facilities and know-how to turn the concept into a pill (Rosenfeld, 1986). (Baulieu was ineligible for financial rewards from any commercial sales.) He also suggested to the Roussel chemists that they try to graft a molecular cluster onto a progesterone-like molecule. In 1980, George Teutsch succeeded.

Clinical tests of the pill, dubbed R(oussel)U(claf)-486, began in Switzerland in 1982 under the direction of Walter Herman, a long-time friend of Baulieu (Rosenfeld, 1986). In 1983 Gilbert Schaison and Beatrice Couzinet at Bicêtre Hospital in Paris also began tests. There was little opposition to the tests because they had been cleared by the French national bioethics committee (Nayeri, 1987).

The drug rapidly showed promise. Eighty-five of the 100 women taking the drug had complete abortions. Subsequent tests showed that the drug should be followed with prostaglandins to raise the effectiveness rate from 80 percent to 96 percent.

Sakiz quickly became an enthusiastic supporter of RU-486. The discovery was hailed as a breakthrough, especially for developing countries where physicians and sanitary conditions are in short supply. Further research was initiated, although it remained almost exclusively in Europe because of a generally hostile climate for contraceptive innovation in the United States.

The most striking recent victim of this hostility was Depo-Provera, an injectable contraceptive developed by the Upjohn Company. Despite favorable test results, the compound showed some minimal indications of a tendency to induce cancer in certain laboratory animals when given in extremely high doses (Rosenfield et al., 1983). The result was a tortuous FDA regulatory review. Its problems were also attributable in part to an article in the journal *Women and Health* asserting that the U.S. Agency for International Development (USAID) was dumping dangerous contraceptives, most notably Depo-Provera, on markets in developing countries. This and other articles asserted that Depo-Provera was just the latest in a series of contraceptives that were being tested and marketed in developing countries with little regard for the health of the women using them (Gordon, 1976; Minkin, 1980; Seaman and Seaman, 1977).

Others argued that the charges being leveled at Depo-Provera were unfounded. They cited safety data and noted that USAID was not distributing the drug in developing countries. At least half of all Depo-Provera distributed abroad from any source, they maintained, had been directed to the markets of developed countries (Rosenfield et al., 1983).

Nevertheless, the *Women and Health* article was widely distributed to ministries of health in developing countries. A cover letter signed by a number of physicians maintained that Depo-Provera was unsafe (Rosenfield et al., 1983). Unpersuaded by these assertions, some U.S. politicians began lobbying FDA to approve the drug. House Agriculture Research and Environment Subcommittee Chairman James Scheuer wrote to FDA Commissioner Frank Young, expressing his surprise that Depo-Provera, approved in the United Kingdom, Sweden, and West Germany, was not being approved by the FDA (F-D-C Reports, Inc., 1985a).

Despite congressional interest, however, FDA rejected Upjohn's efforts to compare Depo-Provera carcinogenicity data with data for oral contraceptives that had already been approved. It strongly criticized Upjohn's reliance on World Health Organization (WHO) studies, calling them "seriously flawed" (F-D-C Reports, Inc., 1985b). In August 1986 the FDA refused to reopen its Public Board of Inquiry record so that new data could be submitted. To justify the action, Commissioner Young asserted that Upjohn had failed to show that additional studies were relevant. Finally, in October 1986 Upjohn announced it would seek a wholly new approval procedure. That, too, eventually failed (F-D-C Reports, Inc., 1986).

The long, expensive, and ultimately unsuccessful effort to get Depo-Provera approved helped fuel charges that the U.S. regulatory system and the women's health movement made this country a hostile environment for contraceptive research and development. Contraceptive and abortion research continued in Europe, however. In December 1984, Baulieu and his Swedish colleague Mark Bygdeman of the Karølinska Institute in Stockholm reported that their method of combining RU-486 with follow-up prostaglandin treatments resulted in a "100 percent" success rate for inducing abortions and, further, that there were no significant side effects (Reuters North European Service, 1984).

During this time, RU-486 was billed as a sort of "morning-after" pill (Reuters North European Service, 1984) that acted as a "contragestive" as opposed to a contraceptive. Within a month, newspapers reported that the inventors had suggested RU-486 might become a once-a-month contraceptive. "Its main target is the one billion women in Third World nations who should be using birth control," the *Washington Post* quoted Baulieu as saying. "Eventually it could be used protectively in developed nations, like a monthly contraceptive pill" (Berg, 1985).

COMMERCIAL INTEREST IN RU-486

By the spring of 1985, the commercial and political potential of RU-486 was being discussed in popular business magazines. *Business Week*, for example, ran a piece on Roussel's RU-486 and Sterling's Epostane (a progesterone formation inhibitor), describing the clinical trials that were being conducted in the United States (under the guidance of Daniel Mishell, Jr., chair of the obstetrics and gynecology department at USC), and in China, India, and Europe (Rhein et al., 1985). Other European companies were working on similar products. Schering, a German company, had been working on two antiprogestins called ZK 98.734 and ZK 98.299. Only the former, however, had been tested in animal and human trials (Klitsch, 1989).

Portraying RU-486 and Epostane as morning-after pills, the *Business Week* article said they were better than three Upjohn prostaglandin products that could be used for abortion. (Those drugs, unlike Epostane and RU-486, produced severe uterine contractions and other side effects.) Sterling's senior vice president for medical and scientific affairs, Monroe Trout, discounted reports of nausea caused by Epostane: "It's possible it was morning sickness." Similarly, Baulieu discounted reports of excessive bleeding associated with RU-486: "While bleeding can sometimes be excessive, in most cases it is the same as a regular period or a spontaneous abortion" (Rhein et al., 1985). (Discounting complaints of side effects brought on by contraceptives was nothing new: it had also been a problem associated with the birth control pill and the IUD, or intrauterine device.)

Both companies saw a major market for their drugs as an alternative to approximately 50 million surgical abortions each year, including the nearly 1.5 million abortions in the United States. Securities analysts thought RU-486 and Epostane could also compete in the $697 million oral contraceptive market. In 1985, this market was the exclusive domain of Ortho Pharmaceutical's Ortho-Novum and Wyeth Laboratories' Ovral (Rhein et al., 1985).

Analyst David Crossen noted that safety fears had caused a 2 percent decline (to 51.7 million) in birth control pill prescriptions in the early 1980s (Rhein et al., 1985). RU-486 might suffer fewer problems. In January 1987, the *New England Journal of Medicine* published the results of a study led by Lynette Nieman of the National Institute of Child Health and Human Development. The study confirmed that RU-486 had few serious side effects (Stein, 1987).

Roussel officials, even before all the necessary dosage studies were completed, were optimistic about French government approval. "The Ministry [of Health] will examine the question on a scientific basis, not on a moral basis, because abortion is already legal in this country," said Maurice Ullman, who supervised clinical studies at Roussel (Nayeri, 1987). Analyst David Crossen concluded that "the oral contraceptive market is clearly tremendously ready for an alternative." Thinking of RU-486 as an at-home morning-after method of contraception, Crossen estimated that at $2.50 to $3.50 per pill, a $1 billion market for the drug would be created in the United States alone (Rhein et al., 1985).

But the United States was not an open market: political and religious opposition managed to keep that market closed. At the end of 1986, Congressman Robert Dornan (R-Calif.) called RU-486 a "death pill" (Rosenfeld, 1986). John Willke, NRLC's president, worried about the pill's effect on his organization's campaign. "We're really a very simplistic, visually-oriented people. And if what [abortions] destroy in there doesn't look human, then it will make our job more difficult" (Rosenfeld, 1986). Cal Thomas, former associate of televangelist Jerry Falwell, publicly urged the FDA to reject RU-486 partly because "the United States has never had a national debate on abortion." This was angrily denied by several readers of the *Los Angeles Times* (January 17, 1989), who complained in "Letters to the Editor" that antiabortion forces had long dominated the political scene.

Baulieu was nevertheless ready to enter the fray. He chose what he saw as the high road of scientific objectivism: "I believe to work scientifically and to bring this thinking to the debate is very important," he said. "People know that scientists make a point to remain basically honest, because if you cheat in science you are dead. . . . So if people give us the credit that we are fair, I am ready to use that credit for a cause of this sort" (Rosenfeld, 1986).

Using that credit, Baulieu argued that preimplantation interference with reproductive processes cannot be characterized as abortion. Pregnancy, he argued, does not commence until full implantation of the fertilized egg in the uterine wall. (This view is held by most U.S. scientists and has been adopted by the U.S. government for the purpose of defining "fetus" in its regulations governing research on human subjects [U.S. Congress, Office of Technology Assessment, 1988].) The result, according to Baulieu, is that, for the sake of public discussion, "the whole concept of abortion must change" (Rosenfeld, 1986).

The hope that RU-486 might become a once-a-month contraceptive led gynecologist Raymond Faraggi to predict: "If it works, it will be the end of contraceptives and the end of abortion. No more daily pills, no more IUDs, you take a pill on the 25th to 28th day of your menstrual cycle regularly, every month. It means the end of abortion, anyway, and an end to all our problems" (Nayeri, 1987). William Crowley, Jr., an endocrinologist at Harvard Medical School, hoped RU-486 would lessen opposition from antiabortionists. "If you look at drugs that have changed the history of society," Crowley said, ". . . I think RU-486 is another significant advance" (Stein, 1987).

THE GROWING THREAT OF ANTIABORTION GROUPS

Viewing RU-486 as a once-a-month pill or a menstrual regulator did not lessen opposition from antiabortion organizations. In mid-June 1987, antiabortionists held a three-day conference in New Orleans at which they attended workshops on, among other things, political action strategies for resisting RU-486 (Emiling, 1987). Among these strategies was a plan to lobby Congress to stop the FDA from authorizing clinical trials of RU-486, such as those under way at USC under the auspices of the not-for-profit contraceptive research organization the Population Council (Sheler, 1987). On June 12, 1987, the NRLC proposed guidelines for amending FDA regulations for testing contraceptives. They recommended that no FDA funds be used "to perform any function with respect to" the investigational new drug application in effect for RU-486. In another effort to slow RU-486 development, they also recommended that all oral contraceptives and devices have mandatory 7- and 10-year dog and monkey trials prior to initiation of clinical trials (F-D-C Reports, Inc., 1987).

In February 1988, a WHO task force announced the results of clinical studies in Britain, China, France, and Sweden. They found that RU-486, when administered in conjunction with prostaglandin therapy, was 95 percent effective and free of significant side effects (Steinbrook, 1988). Sensing a growing enthusiasm for the drug, the NRLC and other antiabortion organizations threatened to boycott any drug company that decided to develop the drug—just as Upjohn had been boycotted several years earlier for its development of prostaglandins that had abortifacient qualities (Kolata, 1988b). Publicly, pharmaceutical companies claimed they were not concerned by the boycott threat. Privately, however, according to the *New York Times*, the message was different. "The reasons are obvious," said one unnamed company executive, "and we don't want to get into it" (Kolata, 1988b).

One strategy that might have been employed to avoid the public relations problems raised by developing and marketing RU-486 for early abortions would be to approve it in the United States under another guise, for example, as a drug to widen the cervix and help avoid cesarean sections. Once a drug is approved for marketing by the FDA, it can be prescribed by physicians at their discretion for any condition. But NRLC's education director Richard Glasow said his group would not be fooled by such an action. The group's thousands of local chapters, he said, would organize to boycott any company making the drug—unless it were the only drug available to treat a life-threatening disease. "Our basic position," said Glasow, "is that death drugs designed to kill babies have no place in America" (Kolata, 1988b).

The boycott threat was real because previous boycotts had been effective. In 1985, after NRLC had boycotted Upjohn products for two years, the company stopped all research on drugs to induce abortions or prevent pregnancy. An Upjohn spokesman said that the company decided to stop because of the "adverse regulatory climate in the United States" and the "litigious climate." Glasow, however, insists it was the boycott (Glasow, 1988b). Wayne Bardin, vice president and director of biomedical research at the Population Council, and several others agree (Kolata, 1988b).

In light of this history and the threats to boycott companies involved with RU-486 development, Irving Spitz of the Population Council characterized the power of U.S. antiabortion groups as "very upsetting": "Because of the possible political backlash, we have kept a low profile. We have not really encouraged studies in this country. We feel that our hands are tied. It's a question of political realities" (Kolata, 1988b).

Ironically, little more than a month later the NRLC joined forces with women's groups and consumer activists to oppose certain provisions of proposed legislation that would reduce manufacturer liability for defective products. Consumer groups opposed the entire bill; NRLC encouraged an amendment, sponsored by Congressman Gerry Sikorsky (D-Minn.), that would have removed all drugs or medical devices used as contraceptives or to facilitate abortions from the broad protections of the bill. In its efforts on the amendment, NRLC sent letters to members of Congress complaining that the original version of the bill "would severely curtail the ability of women to obtain recompense for injuries inflicted on them and on their unborn children" (Gladwell, 1988b). Uppermost in NRLC's thinking was RU-486. "It's in our interest to keep the law the way it is," said Douglas Johnson, legislative director for NRLC. Without limitations on liability, the 5 percent failure rate posed a problem for the drug's manufacturers (Gladwell, 1988b). Should the drug fail to terminate a pregnancy, and the mother then decide to carry the child to term rather than seek a surgical abortion, the manufacturer could be exposed to enormous liability if the child were born with health problems traceable to RU-486 exposure. Although exceedingly unlikely, the magnitude of the liability and "bad press" that might be associated with even one such birth defect might be enough to curtail serious interest in the drug.

Women's groups also opposed the original version of the bill, not to hinder RU-486 production but rather for the very reasons stated in the NRLC letter: fear of restricting women's access to damages for injuries resulting from contraceptive use. Not wishing to join too closely with NRLC, women's groups fought the entire bill on the ground that it was unfair to consumers. NRLC set its sights much lower and aimed only to pass the Sikorsky amendment. Passage of the amendment would make the bill fairly useless to pharmaceutical companies and help break the business coalition supporting overall product liability reform (Goodman, 1989). With this kind of opposition, the bill was eventually defeated in Congress.

NRLC's public statements of concern for women's safety did not end with the fight over the product liability bill. In his April 23, 1988, letter to the editor, for example, Richard Glasow protested the *New York Times* editorial stance in favor of the drug. Comparing it to the ill-fated Dalkon shield, he noted that IUDs had also been viewed as safe and effective when they first were put on the market. NRLC asserts that RU-486 might cause cancer, citing a chemical structure with some similarities to the carcinogenic compound diethyl stilbestrol, or DES (Harris, 1991). The claim is dismissed as preposterous by David Grimes of the USC Medical School (Stein, 1988).

The NRLC letter to the *New York Times* concluded as follows: "[Our] opposition to RU-486 arises out of a concern for the life of the unborn child and the life and health of the mother. If any pharmaceutical company attempts to manufacture or market such a killer drug in the United States, it would face so massive a boycott by right-to-life organizations, church groups, and pro-life hospitals that RU-486 profits would be swallowed up many times over by the loss of other business. American women aren't looking for a chemical Dalkon Shield. Neither are we."

NRLC continued to draw connections between RU-486 and the failed IUD when it critiqued a peer-reviewed study of the drug: "The French study . . . offered nothing to calm fears about the possibility of long-term adverse side effects, such as damage to the aborted woman's later children. This is especially important in light of the abysmal track record many of those advocating RU-486 in the United States (such as Planned Parenthood) had in promoting such dangerous products as the Dalkon Shield IUD" (Glasow, 1990a).

By May 1988, RU-486 was making its way into the general public's debate over abortion rights. A Virginia mail handler, for example, wrote in *The New Republic* (Fagen, 1988) that:

> [P]ro-lifers like to compare their struggle with the fight against slavery. In fact, it has more in common with prohibition. . . . Abortion is like alcohol abuse—it pervades our whole society. . . . The idea that abortion can be stopped by reversing Roe is prohibitionist romanticism, as naive and foredoomed as that of the Anti-Saloon League. . . . The issue is not whether women theoretically should be the ones making abortion decisions. As a matter of fact they are, and in the future, with RU-486 or the equivalent, their decision making capacity is likely to increase. Faced with this reality, the only practical way to decrease abortion is to influence the decisions they make.

There is no way to overstate the anger that abortion, and RU-486, can generate. When asked whether he'd prefer his daughter be forced to use the riskier suction technique rather than use RU-486 should she become pregnant, one antiabortion demonstrator said "I don't think it makes much difference if she kills her baby or kills herself" (ABC News, 1990).

The political controversy surrounding RU-486 soon took its toll on Roussel. By June 1988, Sakiz's support for RU-486 began to wane in the face of taunts outside his window and as many as 25 threatening letters a day. The protesters claimed he was "changing the uterus into a death oven" (Greenhouse, 1989b). "Assassins, stop your work of death," read some letters. Others contained threats: "Your pill kills babies and you will suffer the consequences." Handbills were distributed calling RU-486 a "chemical weapon" that would "poison a billion third world children."

In addition, other pressures began to build. On June 22, 1988, the eve of Roussel Uclaf's annual meeting, NRLC executive director David O'Steen released a letter the organization had sent to the French ambassador (PR Newswire, 1988b) protesting the French government's involvement with RU-486 through its minority shareholder position in Roussel Uclaf:

[A] lethal drug has no place in America or anywhere else. We are especially incensed that the abortion pill's proponents have announced that they intend to make women of Third World countries a special target for the death drug's use. . . . If Roussel Uclaf or any other pharmaceutical company attempts to manufacture or market RU-486, [the] National Right to Life Committee would seriously consider joining with other pro-life groups around the world to initiate a boycott of the products of Roussel Uclaf and firms affiliated with it through the parent company Hoechst.

This letter, like the congressional lobbying over the product liability legislation, demonstrated NRLC's ability to borrow arguments and language from the women's health movement. This movement often cited inadequate testing of new products and exploitation of women in developing countries as reasons to oppose many contraceptive innovations. The promise of RU-486 was so great, however, that it encouraged the women's health movement to join with the "population controllers" whom they bitterly opposed—Planned Parenthood Federation and the Population Council—in support of the drug (Fraser, 1988).

Now ambivalent about RU-486, Sakiz arrived at Roussel's annual meeting on June 23, 1988, to be met by hundreds of abortion protesters on the Boulevard des Invalides. Instead of focusing on the company's recent increase in profits, the meeting was dominated by anatomy professor and abortion opponent Xavier Dor, who excoriated Sakiz for 20 minutes (Greenhouse, 1989a). Yet despite this growing internal and external pressure, Sakiz was unwilling to repeat the company's mistake of the 1960s, when it chose not to produce oral contraceptives for fear of a public and religious backlash. He hoped that the protests would disappear after France's minister of health, Claude Evin, ruled on Roussel's application to market the drug. He believed the protests were directed more at the government than at the company (Greenhouse, 1989a). Meanwhile, Baulieu also lobbied colleagues within the company, urging them not to give in to the right-to-life movement and to support the clinical trials beginning in Great Britain (Facts on File, 1987).

CORPORATE PRESSURE FOR WITHDRAWAL

Although antiabortion forces clearly were having some effect on Sakiz, they were having their greatest effect on Roussel's parent company. A spokesman for Hoechst acknowledged that the company had received threats of boycotts against all of its products and that the director had "decided it [proceeding with RU-486] was simply not worth the risk" (Ricci, 1988).

According to the following excerpt from a *New York Times Magazine* article (Greenhouse, 1989a) written by Paris-based reporter Steven Greenhouse on the basis of interviews with unidentified Roussel employees and their friends (S. Greenhouse, personal communication, February 6, 1991), it was the resulting intra-company pressures that finally persuaded Sakiz to withdraw support for the drug.

> Sakiz's friends say it was not the anti-abortion protestors but intra-company pressures that finally caused him to cave in. Roussel, after all, had a parent company to answer to. Hankering for what the French call a "petite danseuse," a little dancer, Hoechst A.G., the stolid West German chemicals giant, had first bought a stake in Roussel in 1968; it has since grown to 54.5 percent. Hoechst was attracted by the smaller company's expertise in biochemistry, and by its creativity and impulsiveness. But in the RU 486 affair, it appeared that Roussel was too creative and impulsive. Hoechst made it clear that RU 486 was no longer welcome, when the company's chief executive officer, Wolfgang Hilger, stated that an abortion pill violates the company's credo to support life.

> Hoechst also feared that boycott threats by the American anti-abortion movement could cripple Hoechst's $6-billion-a-year American subsidiary. "Officials at Hoechst's American subsidiary asked headquarters to get Roussel to cease and desist," says Sheldon Segal, director of population sciences at the Rockefeller Foundation and a hard-fighting advocate of RU 486.

> Privately, Roussel officials said colleagues at Hoechst were dismayed by the right-to-lifers' taunts that Hoechst and Roussel were doing to fetuses what the

Nazis had done to the Jews. I.G. Farben, Hoechst's ancestor company, manu-
factured cyanide gas for the death camps.

The key development that seemed to force Sakiz's about-face came when
Alain Madec, an ambitious 41-year-old executive vice president, the No. 3 man
at Roussel, announced that he was against RU 486. He was the third of Roussel's
five-man executive committee to throw his weight against the pill, joining
two other executive vice presidents. Sakiz had withstood their opposition be-
cause they were due to retire soon. But with Madec's announcement, he began to
worry that Madec might be currying favor with Hoechst to stage a palace
coup. (Greenhouse, 1989a)

Still, Sakiz held out. On September 23, 1988, French Minister of
Health Evin approved the pill for marketing (Foreman, 1988a). But
instead of the protests dying down, as Sakiz had hoped, they escalated.
The influential Archbishop of Paris Jean-Marie Cardinal Lustiger
condemned the pill (Greenhouse, 1989a). Even Judy Norsigian of the
National Women's Health Network in the United States was less than
completely supportive of the decision: "Women think this is a great
idea and it does offer an option to women ambivalent about abortion,
but it's too early to say if it is a good thing until it has been around
longer" (Foreman, 1988a).

Norsigian's ambivalence was noted and her remarks repeated in the
National Right to Life News (Glasow, 1988c), in which NRLC's education director Richard Glasow echoed this safety theme: "We are opposed
to marketing of RU-486 in the U.S. or any other country because it kills
unborn babies and it can injure if not possibly kill women. It is a very
dangerous drug. It causes every woman who takes it to experience a
miscarriage with excessive bleeding. Women in the United States and
other countries should not be guinea pigs to determine its long-term
adverse side-effects" (Foreman, 1988a). These were the same kinds of
charges made earlier by women's groups who opposed Depo-Provera,
and they reflect the continued mistrust generated by the early birth
control pill trials.

In the week that followed, Dutch researchers announced that another
drug, Epostane, was about 84 percent effective at inducing abortions.
Glasow announced that NRLC opposed Epostane as strongly as it opposed RU-486 (Stein, 1989).

With attention beginning to focus on prospects for U.S. marketing of
either Epostane or RU-486, U.S. pharmaceutical companies, seemingly
in an effort to ward off boycotts and bad publicity, began to deny interest or involvement. John Wood, vice president for public affairs at Searle,
which owned the rights to Epostane in the United States, announced
that the company had no plan to market it. "The drug is not a suitable
candidate for our overall objectives," he said (Stein, 1989). GynoPharma,

a New Jersey company, announced that, despite Roussel's statements that discussions were taking place between the two companies (Technology Newsletter, 1988), it did "not have an agreement, nor is the company involved in negotiations with Roussel Uclaf" (Foreman, 1988c). Glasow of NRLC asserted that GynoPharma had "backpedaled immediately, pull[ing] itself out of this debate" following the French government's approval of the drug (Foreman, 1988c).

In an October 6, 1988, editorial entitled "Pills and Parallels," the *Boston Globe* noted the parallels between the introduction of the birth control pill and the introduction of RU-486:

> *Historic parallels between the two pills are remarkable in the extent to which American pharmaceutical companies fear political and religious backlash against the new abortifacient, just as they did 30 years ago against the contraceptive. Such fears about "the pill" turned out to be groundless, as they should about the abortifacient.*
>
> *To test the waters of social acceptance, the contraceptive pill was first presented as a medicine for menstrual regulation, a legitimate use but not the pill's primary purpose. The same ruse—menstrual regulation—is being used today to try to gain approval of the abortion pill. . . .*
>
> *In the 1950s, America's mightiest drug companies did not dare to market the contraceptive pill, fearing they would become the target of boycotts over the "immorality" of birth control. The identical fear now—of a vast boycott threatened by the National Right to Life Committee over the "immorality" of abortion—has cowed the pharmaceutical industry. No United States company is seeking federal permission to market RU-486 as an abortifacient or for any other medical purpose.*
>
> *The presumed power of anti-abortion groups . . . should be challenged. When the G.D. Searle company finally plunged ahead with the marketing of the contraceptive pill, it experienced no adverse reaction. . . .*
>
> *History's lesson is that society was way ahead of politicians, federal agents, and socio-religious groups in its acceptance of the birth control pill. Today, Americans widely approve the option of abortion; the earlier, the better.*

The editorial's point about public attitudes was accurate. A Louis Harris survey, released on October 12, 1988, found that 82 percent of Americans supported government spending on research and development of new contraceptives and 59 percent thought that RU-486 should be made available in the United States (PR Newswire, 1988d). Even America's oldest advice columnists, Abigail Van Buren and Ann Landers, supported the drug. At an October 17 dinner to honor them with Planned Parenthood's 1988 Margaret Sanger Award, Van Buren said: "[RU-486] is said to be safe and effective. Hallelujah sisters. But what will the politics of this medication be? Will the FDA approve it? And who's going to manufacture it? Between my sister and me I am told we are read by an estimated 100 million people daily. Thank God," she continued (borrowing the religious rhetoric of the antiabortion movement), "we are on the right side of this issue" (PR Newswire, 1988c).

Nevertheless, despite this evidence of public support in the United States, corporate pressures and local demonstrations began to take their toll on Roussel's Sakiz. Roussel had been inundated with letters of protest and threats of boycotts (Associated Press, 1988); Hoechst, with 25 percent of its $23 billion in sales located in the United States, made it clear that it strongly favored suspending sales of the drug (Greenhouse, 1988b). On October 21, 1988, Sakiz called a meeting of the management committee. After two hours, he called for a vote, and he raised his hand to withdraw RU-486 from the markets both in France and abroad (Greenhouse, 1989a), despite having already contracted with China, Spain, Britain, and the Scandinavian countries to supply the pills (Tempest, 1988b). "We have a responsibility in managing a company," he explained in an interview. "But if I were a lone scientist, I would have acted differently," thus summing up the conflicting priorities of business and science (Greenhouse, 1989a).

Baulieu was traveling and did not hear of the decision until the following week. When he did, he returned to Paris to protest privately, in Sakiz's office. Reportedly, Baulieu's Roussel colleagues felt at times that he was too outspoken, as when he suggested investigating the use of RU-486 as a once-a-month pill, thus blurring the lines between contraception and abortion. Nonetheless, Sakiz encouraged Baulieu to go public. "You're independent," he said, "you can go out and speak freely" (Greenhouse, 1989a).

The next day, October 26, 1988, Roussel informed the press it was pulling RU-486 off the market because of the "outcry of public opinion" and the "polemic" surrounding the pill. "Side effects were in no way a problem," said Arlette Geslin, director of medical relations for Roussel Laboratories. "The problem was that there were protests, letters threatening to boycott, and demonstrations in front of our headquarters. We didn't want to get into a big moral debate" (Greenhouse, 1988a).

Roussel vice chairman Pierre Joly commented, "We believed that after the French government approved the product, everybody would be influenced by that decision and we could forget the problem. But that was not true. The trend, the threats kept increasing" (Tempest, 1988c). For example, a militant French antiabortion group, the Committee to Save Unborn Children, called for the "destruction of all stocks of the chemical weapon RU-486" (Tempest, 1988c).

Roussel officials were concerned about protests not only in France but in the United States, citing the NRLC letter to the French ambassador and American threats of boycotts against all Roussel and Hoechst products (Greenhouse, 1988a). "We witnessed an orchestrated campaign that became more and more powerful," said Joly (Greenhouse, 1988c).

There have also been personal threats. Baulieu once traveled with a bodyguard during a U.S. visit (United Press International, 1988). David Byrd (a Scottish researcher), Joly, and a number of Roussel officials also received threats (Atwood, 1988; Gruhier et al., 1988; Reuters, 1988). Minister of Health Evin later commented, "Their children and their wives were threatened through anonymous letters. This is totally inadmissible and utterly cowardly. It is difficult to say who these people are, since they are acting anonymously, but they are basically those same religious fundamentalists who in the early 1970s campaigned against the abortion law" (Naughton, 1988b).

U.S. pressure was particularly influential. "The pressure groups from the United States are very powerful, maybe even more so than in France," said Pierre de Rible, Roussel's deputy financial director. "We see that in the American presidential campaign, abortion is a major subject of debate, but in France people speak less and less of it" (Greenhouse, 1988c). But, he added, the introduction of the abortion pill had begun to revive that debate in France (Greenhouse, 1988c). French physicians were writing to the company, threatening not to prescribe any of its products to their patients (Laurenson, 1988).

NRLC agreed that public pressure must have caused Roussel to take RU-486 off the market. "Roussel Uclaf expended millions of dollars to promote their abortion pill," said John Willke, president of NRLC. "If they've decided to halt their distribution, we can be sure the 'public outcry' must have been massive and worldwide. They evidently concluded that peddling death drugs was not in their best interests" (PR Newswire, 1988a).

One unnamed Roussel employee said, "We cannot put the group's development at risk. Public opinion is not ready for this product" (Naughton, 1988a). Although Roussel's exports to the United States represented only 7 percent of its annual $1.7 billion in sales, financial analysts said the company was worried that a boycott over RU-486 might cripple its ambitious plans to increase American sales.

According to another Roussel employee, concern about its international image had been more important than the short-term economic effects of a boycott when Roussel made its decision to pull the drug from the market. "We decided more than five years ago that we didn't want to make money on RU-486," said Joly. "We decided to sell it at cost" (Tempest, 1988c). Although protests in France itself had been fairly weak, NRLC asserted that there had been demonstrations against the drug at 40 French embassies worldwide. Although Agence France Presse reported it had no such information (Foreman, 1988d), "the company acted to preserve its image abroad," according to a Roussel employee (Tempest, 1988c).

Roussel's decision met with mixed reactions within the French government. Michèle André, minister for women's rights, called the decision disagreeable. Junior Minister for Family Affairs Hélène Dorlhac, however, said, "I am pleased by this withdrawal, as by the decision to take pornographic films off prime-time television" (Greenhouse, 1988c).

Roussel's decision came at a time of tension in France during which religious conservatives and the secular society were publicly and privately at odds. For example, the Roussel announcement was made three days after a firebombing of a Paris cinema showing the film "The Last Temptation of Christ." A Hoechst spokesman denied any connection between the cinema fire and the decision to stop making RU-486. He did say, however, that both events "stemmed from the same thinking" (Ricci, 1988).

The French Movement for Family Planning issued a statement drawing attention to the link between the political opposition to RU-486 and the political opposition to the film: "After setting the fires of intolerance with the Scorsese film, the traditionalists and Catholic reactionaries want to impose their outdated laws on women. When will we start seeing women burned alive at the stake as in the Middle Ages?" (Ricci, 1988). Scientists and leftist politicians also drew parallels between the withdrawal of the drug and a Catholic fundamentalist campaign to drive the controversial film from theaters. Only one Paris cinema showed the film after the protests and arson attack (Naughton, 1988a).

THE RETURN OF RU-486

On the same day Roussel announced its decision to withdraw RU-486 from the market, nearly 10,000 physicians and researchers were gathered in Rio de Janeiro for the World Congress of Gynecology and Obstetrics. Roussel's decision turned the meeting into a rally to rescue the drug. It could appear that Roussel had timed its announcement to coincide with this meeting to generate support for the drug, and to lay the groundwork for subsequent events that allowed Roussel to market the drug without appearing to endorse its development or use.

The Roussel decision was widely criticized at the Rio meeting. Sheldon Segal attacked Roussel for "betraying its partnership with the medical profession" (Greenhouse, 1989b). Elisabeth Aubény, a Parisian gynecologist, carried a 2,000-name petition of protest back to France. Baulieu called for women to organize: "It's not enough for women to show a simple desire for the pill. There must be a public mobilization to demand it be made available" (Reuters Library Report, 1988). He also said, "Sakiz told me he hopes there is pressure to counteract this decision" (Simons, 1988). Indeed, such pressure was building. A group of American and European university professors began preparing a list of Roussel's products and said they would ask physicians to boycott them. A protest campaign was planned that included placing advertisements in newspapers and sending letters to Hoechst. "Medical groups and family planning clinics should protest the decision to show that we too have a voice, not only right-to-life groups," one professor said (Simons, 1988).

Other organizations also issued statements of protest. The National Abortion Rights Action League (NARAL) said, "A fringe group of anti-choice extremists, having failed to halt legal abortions through the courts and the legislature, is holding a large multinational drug company hostage" (Ricci, 1988). The French minister of women's rights, Michèle André, said the action might encourage an attack on abortion rights in general: "We are witnessing a return to morality. And who are the victims of morality?—women. Always. It's as old as the world" (Naughton, 1988a).

An October 28, 1988, *New York Times* editorial entitled "Abortion, Intimidation, and Death" also focused on the women who would be affected by the decision: "By capitulating to activists who regard abortion as immoral, a French company called Groupe Roussel Uclaf may be committing a larger immorality, ordaining the death of tens of thousands of women around the world. . . . It is they, and not a corps of noisy intimidators, who should have the company's ear."

Planned Parenthood Federation called Roussel's move a "tragic display of cowardice and a shocking blow to women around the world" (PR Newswire, 1988d). It accused Roussel of "buckling to the political pressure exerted by a small but vocal anti-family planning minority, with total disregard for the health benefits this drug could have had for millions of women worldwide. . . . We hope that another manufacturer, one truly devoted to improving the health of the world's people, will step in and make available this much-needed product" (PR Newswire, 1988d).

In fact, physicians, scientists, feminists, and family planning organizations began to work almost immediately to bring RU-486 to market without Roussel. "We're worried about the rise of Catholic fundamentalism and the blackmail exercised against Roussel," said Catherine Lesterpet, the national coordinator of the French Family Planning Association (PR Newswire, 1988d). One suggestion was to set up a nonprofit company to buy the patent because, as a single-product enterprise, retail boycotts could not harm it. Another suggestion was to have China, the only country besides France to approve the drug, buy the patent and manufacture the pill for the whole world. A third suggestion was that WHO, which had sponsored many tests of RU-486's safety and effectiveness, distribute the pill (Greenhouse, 1988a). But WHO would face problems in manufacturing and marketing on such a scale, asserted José Barzalatto, then director of WHO human reproduction research, "because we are not a pharmaceutical company" (Greenhouse, 1989b). In addition, obtaining the patent from Roussel would not be easy because of the drug's promising uses in other areas, such as fighting breast cancer or dilating the cervix to avoid cesarean sections in cases of prolonged labor.

There was also the chance Roussel might change its mind. Pierre Joly, Roussel's vice chairman, hinted at this the day following the announcement: "We might resume distribution of RU-486 if the atmosphere becomes peaceful again" (Greenhouse, 1989b). Within the French government, efforts were under way to force Roussel to make such a change. Michèle Barzach, former health minister under conservative Jacques Chirac, was the first to attack the company's decision and to criticize the Socialist government for remaining silent (Izbicki, 1988). Two days later, Claude Evin summoned Joly to his office. Evin was angry that the company had pulled RU-486 only four weeks after the government had defied the Church and antiabortion pressure groups and approved the drug. "[I am] astonished by such a decision, which is contrary to the industrial policy pursued up to now on this product," he said (PR Newswire, 1988a).

Evin feared that if the antiabortion movement was triumphant in its crusade against Roussel, it would begin fighting for a repeal of the 1975 French law legalizing abortion. The government did not wish to enter such a fray. Bitter controversy had preceded passage of the 1975 law, as well as the 1984 Socialist government decision to reimburse abortion costs under the national health plan (Naughton, 1988a). "I was doing what I could," said Evin, "to make sure France did not surrender to pressure groups animated by archaic ideologies" (Greenhouse, 1989a). Roget Bouzinac, a distinguished French commentator writing in Le Var, pointed to another aspect of the controversy. Noting the violence surrounding "The Last Temptation of Christ" and RU-486, he asked whether France might not be on the verge of another religious war. "We must be careful that the affair of this abortion pill does not recreate the anti-clerical movement which at another period did our nation so much harm" (Izbicki, 1988).

Evin told Joly that, if necessary, the French government would use its status as 36 percent owner of Roussel (and some special provisions of French law) to transfer the patent to another company in order to serve the public good. In light of this threat, Roussel issued a statement on October 28, agreeing to put the drug back on the market (Associated Press, 1988). Explaining his decision to force the company to change its mind, Evin said, "I could not permit the abortion debate to deprive women of a product that represents medical progress. From the moment Government approval for the drug was granted, RU-486 became the moral property of women, not just the property of the drug company" (Greenhouse, 1989a, 1989b).

Baulieu echoed this sentiment: "It is a good reaction in the face of demonstrations of intolerance that constituted a grave precedent. Medicine is at the service of patients and goes beyond other considerations" (J. Phillips, 1988b). He added, "Intolerance cannot be introduced into choices made between a patient and her doctor. That would be something of incalculable consequences" (Atwood, 1988).

Prime Minister Michel Rocard's Socialist Party praised Evin's decision: "This is in accord with the morals, needs, and mentality of medical science. The majority of public opinion, and especially most women, expected it" (J. Phillips, 1988a). This perception was accurate: an October 1988 survey found 64 percent of the French public in support of the drug. Fifty-six percent believed that Roussel had violated women's rights by withdrawing it (Gruhier et al., 1988). Representatives of conservative parties disagreed: "It is in the interests of public health to favor life, not to kill it with a chemical product" said Christine Boutin, a deputy of former President Valery Giscard d'Estaing's Union of French Democracy federation (J. Phillips, 1988a).

The French government's stance was also supported by interested medical and political groups around the world. José Pinotti, president of the International Gynecological and Obstetrics Federation, said, "France has made a courageous decision, one that shows science cannot be blocked by narrow-minded politics" (Atwood, 1988). Scottish gynecologist David Byrd called the decision a "mature response to pressure from people who are not opposed to this drug but to any kind of abortion" (Atwood, 1988).

Sakiz was delighted with the government order because it took the onus off his company and shifted responsibility to the Ministry of Health. "The Government's order helped us," he said, "because it showed the Government was on our side." Joly added, "We are relieved of the moral burden weighing on our group. For us, the problem is now solved" (Greenhouse, 1989a). Some opponents suggested that Evin and Sakiz had orchestrated the series of events to shift blame from Roussel to the government, but both men denied the charge (Greenhouse, 1988a, 1989b; Gruhier et al., 1988).

Hoechst, however, also denied any allegation of collusion: "This is a purely political decision of the French government and we have always said that we would respect such political decisions" (Naughton, 1988b). The Hoechst spokeswoman also sought to distance the company from events by noting that "Roussel Uclaf is totally independent and the decision they made has nothing to do with whatever Hoechst thinks" (Foreman, 1988b). But, she added, the pill would not be put on the market in West Germany.

The leading French weekly *Nouvel Observateur*, however, hinted at collaboration between the government and the company. It noted that Roussel had responded far more quickly to the government threat than would be expected, especially in light of the legal questions raised by the government's minority stockholder status (Gruhier et al., 1988). (France would sell its shares in July 1990 to Roussel's competitor Rhône-Poulenc, for $700 million) (Dawkins, 1990; Glasow, 1990d, 1990e). American observers agreed. Based on conversations with Sakiz, the director of population policy work at the Rockefeller Foundation, Sheldon Segal, said: "I personally believe that this was a joint decision on the part of Groupe Roussel and the Ministry of Health" (Tempest, 1988c).

The antiabortion movement also rejected Hoechst's denials of collusion. Judie Brown, president of the American Life League, said she was not surprised by the French government's decision: "We originally thought the whole thing was a public relations gimmick" (Tempest, 1988c). The NRLC stated that "the withdrawal was all for show, a carefully staged ploy to take the heat off of the manufacturer by placing the blame on the French government" (Glasow, 1988d). Its president, John Willke, said, "We hold Roussel-Uclaf and its parent company, Hoechst AG in Germany, 100 percent responsible" (Glasow, 1988d). In another interview he said: "We cannot rule out a massive worldwide boycott against Hoechst . . . and every other subsidiary. The attempt by the French minister to take the blame and absolve the company is a charade and we will directly hold the company totally responsible for release of this drug" (Foreman, 1988b).

These organizations and the Catholic Church denounced the French government's move. Msgr. Albert Decourtray, president of the French Bishops Conference, called it "a victory for savage liberalism" (United Press International, 1988). He also asserted that the reason for the government's intervention was financial, not ethical: "There are huge sums at stake and I am afraid that economic considerations weighed heavily in this decision" (Tempest, 1988a). In Washington, Victoria Leonard, executive director of the National Women's Health Network, said she was "relieved" by the French government's decision. She called it courageous and predicted that "this drug's entry into the United States is inevitable" (J. Phillips, 1988b).

THE CONTINUING OPPOSITION

With the drug's marketing in France assured, concern switched to the possibility of a dangerous black market in RU-486 in countries where the drug was not available. Evin said that precautions to prevent abuse and black market sales had been taken. "These pills will only be administered in the presence of a doctor and sales will be subjected to the same rigorous restriction as those which apply to hard drugs," he said (Reuters, 1988). Others, however, like Louise Tyrer of Planned Parenthood, predicted that a black market would appear in the United States (Thomas, 1988). "It's coming," agreed Planned Parenthood president Faye Wattleton. "The question is whether it will come unsupervised and unsafe, or supervised and safe" (Goodman, 1988a). Joseph Speidel and Victoria Leonard also thought that women would smuggle the drug to obtain it. "Women smuggle contraceptives into Ireland, where they are illegal, and women are going to smuggle RU-486 into this country," said Leonard (Stein, 1988).

The feminist leadership were concerned that a black market in RU-486 would make lay abortions dangerous. Recently, a number of groups have sprung up to teach women to do lay abortions using the relatively safe suction technique lest the medical community become unwilling or unable to provide the service (Japenga and Venant, 1989; Kolata, 1989). Some have already talked of trying to smuggle in RU-486, although none as yet have been successful. But if taken too late by someone with contraindications, or without follow-up prostaglandin therapy, RU-486 could produce complications. To prevent a black market from developing, feminists began working to get the drug into the country, either through an established company or by organizing a new company (Goodman, 1989). The groups began by visiting Roussel in Paris and its New Jersey subsidiary, hoping in both instances to get the companies interested in U.S. marketing. To date, they have been unsuccessful (Sherman, 1989).

Legal access to RU-486 in the United States does not appear likely in the near future. At the moment, the companies most likely to take on testing and development of the drug are keeping a low profile. In January 1989, Victor Bauer, president of Roussel's U.S. subsidiary, HRPI, asserted that its decision not to pursue testing and licensing of the drug in the United States had nothing to do with "extremist pressures." Rather, RU-486 "lies outside the experience and medical expertise of this company. HRPI does no research in the birth control area" (Savage and Tumulty, 1989).

At this same time, however, controversy began over drugs not destined for the birth control or abortion markets, such as Searle's antiulcer drug, Cytotec. While the drug was under review by the FDA, antiabortion groups began petitioning the federal government to prevent its production because it could be used to induce miscarriages. Richard Glasow of NRLC asserted that the drug would be "on the streets" within days of approval as a black market source for abortifacients, and antiabortion groups threatened to boycott Searle should it market the drug (Kolata, 1988c). Despite these threats, the FDA approved the drug.

SUCCESS OF THE BOYCOTT THREAT

In late 1988, a new opposition group, the RCR Alliance, registered with Congress as lobbyists. The registration stated that RCR was interested in abortion-related legislation. In fact, the group was formed solely to persuade the French government, Hoechst, or Roussel to pull RU-486 off the market (Ciolli, 1989a). Its strategy is partly revealed by its name. The initials stand for Robins-Carbide-Reynolds, referring to three companies that have faced extensive product liability litigation (Sarasohn, 1988).

"We feel the pill is devoid of conscience. It is nothing more than a human pesticide," said Kenneth Dupin, pastor of the Valley View Wesleyan Church in Roanoke, Virginia, and a director of the RCR Alliance (Sarasohn, 1988). Legal abortions in the United States are handled by the medical community, which, according to Dupin, has a conscience. But women in the third world generally would use the drug without such supervision (Sarasohn, 1988).

Although Dupin's RCR Alliance is centered at his church, its membership includes others as well. The church has already organized a boycott of such high-visibility French products as Perrier and Michelin tires. RCR Alliance plans to back the boycott if other efforts at persuasion fail. Its immediate goal, however, is to negotiate with the French government, Hoechst, and Roussel. "We're not trying to be corporate terrorists," Dupin says. "We're willing to compensate this company for its research" (Sarasohn, 1988).

In September 1988, the unknown RCR Alliance tried unsuccessfully to set up a meeting with Hoechst. "We were just another telex," Dupin said (Ciolli, 1989a). So the group tried a more indirect method. With an anonymous donor covering their costs, the alliance spent thousands of dollars in computer time examining documents in Europe and the United States to get a detailed profile of Hoechst and its owners. A source in Frankfurt provided them with the U.S. global money market funds, European banks, and other financial institutions that held stock in Hoechst. RCR then sent a courier to hand-deliver the document to the chairman of Hoechst in Frankfurt with an outline of their three-pronged strategy (Ciolli, 1989b).

First, it would organize a boycott of any U.S. financial firm that was holding Hoechst stock in its international funds. Fearing that Hoechst would divest itself of Roussel to avoid controversy, RCR Alliance sent letters warning against such an action to 75 of the world's brokerage houses able to finance such a sale (Ciolli, 1989b). RCR also said it would solicit media attention through Operation Rescue and threatened to picket Hoechst's New York headquarters and other locations.

The group also said it would focus public attention on Hoechst's South African assets and its predecessor, I. G. Farben, which had produced cyanide gas for the Nazi death camps (Ciolli, 1989b), a threat made good in 1991 with a lengthy article on the drug's "Nazi connection" (Brennan, 1991) in a special issue of the *National Right to Life News*. The article was accompanied by a cartoon depicting shower heads spewing forth both deadly gas on trapped naked victims in a concentration camp and RU-486 pills on a well-developed fetus in utero.

Further, the group threatened to tie Hoechst up in litigation by finding plaintiffs in developing countries where the drug might be distributed. RCR retained a French law firm that was ready to go forward with the litigation. It also identified religious organizations that would look for any woman who could claim to have been harmed by taking the drug (Ciolli, 1989b).

While RCR focused on the private sector, other groups focused their efforts on Washington. At a news conference regarding his confirmation hearings, Health and Human Services Secretary-designate Louis Sullivan was asked specifically whether he would oppose FDA review and approval of the drug. He declined to respond (States News Service, 1988).

In February 1989, Congressman Robert Dornan (R-Calif.) introduced H.R. 619, a bill to prohibit federal assistance for investigation of Roussel Uclaf's antiprogesterone steroid. No federal funds may be used for abortion research, but this bill would have prohibited federal funding even for non-abortion-related applications, such as treatment of Cushing's disease. The bill died in committee (F-D-C Reports, Inc., 1989); however, White House Chief of Staff John Sununu ordered aides to research RU-486 in case a decision was needed about U.S. availability (Walsh, 1989).

In addition to U.S. groups, several international bodies joined the campaign against RU-486. In mid-March 1989, the International Right to Life Federation (IRLF) urged consumers to boycott Roussel and Hoechst (Greenhouse, 1989b; Reuters Library Report, 1989). IRLF said it would join its Canadian affiliate, Alliance for Life, and call for extending the boycott to other French products, such as wine or perfume, if France did not stop its "chemical warfare against unborn children" (Reuters Library Report, 1989).

The IRLF and the Moral Majority, a conservative U.S. political/religious group, asserted that using RU-486 could devastate African populations by drastically cutting birth rates while failing to reduce mortality rates. The statements echoed those charges from the political left that U.S. population policy and family planning programs are a covert form of colonialist genocide. IRLF claimed that "[t]he effect on agrarian cultures could be their very elimination" (Arch, 1989). The statement, however, made no reference to likely rates of use nor to reduced maternal mortality from avoidance of illegal, unsanitary abortions or overly short birth intervals. Each year approximately 500,000 women a year die from pregnancy-related complications, an estimated 200,000 of whom die from illegal abortions (Yinger, 1990).

Later that month, Jerry Nims, president of the Moral Majority, claimed that his group had reached a "milestone" agreement with Hoechst and Roussel to prohibit marketing and distribution of RU-486 outside of France. Nims said the companies also agreed not to begin any new tests, limiting trials to those already under way (Glasow, 1989). Finally, the companies had agreed not to offer the drug to WHO for other medical applications (Arch, 1989). According to Nims, the agreement came after "several months of dialogue" among the companies, the Moral Majority, RCR Alliance, and other antiabortion groups. Nims implied that the threats of economic boycott, picketing, and "social action" by groups currently associated with Operation Rescue "clearly communicated" to Hoechst that they had to be "taken seriously" (Arch, 1989).

The agreement was outlined in a telegram from Hoechst's spokesman Dominik Von Winterfeldt to Nims (Arch, 1989). Von Winterfeldt, however, denied that there was an agreement: "We exchanged various messages since January [1989] and it seems that our last message in which we restated our former policy satisfied them and led them somehow to the conclusion that what they had discussed with us constituted an agreement" (Sachs, 1989). RCR's Dupin replied that Hoechst's freedom to make this claim was part of the agreement (Ciolli, 1989a).

Von Winterfeldt asserted that Hoechst had decided years ago never to sell an abortifacient under its own name because its directors did not want to decide whether abortion was morally correct (Sachs, 1989). "The board . . . does not want the company . . . to get involved in a decision of whether you are interfering with life itself" (Ciolli, 1989a).

THE FEMINIST AND MEDICAL COMMUNITY RESPONSE

U.S. support for legalizing RU-486 was demonstrated again in an April 1989 Associated Press poll. It found that 51 percent of Americans supported legalization, a figure similar to the 59 percent supporting availability in the earlier Louis Harris survey (Associated Press, 1989). Indeed, public support was considered so strong that some pro-choice supporters, such as Congresswoman Pat Schroeder (D-Colo.) were considering legislation to offer federal funding for RU-486 research (Walsh, 1989).

In June 1989, feminist leaders announced a campaign to bring RU-486 to the United States (United Press International, 1989). "We intend to visit the pharmaceutical leaders, the medical health leaders to urge them to rise up against this . . . know-nothing movement that is denying the best of medical research and the best that modern medicine can provide for the modern woman," said former National Organization for Women (NOW) president Eleanor Smeal (Reuters, 1989b). "RU-486 can help save so many lives that we are determined to build a network both nationally and internationally to ensure that its research and development proceeds as fast as possible," announced NOW's current president, Molly Yard (Anderson, 1989).

Following the July announcement of the Supreme Court's decision in *Webster* v. *Reproductive Services*, in which the Court expanded state powers to curtail even privately funded abortion services in state facilities, Eleanor Smeal renewed calls for testing and distribution of RU-486 (Goodman, 1989). An office-based technique such as RU-486 was now more crucial than ever, given the Illinois case concerning restrictive abortion clinic licensing statutes that might drive most clinics out of business (Goodman, 1989). Maintaining that there are no serious side effects from RU-486 and that the new drug was a needed contraceptive option, Smeal added that RU-486 was also promising for the treatment of endometriosis. "The irony is, this [Supreme] Court just said you should favor childbirth, yet RU-486 could help cure one of the leading causes of infertility" (Federal Information Systems Corporation, 1989).

Fury over the *Webster* case fueled the national abortion debate and filled the coffers of abortion rights as well as antiabortion organizations. Pro-choice groups such as NOW and NARAL experienced sizable increases in donations and membership, as supporters felt threatened by receding constitutional protection from legislative action. The American Civil Liberties Union, already relatively flush from the 1988 presidential election, received another wave of support. Antiabortion organizations also began to receive more donations. They started subscription drives to gear up for a push in state legislatures nationwide. The attention given to the abortion issue in the 1989 local elections was extraordinary (Kornhauser, 1989).

When in July 1989 the NOW membership endorsed the idea of a third party, they made abortion rights a centerpiece of that party's platform, and specifically listed bringing RU-486 into the United States as part of their agenda (Black, 1989). Two months later, Eleanor Smeal called on NOW to make RU-486 availability a "top priority." She also urged women to organize counterboycotts and lobby Congress to ensure that the next FDA commissioner (Frank Young had resigned in mid-1989) was not ideologically opposed to the drug (Arnst, 1989a).

The medical community also urged Roussel and the FDA to make RU-486 available in the United States. In June 1990, at its annual policymaking session, the American Medical Association (AMA) unanimously supported testing and possible use of RU-486. "The abortion issue, pro and con, should not interfere with our ability to conduct all kinds of investigations for all kinds of problems," noted Dr. Charles Sherman, who chaired the AMA committee recommending support for RU-486 (St. Paul Pioneer Press, 1990).

INTERNATIONAL RU-486 AVAILABILITY

As a result of the governmental intervention discussed earlier, Roussel is currently distributing RU-486 to 350 hospital clinics in France. Since it was first introduced, more than 40,000 women worldwide have taken the drug (Herman, 1989; Ullman et al., 1990). Projected annual sales in France are $3.3 million (Laurenson, 1988). With RU-486, abortion is a four-step process: (1) an initial interview; (2) after a one-week waiting period, administration of RU-486; (3) administration of prostaglandin therapy several days later; and (4) a follow-up examination approximately one week after that (Klitsch, 1989).

Roussel is not distributing the drug outside France; as Sakiz says, "We're not eager to start a new debate" (Greenhouse, 1989a). Neither the French government nor WHO, which cosponsored clinical trials of the drug, is pressing Roussel to release the drug abroad. WHO, citing data from more than 10,000 women who participated in tests over the past seven years, has confirmed that RU-486 is safe and effective. But the agency, which has the right to commandeer the drug and supply it to developing countries at cost, has cautiously decided to await further trials. It wants the drug to be "discredit-proof" (MacFarquhar, 1988). Some have suggested that WHO fears its U.S. funding would be cut off if it were to promote the drug, just as the United Nations Fund for Population Activities lost U.S. contributions for supporting family planning services in China, which the United States contends has a coercive population policy (Glasow, 1990c).

The most likely market outside France is Britain (Arnst, 1989b), where physicians endorsed the drug in October 1989 (Arnst, 1989a). Roussel filed an application for a license in September 1990, and while denying that the application was "fast-tracked," a Department of Health spokeswoman did say it was "quite high in the pile" (The Independent Staff, 1991). According to the spokeswoman, the application would be going to the Committee on Safety of Medicines by early to mid-1991. It usually takes the committee about 18 months to process an application (The Independent Staff, 1991). The British Society for the Protection of the Unborn has made clear the importance of resisting U.K. approval of the drug, lest it become widely available in Britain and pave the way for introduction in other European Community countries (Françoise, 1991).

Another likely market is China, where the drug is already being used on an experimental basis, and the government need only make a request to the company for supplies to distribute it more widely (Arnst, 1989b). As a nonsignatory to the International Convention on Patents, China could produce the drug on its own. Yet even if it were to become a signatory, it could continue to manufacture the drug for domestic consumption without a license from Roussel (Klitsch, 1989).

Although plans to license RU-486 in the Netherlands and Scandinavia were scuttled in 1988 when Roussel temporarily pulled the drug off the market, research there is continuing. At the Karølinska Hospital in Stockholm, RU-486 is being administered to 30 women over a period of six months to determine if it can be used as a once-a-month contraceptive (Reuters, 1989a). There are indications that Roussel will seek licensing in all European countries that approve the drug (Holmes, 1989).

In Europe, however, the *Webster* decision in the United States is stirring up what generally had been settled debates on abortion. It encouraged renewed activity by antiabortion groups in Britain and Italy that want to slow the introduction of RU-486 (LaFranchi, 1989). In Italy, for example, the deputy party leader of the antiabortion Movement for Life, Christian Democrat parliamentarian Carlo Casini, said his group would consider calling on Italians to boycott Roussel products if the pill were introduced. Roussel's Italian subsidiary consequently has announced it has no plans to introduce the drug—because of a lack of "technical guarantees" (Holmes, 1989).

Elena Marinucci, a Socialist party senator and undersecretary at the Health Ministry, has instead proposed making the pill available. She calls the subsidiary's response an insult to Italy's health service. The secretary of health, Liberal party member Francesco de Lorenzo, has distanced himself from Marinucci's campaign, asserting that it is not the ministry's job to invite drug companies to market their products in Italy (Holmes, 1989).

Commenting on efforts to expand distribution in Europe, NRLC's Glasow wrote: "Roussel-Uclaf's policy of introducing the abortion drug into one country at a time can also be viewed as a test of how pro-life advocates in Europe and America will react. Evidently Roussel-Uclaf and Hoechst A.G. have decided to see how far they can go before provoking retribution by the U.S. right-to-life movement" (Glasow, 1990c).

Outside Europe, Roussel may find easier markets. India's official Bombay Council for Medical Research in 1988 recommended that RU-486 be investigated for use, but use in other developing countries may be limited. The need for physician supervision and for a second office visit to obtain the follow-up prostaglandin may make RU-486 difficult for the millions of women living in countries with poor doctor-patient ratios.

Pharmaceutical industry analysts point instead to Eastern Europe as a potentially huge market. In general, Eastern bloc countries have poor contraceptive availability and abortion is more frequent there than in the West. (The Soviet Union has one of the highest abortion rates in the world.) U.S. protests are unlikely to have much weight should these countries approve RU-486. In fact, opening these markets, say analysts, may provide a sufficient profit motive to get Roussel back into the business of aggressively marketing its discovery (Arnst, 1989b).

GETTING RU-486 TO THE UNITED STATES

In late September 1989, Etienne Baulieu received the Albert Lasker Clinical Medical Research Award, the United States' most prestigious medical award and often a forerunner to a Nobel Prize (Specter, 1989). Scientists and family planning organizations praised the choice; antiabortionists were outraged and accused Baulieu of waging chemical warfare against the unborn (Specter, 1989). "Where does the demented imagination of abortionists end?," demanded R. Alvarez in a letter to the editor of the *Washington Times* on October 18, 1989. Apparently unaware of Hoechst's link with I. G. Farben, Alvarez continued, "With such a mentality, those responsible for making this presentation will next be awarding the Medal of Honor to the developer of Zyklon B gas used to exterminate millions of Jews in Nazi Germany."

With the exception of recreational drugs that could also be used for pain relief, there seems to be no modern precedent for withholding a proven drug on moral grounds. Inadequate return on investment is a far more common reason for such an action, but in the case of RU-486, it is the commercial and public relations consequences of the antiabortion groups' moral outrage that seem to underlie the decision of so many pharmaceutical companies to avoid the drug and of Roussel to limit its distribution and licensing. Hoechst continues to deny that it is concerned about a boycott. Its chairman says that it simply is not Hoechst policy to sell abortifacients. Company insiders suggest that Hoechst directors may have agreed to the research because they never expected it to succeed. They are now torn between pride in the discovery and their own antiabortion sentiments. "What we need is a company psychiatrist," says one researcher (MacFarquhar, 1988).

Yet concern about the financial aspects of marketing RU-486 can have played only a small role in the decision to withhold the drug. There is little doubt that it could be a moneymaker. At $100 per treatment, RU-486 could generate $8 million in sales by replacing only a third of France's annual 250,000 surgical abortions. Globally, it could become one of the few billion-dollar drugs (MacFarquhar, 1988). NRLC knows this: "Our weapon in a democracy is to sting them financially and make it unprofitable for them. . . . If we can keep them from making money they won't market it," says Willke (ABC News, 1990).

There are ways to circumvent Roussel's self-imposed ban on exports. Some countries, such as Britain, have compulsory licensing laws to deal with reluctant pharmaceutical manufacturers. If necessary, the government can give away an unused patent for the public interest. The catch is that Roussel cannot be compelled to produce its testing data, which is necessary for licensing approval. A would-be distributor would have to repeat Roussel's trials to get the drug approved, which would take about two years (MacFarquhar, 1988).

Another route is moral suasion. This strategy seemed to help in October 1988 when the scientists and physicians at the Rio conference joined to denounce Roussel's decision to pull RU-486 off the market. But Roussel says it will respond only to direct appeals from foreign governments. The most likely country to make such an appeal is China. Beijing has had the largest clinical trials—more than 3,000 women— outside France; it also runs the world's largest national abortion service, with more than 11.5 million abortions performed annually (MacFarquhar, 1988). China has approved the drug but has not yet asked Roussel for supplies (Herman, 1989; MacFarquhar, 1988). Private groups can also appeal. In 1990, the Fund for the Feminist Majority sent a delegation to Roussel carrying 115,000 petitions and a list of 250 medical researchers supporting RU-486 importation to the United States.

It may be possible to obtain the drug in the United States with a prescription from a French physician who perhaps has been contacted by a sympathetic American doctor. But U.S. customs and postal officials can intercept drugs for examination by the FDA, and current FDA policy has authorized inspectors to seize RU-486 because the agency considers it dangerous (Lunzer, 1989). In the past, FDA has issued regulations allowing patients to ship unapproved drugs into the country to treat life-threatening conditions. On September 26, 1988, however, it announced that these regulations do not apply to RU-486 (Kolata, 1988a).

In May 1989, noting that RU-486 was omitted from the list of drugs specifically excluded from the United States, Congressman Robert Dornan (R-Calif.) and a group of his antiabortion colleagues in the House wrote FDA Commissioner Frank Young requesting clarification, and expressing concern that importation of RU-486 and other abortifacients might be occurring (letter from Congressman Robert Dornan to Dr. Frank Young, commissioner of FDA, May 5, 1989).

Young responded by updating the import alert on June 6, 1989, instructing field personnel to prevent the importation of unapproved abortifacient drugs such as RU-486. He explained: "[U]napproved drugs may be imported only if there is no unreasonable safety risk or evidence of fraud, and other criteria are met relating to personal use, quantity, and other factors. We do not believe this policy can be appropriately applied to the importation of RU-486 because use of the product could present unreasonable safety risk. . ." (letter from Dr. Frank Young, commissioner of FDA, to Congressman Robert Dornan, June 9, 1989). Young did not explain how a drug with such a low incidence of side effects might be considered unreasonably dangerous.

Congressman Ted Weiss (D-N.Y.) became so concerned by the appearance of inappropriate political judgments entering FDA's scientific evaluations of RU-486 (Diana Zuckerman, staff member, Subcommittee on Human Resources, Committee on Governmental Operations, personal communication, August 6, 1990) that he asked the agency for a formal explanation of its findings. Meanwhile, however, the drug cannot be legally brought into the United States, even with a French prescription and under an American doctor's supervision.

Although seemingly aimed only at users, the import ban also affected researchers studying nonabortion uses of RU-486 (Hilts, 1990a). Testifying at a November 19, 1990, hearing held by Congressman Ron Wyden (D-Ore.), chair of the Small Business Subcommittee on Regulation, Kathryn Horwitz (a breast cancer and hormone specialist at the University of Colorado) said that an FDA official had told her she could no longer import the drug by mail or in person for her breast cancer research (Hilts, 1990b). Federal researchers at the National Institutes of Health (NIH) announced they were shutting down research on RU-486 treatment for Cushing's syndrome, a potentially fatal illness affecting 5,000 Americans, because they could no longer be assured a supply of the drug (Hilts, 1990a). An NIH official said, "It is wrong to say that politics were the only reason to stop the work, but that was a major factor in our decision" (Hilts, 1990a).

At the Wyden hearing, FDA blamed the application of the import ban to researchers on "poor communication," and said researchers need only ask for permission (Hilts, 1990b). Roussel, however, appears to be hesitating to guarantee supplies even for non-abortion-related research due to the FDA's evident opposition to abortion and continued pressure from antiabortion forces who support the import ban (Hilts, 1990a, 1990b). NRLC, however, maintains that the hearings were biased and failed to document the side effects of RU-486 and prostaglandin therapy or to emphasize the preliminary nature of the data supporting its nonabortion applications (Glasow, 1991a). NRLC also charges that interest in the drug's nonabortion uses is simply an effort to provide political cover for those physicians and politicians who want it brought to the United States (Glasow, 1991b) and not part of an overall strategy to discuss the drug on all its merits (Ciolli, 1990).

Congressional interest following the Wyden hearings remained strong. In early February 1991, Wyden introduced H.R. 875 to rescind the FDA import ban. Two days later, Congressman Dornan introduced H.R. 798 to prohibit use of federal funds to investigate any aspects, abortifacient or otherwise, of RU-486. His bill also proposed that drugs derived from materials from human fetuses be labeled as such, and set forth a scheme for regulation of storage and interstate transportation, importation, or exportation of human fetal tissue.

Of course, there is always smuggling and patent infringement. The Chinese could re-create the drug quite easily, but their manufacturing facilities are inadequate. Black markets in RU-486 pose the danger of unsupervised use without the necessary follow-on prostaglandin therapy and backup availability of surgical abortions. The only way to prevent this situation may be to make the pill legally available under a less threatening name (e.g., as a menstrual regulator) in countries where it is likely to be controversial (MacFarquhar, 1988).

Currently, Roussel is holding discussions with nonprofit organizations from the United States, Great Britain, and Sweden that would like to buy the pill at minimum cost and distribute it in their home countries. Of course, the appeal of this arrangement is that these organizations, rather than Roussel, would become the target of activities by antiabortion groups. In the United States, however, RU-486 also faces the hurdle of FDA approval, a process that takes five to seven years at best. With a strong antiabortion lobby supported by the administration, many supporters of the pill worry that the FDA will never approve the drug.

Nonetheless, research continues at USC under the original Population Council permit, which is the only ongoing work on RU-486 in the United States (Ciolli, 1989b). In December 1988, USC researchers announced that a single dose of RU-486 alone could provide an effective chemical abortion for 81 to 100 percent of women using it within 49 days of their last menstrual period. Effectiveness was 100 percent with further dose adjustment (Grimes, 1988). In the past four years, 300 women have used RU-486 alone, and another 30 have tried it with follow-on prostaglandin therapy. USC researchers used the last of their supplies of the drug on a study of 16 women (Stein, 1990). It demonstrated that women taking RU-486 alone were no more likely to experience cramps, heavy bleeding, nausea, vomiting, or other side effects than the control group of women taking Tylenol (Stein, 1990).

Another possible route toward U.S. introduction of the drug is through individual states. Although states usually cannot review or approve a drug independent of the FDA, there are exceptions. In California, for example, there is a Food and Drug Bureau, a so-called mini-FDA, that was set up in 1987 to bypass the FDA so that AIDS drugs could be tested more rapidly in the state (Miller, 1990). Under state law, the bureau can approve the sale of drugs not approved by the FDA provided they have been tested and are manufactured and distributed solely within California (Miller, 1990).

In early March 1990, Attorney General John Van de Kamp, then candidate for the Democratic nomination for governor, publicly called on the state's health department director, Kenneth Kizer, to authorize importation and testing of the drug (Scott, 1990) and to resist "nonmedical political pressure" (Van de Kamp, 1990). His campaign opponent Diane Feinstein questioned his motives, asserting he was just "trying to one-up me with the female vote" (Scott, 1990), a view that reportedly was held even by some of those close to the campaign (V. Rideout, Issues Director, Van de Kamp for Governor Campaign, personal communication, February 19, 1990).

Abortion opponents were also angry, with NRLC's associate western director Jan Carroll calling it a "desperate political maneuver to out-pro-abort two other pro-abortion candidates . . ." (Glasow, 1990b), and education director Richard Glasow writing that "right-to-life supporters should recognize that preventing U.S. tests of the abortion pill [is] a very important objective. Without testing in the U.S., it will be much more difficult to have the death drug licensed and marketed here" (Glasow, 1990b).

The head of California Right to Life, Camille Giglio, sent a letter to Kizer opposing California review of the drug in the strongest possible terms, once again connecting the drug with concerns about genocide. "The RU-486 is a radical departure from the normal routes to controlling the size of one's family. Does your department consider the human population of this state to be such a threat to the environment that the procreation of human babies must be prevented with such a sweeping pesticide approach to reducing the size of the human population . . . . Is this the Health Department's 'medfly approach' to the human condition?" (PR Newswire, 1990).

While Van de Kamp did not go on to win the nomination nor did the health department accede to his request, he was not alone in this idea. Carol Ruth Silver, a former member of the San Francisco Board of Supervisors, formed an organization called "Every Child a Wanted Child," devoted solely to bringing RU-486 to the United States (Miller, 1990). The medical advisory group for the organization was formed from among those interested in testing the drug, and on April 2, 1990, a group of doctors unveiled a plan to test the drug in San Francisco (Herscher, 1990). Board of Supervisors member Terence Hallinan introduced a resolution calling on the governor and the state legislature to pay for the tests and support clinical trials with 200 women subjects at San Francisco General Hospital, Children's Hospital, and the University of California at San Francisco (Herscher, 1990). The cost was estimated at $60,000 to $100,000 for three months of work.

The California state regulators reportedly looked favorably on the proposal, but were unable to give final approval without information about the drug that only Roussel could supply. Roussel, still unpersuaded that the political climate was receptive, continued to refuse to ship the drug to the United States for abortion-related clinical trials (Glasow, 1990g). Marie Bass, codirector of the Reproductive Health Technologies Project, a Washington-based organization working to promote RU-486, emphasized in the press and technical journals that with legislative and private sector support in place, grassroots political pressure was now needed to persuade Roussel to take a chance on licensing the drug in the United States (Glasow, 1990g).

The California example did not go unnoticed. By November 1990, New York City was discussing the same tactic. Mayor David Dinkins was receiving "options memos" from Deputy Mayor Steisel, Consumer Affairs Commissioner Green, Health Commissioner Myers, and Hospital Commissioner Carillo because, as Green said: "The federal government, the natural jurisdiction on this issue, is so anti-choice that it's forcing a congressional-urban alliance to cut this Gordian Knot" (Carroll, 1990). Within weeks, Green and mayoral advisor Rivera had developed a plan for Dinkins and other U.S. mayors to lobby everyone from George Bush to FDA to WHO on the issue of RU-486 (Barth, 1990), and to bring the drug to New York City under a state law that would allow testing (although not sales) of non-FDA-approved drugs (Barth, 1990). While Linda Sachs, spokesperson for Green's office, told the *National Right to Life News* that the health and consumer affairs departments were merely "evaluating" their options (Glasow, 1990f), she was quoted in the *Village*

Voice as saying that the departments are researching the drug to "come up with a possible plan to provide for the women in New York City" (Hancock, 1990).

Oregon, too, has considered taking an independent stance, although there the proposals are coming with a different political flavor. Then Governor Neil Goldschmidt released a December 1990 report of the Oregon Task Force on Pregnancy and Substance Abuse, recommending that RU-486 be offered to welfare-dependent women who have a history of drug abuse (Rarick, 1990). Goldschmidt endorsed the proposal (Seattle Times Staff, 1990). The 10-member board of lawyers, doctors, and state legislators also recommended that the state encourage such women to use Norplant, a recently approved five-year implantable contraceptive, and that it relax restrictions on the ability of doctors to perform publicly funded sterilizations (Rarick, 1990). Newly elected Governor Barbara Roberts, while not commenting on the merits of the proposal, did say that Oregon could pass legislation permitting RU-486 testing if it wished: "We believe that if California can do it, Oregon can do it" (Rarick, 1990).

Under the auspices of the American Society of Law and Medicine, David Grimes, of USC, and Rebecca Cook, of the University of Toronto Law School, are organizing a December 1991 conference on RU-486. With presentations on its latest safety and efficacy data for abortion and nonabortion uses, explanations of regulatory issues by FDA officials, and discussions by Congressman Wyden, Weiss, and Dornan on its political repercussions, the meeting is likely to create the most complete public record to date on the prospects for this drug in the United States (personal communication with Rebecca Cook, November 2, 1990).

INDUSTRY CONSTRAINTS ON RU-486 DEVELOPMENT

No matter how much good research is done in the United States on RU-486, certain pharmaceutical industry constraints will slow or prevent its production and distribution. One of the most important such constraints is corporate profitability. Even such strong supporters as Edouard Sakiz view corporate responsibility to maximize profits for shareholders as a paramount consideration. To that end, pharmaceutical companies examine the profitability of a new drug like RU-486 from four standpoints: (1) the size of the market and the likely price of the product; (2) the difficulty and expense of obtaining FDA approval; (3) the costs associated with product liability claims; and (4) the costs associated with loss of public good will.

Market Share and Price

Early presentations to security analysts misrepresented RU-486 as a "morning-after" pill to be taken at home in lieu of contraception prior to intercourse. Characterized as such a product, the drug would be aimed at the global birth control pill market of 51.7 million users. Later statements made it clear, however, that RU-486 could at best replace first-trimester surgical abortions, which are performed at the annual rate of a little under 1.5 million in this country. This distinction is important. "If drug companies don't see it as enough of a moneymaker to offset their liability costs, they aren't interested," says Allan Rosenfield. "The pill makes lots of money, so companies make it. The IUD doesn't, so we have a new FDA approved IUD, the best ever made, that no one will make" (Rosenfield et al., 1983). Joseph Speidel, vice president of the Population Crisis Committee, commented, "It is ironic that the American consumer is denied the IUD, which costs less and is generally safer than the pill, principally because IUD sales in the U.S. have totaled only about $12 million annually whereas the pill generates about $600 million."

Because RU-486 would be taken at most for a few days a year, potential profits are probably less than from the daily contraceptive pill—that is, unless the drug were priced extremely high. Such markups are not unheard of, of course. (The U.S. government, buying in bulk shipment for distribution overseas, can obtain a month's supply of birth control pills for about 18¢, whereas consumers pay $12.) Another option is for companies to wait until patent protection on RU-486 expires in 1999. U.S. companies could then manufacture the drug and save a considerable amount of money by avoiding licensing fees (Klitsch, 1989). The hurdle of FDA review would still, however, pose a substantial disincentive.

FDA Review

Upjohn tested RU-486 in its laboratories but has no interest in pursuing it (Rosenfeld, 1986). "FDA standards are so high, and the chances of getting something approved are so low, it just isn't worth it," said a company representative (Rosenfeld, 1986). Upjohn, it may be recalled, was unable to get FDA approval for Depo-Provera. Having already experienced the difficulties that arise from the combination of a politically sensitive drug and the lengthy review required for contraceptive products, it is unlikely to enter the fray.

As an editorial in the October 28, 1988, edition of the *New York Times* noted, even working with an already developed and tested drug, FDA approval can cost as much as $50 million over the four- to seven-year process required for action. The agency's notoriously slow and methodical review process has been cited with approval by many who recall that thalidomide, which caused thousands of birth defects in Europe, was never approved for use in the United States. But pharmaceutical industry spokespersons complain that FDA is too slow and too unwilling to accept studies and government approvals from other countries. However, in the case of RU-486, even if FDA were to accept foreign test data, it would be necessary to run extensive clinical trials using prostaglandins available for use in the United States because the European prostaglandins used in the French and WHO-sponsored trials are not licensed for use here (Klitsch, 1989).

Product Liability

Liability for injuries caused by contraceptive drugs and devices has also generated considerable concern among pharmaceutical companies. Many of them assert that this is the single most important factor in their decisions to leave the field of fertility control. Jacob Stucki, vice president for pharmaceutical research at Upjohn, said his firm, like several other major pharmaceutical firms, has discontinued all fertility control research because liability insurance is so expensive. Fifteen years ago, there were 19 firms with research staffs working on birth control. Today, there is one. There is also 25 percent less money available for contraceptive research than there was in the 1970s (Goodman, 1988b; Institute of Medicine, 1990).

The IUD has been the object of much of the recent liability activity, and manufacturers have responded accordingly. G.D. Searle & Company pulled its IUDs off the shelves in 1986, although it continues to manufacture birth control pills. The firm dropped its IUD line after what it perceived as unwarranted lawsuits over its products following the uproar over the A. H. Robins Dalkon shield. "It's not conducive to making you think of developing new things in an area where there is so much interest in litigation," said Kay Bruno, Searle's senior director of public affairs (M. Phillips, 1988). Other companies, however, cite different reasons for avoiding contraceptive research and development: a saturated and well-served contraceptive market (Syntex Corp.), availability of European research and patents (Warner-Lambert Co.), and lack of any truly revolutionary innovations (GynoPharma, Inc.; M. Phillips, 1988). Henry Gabelnick, director of extramural programs and product development of the Eastern Virginia Medical School's Contraceptive Research and Development (CONRAD) program, however, supports Searle's view: "The reason the major companies have pulled out is quite simple:

dollars. They are afraid to take the risks because of the giant lawsuits that have come up" (M. Phillips, 1988).

Until recently, ALZA Corporation was the only remaining U.S. company to sell IUDs (Gladwell, 1988a). Furthermore, ALZA seemed unenthusiastic about its sudden monopoly following Searle's 1986 withdrawal from the market. With the Searle exodus, ALZA narrowed the focus of its marketing, suspended much of its contraceptive research effort, raised the price on its product, and began to insist on informed consent by users (all purchasers had to read and sign an eight-page statement concerning the risks and benefits of the IUD) at least in part to protect the company from liability claims. These seemingly un-business-like decisions reportedly were aimed at "avoiding new people and more problems" (Gladwell, 1988a).

In this cautionary climate, RU-486 was viewed warily by most firms. "We never even got to a serious examination of the [RU-486] pill's properties," said one pharmaceutical company executive. "As soon as our attorneys learned that it is only 95 percent effective, they began to scream. The other five percent could involve defective children—and that, in terms of liability suits, could blow us out of the water. They wouldn't let us touch this product" (Abrams, 1988). Although three children have been born without health problems following in utero exposure to RU-486, physicians acknowledge that if a woman carries her pregnancy to term following an unsuccessful attempt to abort with RU-486, the child might suffer birth defects (Abrams, 1988; Klitsch, 1989).

Even producers of good products with few side effects are fearful, according to Louise Tyrer of Planned Parenthood. Consumers are willing to take risks when they are sick and in need of medicine, but they are outraged by any side effects to contraceptives, which are taken when they are healthy (M. Phillips, 1988). And manufacturers' concerns on this score are not ill founded; Ortho, for example, lost a $4.7 million jury decision in Atlanta in a 1987 case brought by a woman claiming, on very weak evidence, that her child's birth defects were caused by Ortho Gynol spermicide.

Public Relations

Ortho, the only company currently conducting research on a wide range of contraceptive products, wants nothing to do with RU-486. "I cannot elaborate on our decision," said spokesman Richard Salem, who noted that the 40-year-old company intends to stay in existence. "It is a matter of proprietary information" (Abrams, 1988). However, Neil Sweig, drug industry analyst for Prudential-Bache Securities, says "it just isn't worth the hassle. The market for a manufacturer of RU-486 in this country would be between $200 and $250 million annually. And that is minuscule compared to the markets for antibiotic, antihypertensive and anti-arthritic drugs. Those markets are worth billions, and they don't involve political controversies and other problems created by social or religious groups" (Abrams, 1988).

NRLC's president John Willke builds on that equation. "We have told them that if one of these companies gives a license to any company in the United States, we will unleash a boycott, supported by tens of millions of people. It will have the support of all 50 state and 3,000 local right to life groups, of major church bodies etc. It will include every product produced by any of these companies. . . . It is this, plus the threat of medical liability law suits, that has kept the pill out of the United States so far" (Willke, 1990).

With both abortion foes and women's rights groups highly critical of new contraceptives, firms have begun to view the field of reproductive health as a public relations nightmare. "There's a lot of pressure that builds over time to devote research money where you gain positive public image," says Roderick MacKenzie, former president of Ortho and current chairman of GynoPharma (M. Phillips, 1988). "I've looked at the books," he said, "and people have not been driven out of this business by financial reasons. It's simply that the companies working in this field have become exhausted by the continuous stream of . . . adverse publicity in the press. They've decided to direct their marketing efforts and research dollars toward areas that don't result in such negative publicity" (Gladwell, 1988a).

"Look," said one drug company executive of RU-486, "if this is going on in France, do you have any idea what will happen in the United States if the drug were being distributed? The market is potentially huge and the drug appears worthy. But who needs the headaches?" (Specter, 1988).

Thus, contraceptive research these days is largely found in European pharmaceutical companies, in U.S. or European government-sponsored programs, and in small firms such as GynoPharma, which recently introduced a copper IUD (ParaGard) in the United States. It may be that only smaller companies will find working with abortifacients to be worth the risk. As Forrest Greenslade, senior consultant to the Population Council, says, "There are entrepreneurial opportunities there" (Kolata, 1988a). If a company markets a drug developed abroad or by a nonprofit organization, the need for long-term capital investment in research and development is vastly reduced. Moreover, although profits may be small for a pharmaceutical giant, they might be quite significant for a small, one-product company. Finally, by focusing on one product, the company is immune to boycotts against collateral product lines (Kolata, 1988a).

At present, except for Johnson & Johnson's Ortho, responsibility for developing new forms of contraception is almost entirely in the hands of nonprofit, government-funded research institutions, whose budgets are far smaller than those of for-profit drug companies. The combined budget of the three most important nonprofit companies doing contraceptive research, the Population Council, Family Health International, and CONRAD, is only $16 million. From $60 million to $100 million are routinely spent by major drug companies to bring a new product to market. ParaGard was developed by the Population Council, a New York nonprofit firm that receives considerable funding for contraceptive research from, among other sources, the U.S. Agency for International Development. It then licensed the technology to GynoPharma (Abrams, 1988).

But even this solution has its limitations. "We can spend money developing products, but eventually to make the products available to the public, we have to entice manufacturers to do so," said CONRAD's Gabelnick, whose program is funded entirely by the USAID. "It ends up with things that have reached a certain point, and are ready to be tested more widely, sitting on the shelf" (M. Phillips, 1988).

AMERICAN ACCESS TO RU-486 IN THE 1990s

RU-486 is a drug with substantial market potential that is not likely to be available in the United States in the near future. This delay in access to what many consider a proven drug is primarily due to the vociferous boycott threats and effective private and public sector lobbying of U.S. antiabortion organizations. Product liability exposure and frustration with FDA review procedures are also obstacles to development and marketing, but these factors are only background to the public relations nightmares and boycott possibilities that loom large as serious disincentives to production.

RU-486 is not the only contraceptive drug held hostage to the abortion debate. The most advanced contraceptive, HCG vaccine, has been tested by WHO in Australia, the Dominican Republic, Finland, and India. It has not been tested in the United States because it acts by stimulating the immune system to attack the outer cells of a pre-embryo. Thus, abortion opponents classify it as an abortifacient rather than a contraceptive, although it works on embryos prior to implantation (Foreman, 1989).

RU-486 has many promising applications: dilating the cervix, to help avoid cesarean sections; treating certain breast cancers that grow in response to sex hormones; treating endometriosis, the third leading cause of infertility in the United States; and controlling Cushing's syndrome, a hormonal disorder in both men and women that is currently treated by removing the adrenal glands. Forrest Greenslade says, "There obviously are all kinds of major hurdles to overcome in producing and marketing this drug . . . [but] somebody almost certainly will be willing to take a chance" (Abrams, 1988).

And who will that be? "Somebody with guts," said a high-ranking official at NIH. "Somebody who will see the need, step in, and without describing himself as the savior of American women, simply do the work. But at present, I don't know anyone who would do it" (Abrams, 1988). Neither does Joseph Speidel, who thinks the immediate prospects are pretty dim. "But," he continued, "the potential for this product is so great . . . that I have to believe an American distribution eventually will come" (Abrams, 1988).

Some think that the people "with guts" are already out there. USC researcher David Grimes says at least half a dozen groups of financiers have discussed production with him. Cindy Pearson of the National Women's Health Network says that the women's health community is serious about forming a company to develop and market the drug. And Erin Van Heenin of Planned Parenthood Federation of America says the financing, the personnel, and the will are there.

But Roussel refuses to license RU-486 to any company in the United States because it considers the drug to be a political and commercial minefield. Nothing short of governmental intervention seems capable of persuading the manufacturer to change this policy. Planned Parenthood and other family planning groups will continue their campaign to persuade Roussel to license the drug here. If they are unsuccessful, it will be years before the patent expires. Even then, the domestic obstacles of public pressure, regulatory review, product liability, and inadequate revenue will make the introduction of RU-486 into the American market a risky business. For the moment, then, politics seem more likely than medical merit to determine the availability of this particular drug aimed at enhancing women's choices and women's health.

REFERENCES

ABC News. 1990. World News Tonight with Peter Jennings. May 8.

Abrams, A. 1988. Politics, profits and a new pill. Newsday, December 13, at sec. "Discovery," p. 1.

Anderson, D. 1989. Feminist leaders mount campaign for abortion pill. United Press International, June 1.

Andrusko, D. 1991. The distortion factor. National Right to Life News, January 8, p. 4.

Arch, M. 1989. Moral majority strikes deal to restrict abortion drug. United Press International, March 24.

Arnst, C. 1989a. British doctors backing acceptance of French abortion pill. Reuters, October 26.

Arnst, C. 1989b. French abortion pill gaining support from world's doctors. Reuters, November 7.

Associated Press. 1988. France orders drug firm to market abortion pill. As reprinted in the Los Angeles Times, October 30, part 1, p. 1, col. 5.

Associated Press. 1989. An abortion ban would accomplish little. As reprinted in the Chicago Tribune, April 18, p. 4.

Atwood, R. 1988. Doctors laud French order to go ahead with abortion pill. Reuters, October 28.

Aubény, E., D. Cossey, and M. Tearse. 1990. The French experience with RU-486 and the outlook for Great Britain. A report to the Reproductive Health Technologies Project, Washington, D.C., August.

Barth, I. 1990. Fear and politics versus a safe abortion pill. Newsday, December 17, p. 74.

Berg, P. 1985. New pill would be taken after conception. Washington Post, January 16, at sec. "Health," p. 5.

Black, C. 1989. NOW backs call to form a feminist party. Boston Globe, July 24, p. 1.

Brennan, W. 1991. Chemical warfare on the unwanted: The I. G. Farben-Hoechst connection. National Right to Life News, January 8, p. 6.

Carey, J. 1990. Can the 'abortion pill' save lives? Business Week, December 17, p. 56.

Carroll, M. 1990. Abortion issue a bitter pill for Dinkins? Newsday, November 23, p. 19.

Ciolli, R. 1989a. U.S. school expands abortion pill research. Newsday, February 28, at sec. "News," p. 2.

Ciolli, R. 1989b. The abortion pill controversy. Newsday, May 29, at sec. "News," p. 6.

Ciolli, R. 1990. Campaign for abortion pill. Newsday, July 2, p. 4.

Contraceptive technology: Promises and politics. 1990. A workshop at the Annual Meeting of the American Public Health Association, October 2. (Session 3063, transcribed from audio tape by Mobiltape Company, Valencia, California.)

Dawkins, W. 1990. Rhône-Poulenc raises 4.7 billion French francs. The Financial Times, July 16.

Emiling, S. 1987. Anti-abortionists see graphic film. United Press International, June 18.

Facts on File. 1987. Other medical news. World News Digest, December 31.

Fagen, C. 1988. Fetal distraction: Pro-lifers reconceived. The New Republic 198(22):21-25.

F-D-C Reports, Inc. 1985a. The Pink Sheet: Trade & Government Memos 47(8):T&G-10.

F-D-C Reports, Inc. 1985b. The Pink Sheet: Trade & Government Memos 47(18):T&G-4 to T&G-5.

F-D-C Reports, Inc. 1986. The Pink Sheet: Trade & Government Memos 48(40):T&G-2 to T&G-3.

F-D-C Reports, Inc. 1987. The Pink Sheet: Trade & Government Memos 49(July 20).

F-D-C Reports, Inc. 1989. The Pink Sheet: Trade & Government Memos 51(February 27).

Federal Information Systems Corporation. 1989. Press conference on the Webster decision with Molly Yard and Eleanor Smeal, July 3.

Foreman, J. 1988a. France OK's use of new abortion pill. Boston Globe, September 24, p. 1.

Foreman, J. 1988b. New drugs could change US debate on abortion. Boston Globe, October 2, p. 1.

Foreman, J. 1988c. Under fire, French firm halts distribution of new pill. Boston Globe, October 27, p. 1.

Foreman, J. 1988d. France orders sale of abortion pill. Boston Globe, October 29, p. 1.

Foreman, J. 1989. Abortion: An American divide. Boston Globe, April 23, p. 1.

Françoise, C. 1991. Pro-lifers overseas gear up to fight RU 486: Great Britain next target. National Right to Life News, January 8, p. 6.

Fraser, L. 1988. The abortion pill: Why America trails Europe. Newsday, July 5, at sec. "Viewpoints," p. 49.

Gladwell, M. 1988a. Enemies join hands to gut provisions in bill. Washington Post, April 10, at sec. H, p. H4.

Gladwell, M. 1988b. Birth control makers weary of controversy. Los Angeles Times, May 3, at part 4, p. 15, col. 1.

Glasow, R. 1986. Heavy reliance on new abortion pill marks shift in pro-abortion strategy and rhetoric, National Right to Life News, March 27. As reprinted in Omen of the Future?: The Abortion Pill RU 486, R. Glasow and J. Willke, eds. (Original copyright: National Right to Life Committee, 1986; recent copyright: National Right to Life Educational Trust Fund, 1989.)

Glasow, R. 1988a. Abortion pill advocates map new strategy in 1987 and 1988 to win U.S. approval of RU 486; hurdles remain (part 1). National Right to Life News, June 2. As reprinted in Omen of the Future?: The Abortion Pill RU 486, R. Glasow and J. Willke, eds. (Original copyright: National Right to Life Committee, 1986; recent copyright: National Right to Life Educational Trust Fund, 1989.)

Glasow, R. 1988b. Abortion pill advocates map new strategy in 1987 and 1988 to win U.S. approval of RU 486; hurdles remain (part 2). National Right to Life News, July 7. As reprinted in Omen of the Future?: The Abortion Pill RU 486, R. Glasow and J. Willke, eds. (Original copyright: National Right to Life Committee, 1986; recent copyright: National Right to Life Educational Trust Fund, 1989.)

Glasow, R. 1988c. Abortion pill RU 486 approved for use in France, China; pro-life spokesmen condemn death drug. National Right to Life News, October 6. As reprinted in Omen of the Future?: The Abortion Pill RU 486, R. Glasow and J. Willke, eds. (Original copyright: National Right to Life Committee, 1986; recent copyright: National Right to Life Educational Trust Fund, 1989.)

Glasow, R. 1988d. French abortion pill backers' ploy keeps death drug on market. National Right to Life News, November 17. As reprinted in Omen of the Future?: The Abortion Pill RU 486, R. Glasow and J. Willke, eds. (Original copyright: National Right to Life Committee, 1986; recent copyright: National Right to Life Educational Trust Fund, 1989.)

Glasow, R. 1989. Company claims RU 486 will not be marketed outside France; pro-lifers adopt wait and see attitude, still oppose death pill. National Right to Life News, April 6. As reprinted in Omen of the Future?: The Abortion Pill RU 486, R. Glasow and J. Willke, eds. (Original copyright: National Right to Life Committee, 1986; recent copyright: National Right to Life Educational Trust Fund, 1989.)

Glasow, R. 1990a. Latest abortion pill study finds same adverse side effects. National Right to Life News, March 15, p. 8.

Glasow, R. 1990b. Pro-aborts plans to try to test and market RU 486 outside normal channels in California. National Right to Life News, April 26, p. 9.

Glasow, R. 1990c. Marketing abortion pill outside France key policy shift. National Right to Life News, August 16, p. 5.

Glasow, R. 1990d. RU 486 strategy requires influencing key groups. National Right to Life News, September 17, p. 1.

Glasow, R. 1990e. Three companies manufacture drugs for RU 486 abortion technique. National Right to Life News, September 17, p. 10.

Glasow, R. 1990f. Abortion pill tests proposed for New York City. National Right to Life News, October 2, p. 10.

Glasow, R. 1990g. Advocates turn up pressure to bring RU 486 to U.S. National Right to Life News, October 17, p. 12.

Glasow, R. 1990h. Supporters admit serious underreporting of abortion pill side effects. National Right to Life News, November 19, p. 11.

Glasow, R. 1990i. RU 486: The prostaglandin connection. National Right to Life News, December 13, p. 7.

Glasow, R. 1991a. House hearing used to mask safety concerns over RU 486. National Right to Life News, January 8, p. 4.

Glasow, R. 1991b. Hypothetical 'therapeutic' uses vs. real complications. National Right to Life News, January 8, p. 9.

Goodman, E. 1988a. Birth control goes back to the past for progress. Newsday, May 27, p. 92.

Goodman, E. 1988b. The abortion debate enters a new and climactic phase of conflict. Boston Globe, November 3, p. 17.

Goodman, E. 1989. Abortion: By pill. Boston Globe, July 29, p. 17.

Gordon, L. 1976. Woman's Body, Woman's Right: A Social History of Birth Control in America. New York: Grossman Publishers.

Greenhouse, S. 1988a. Drugmaker stops all distribution of abortion pill. New York Times, October 27, at sec. A, p. 1, col. 6.

Greenhouse, S. 1988b. Maker says pressures could revive pill. New York Times, October 28, at sec. A, p. 9, col. 1.

Greenhouse, S. 1988c. France ordering company to sell its abortion drug. New York Times, October 29, at sec. 1, p. 1, col. 6.

Greenhouse, S. 1989a. A new pill, a new battle. New York Times Magazine, February 12, at sec. 6, p. 23, col. 1.

Greenhouse, S. 1989b. Fears confine pill to France. New York Times, March 26, at sec. 4, p. 18, col. 1.

Grimes, D. 1988. Early abortion with a single dose of the antiprogestin RU-486. American Journal of Obstetrics and Gynecology 158:1307-1312.

Gruhier, F., L. Joffrey, P. Romom, and C. de Rudder. 1988. RU486: Echec a l'intolerance. Nouvel Observateur 1252(November 3-9):49-51.

Hancock, L. 1990. RU 486 hits Manhattan? The Village Voice, September 25.

Harris, C. 1991. RU 486—A chemical time bomb? National Right to Life News, January 8, p. 8.

Herman, R. 1989. In France—oui!; in the U.S.—not yet. Washington Post, October 3, at sec. "Health," p. 12.

Herscher, E. 1990. San Francisco doctors propose testing controversial abortion pill. San Francisco Chronicle, April 3, p. A1.

Hilts, P. 1990a. Abortion link helps to kill research. New York Times (national edition), November 16, at sec. A, p. 12.

Hilts, P. 1990b. FDA says it allows study of abortion drug. New York Times (national edition), November 20, at sec. B, p. 9.

Holmes, P. 1989. French abortion pill sparks storm in Catholic Italy. Reuters Library Report, November 4.

The Independent Staff. 1991. Abortion pill high on list for licences. The Independent (U.K.), January 3.

Institute of Medicine. 1990. Developing New Contraceptives: Obstacles and Opportunities. Washington, D.C.: National Academy Press.

Izbicki, J. 1988. Holy war on abortion pill. Sunday Telegraph, October 30, at sec. "International," p. 9.

Japenga, A., and E. Venant. 1989. Underground army. Los Angeles Times, November 30, at part E, p. 5, col. 2.

Klitsch, M. 1989. RU 486: The Science and the Politics. Washington, D.C.: Alan Guttmacher Institute.

Kolata, G. 1988a. Boycott threat blocking sale of abortion inducing drug. New York Times, February 22, at sec. A, p. 1, col. 3.

Kolata, G. 1988b. U.S. may allow anti-ulcer drug tied to abortion. New York Times, October 29, at sec. 1, p. 1, col. 5.

Kolata, G. 1988c. Any sale in U.S. of abortion pill still years away. New York Times, October 30, at sec. 1, p. 1, col. 1.

Kolata, G. 1989. As new tactic, do-it-yourself abortions taught. New York Times, October 23, at sec. B, p. 12, col. 1.

Kornhauser, A. 1989. Abortion case has been boon to both sides. Legal Times, July 3, p. 1.

LaFranchi, H. 1989. Turbulent forecast: There's a storm brewing over abortion in Europe. Chicago Tribune, September 10, at sec. "Tempo," p. 5.

Laurenson, J. 1988. France mandates drug sale. Chemical Week, November 9, p. 14.

Le Quotidien du Médecin. 1990. RU 486: Roussel adresse une lettre aux gynecologues des centres d'IVG. April 30, p. 11.

Lunzer, F. 1989. When the corner drugstore falls short. U.S. News & World Report 106(6):82.

MacFarquhar, E. 1988. Horizons: Health. U.S. News & World Report 106(3):54.

Miller, M. 1990. Plan to test abortion pill in California sparks fierce debate. Reuters, March 15.

Minkin, S. 1980. Depo-Provera: A critical analysis. Women and Health 5:49-69.

Naughton, P. 1988a. Anger as French Catholics force withdrawal of abortion pill. Reuters, October 27.

Naughton, P. 1988b. French government orders company to go ahead with abortion pill. Reuters Library Report, October 28.

Nayeri, F. 1987. An abortion pill may soon be on the market in France. United Press International, March 28.

Phillips, J. 1988a. Abortpill. United Press International, October 28.

Phillips, J. 1988b. Abortion pill decision stirs debate. United Press International, October 29.

Phillips, M. 1988. Birth control. States News Service, January 3.

PR Newswire. 1988a. National right to life on French abortion pill. June 22.

PR Newswire. 1988b. Planned Parenthood gives Margaret Sanger Award. October 17.

PR Newswire. 1988c. Halt in distribution of new French pill declared. October 26.

PR Newswire. 1988d. Planned Parenthood statement on RU 486 pill decision. October 26.

PR Newswire. 1990. Pro lifers reject tests of abortion pill. March 22.

Rarick, E. 1990. Abortion pill urged to prevent drug abuse. United Press International, December 20.

Reuters. 1988. French government orders company to go ahead with abortion pill. October 28.

Reuters. 1989a. NOW presses for U.S. tests of morning-after pill. June, 1.

Reuters. 1989b. Abortion pill to be tested as contraceptive. As reprinted in the Chicago Tribune, October 3, at sec. "News," p. 5.

Reuters. 1989c. Vatican newspaper says abortion pill a chemical bomb. November 11.

Reuters Library Report. 1988. Abortion pill creator calls for action to get it on the market. October 27.

Reuters Library Report. 1989. Anti-abortion movement calls for boycott of French pill. March 15.

Reuters North European Service. 1984. New substance to induce abortion. December 1.

Rhein, R., D. Hunter, and A. Hall. 1985. A pill that might defuse the abortion issue. Business Week, April 1, at sec. "Medicine," p. 85.

Ricci, E. 1988. Abortpill. United Press International. October 27.

Rosenfeld, M. 1986. Conception and controversy: The French doctor and his pill to prevent pregnancy. Washington Post, December 18, at sec. C, p. C1.

Rosenfield, A., D. Maine, R. Rochat, J. Shelton, and R. Hatcher. 1983. The Food and Drug Administration and medroxyprogesterone acetate: What are the issues? Journal of the American Medical Association 249:2922-2928.

Sachs, S. 1989. Abortion in America. Newsday, April 24, at sec. "News," p. 31.

St. Paul Pioneer Press. 1990. AMA backs abortion pill. June 22, at sec. A., p. 7A, col. 1.

Sarasohn, J. 1988. Oddly named group fights abortion drug. Legal Times, December 5, at sec. "Lobby Talk," p. 4.

Savage, D., and K. Tumulty. 1989. French abortion pill stirs behind the scenes battle. Los Angeles Times, May 14, at part 1, p. 1, col. 5.

Scott, J. 1990. Van de Kamp requests tests of abortion pill. Los Angeles Times, March 15, p. A3, col. 4.

Seaman, B., and G. Seaman. 1977. Women and the Crisis Sex Hormones. New York: Rawson Associates.

Seattle Times Staff. 1990. Task force favors French abortion pill. Seattle Times, December 21.

Sheler, J. 1987. New abortion drug to stir confrontation. U.S. News & World Report, June 1, at p. 31.

Sherman, J. 1989. Molly Yard: New Jersey and Virginia key in abortion battle. United Press International, August 28.

Silvestre, L., C. Dubois, M. Renault, et al. 1990. Voluntary interruption of pregnancy with Mifeprestone (RU 486) and a prostaglandin analogue. New England Journal of Medicine 322:645.

Simons, M. 1988. Doctor's protest company's action on abortion pill. New York Times, October 28, at sec. A, p. 1, col. 1.

Specter, M. 1988. French abortion-inducing pill adds twist to medical ethics debates. Washington Post, October 30, at sec. A, p. 6.

Specter, M. 1989. French researcher wins top U.S. medical award, angering abortion foes. Washington Post, September 28, at sec. A, p. 12.

States News Service. 1988. Sullivan hearings, December 23.

Stein, R. 1987. Drug promising as birth control pill. United Press International, January 22.

Stein, R. 1988. Abortion pill sparks hope, fear, controversy. Los Angeles Times, November 27, at part 1, p. 3, col. 1.

Stein, R. 1989. Abortion pill appears promising. United Press International, September 29.

Stein, R. 1990. Abortion pill 'well-liked' in U.S. study. United Press International, October 1.

Steinbrook, R. 1988. Wide use of non-surgical abortions is called likely. Los Angeles Times, February 4, at part 1, p. 3, col. 1.

Technology Newsletter. 1988. An abortion drug is approved. Chemical Week 143(14):26.

Tempest, R. 1988a. French drug company bows to protest, halts abortion pill. Los Angeles Times, October 27, at part 1, p. 1, col. 5.

Tempest, R. 1988b. Reaction bitter on health of abortion pill. Los Angeles Times, October 28, at part 1, p. 6, col. 1.

Tempest, R. 1988c. France orders company to distribute abortion pill. Los Angeles Times, October 29, at part 1, p. 1, col. 5.

Thomas, O. 1988. New abortion method hit by safety and moral questions. Christian Science Monitor, November 16, at p. 3.

Ullman, A., G. Teutsch, and D. Philibert. 1990. RU 486; drug used to abort pregnancies has many possible applications. Scientific American 262(6):42.

United Press International. 1988. France tells drug firm to resume abortion pill sales. As reprinted in the Los Angeles Times, October 28, at part 1, p. 1, col. 1.

United Press International. 1989. NOW leaders open campaign to bring abortion pill to U.S. As printed in the Los Angeles Times, June 1, at part 1, p. 2, col. 6.

U.S. Congress, Office of Technology Assessment. 1988. Infertility: Medical and Social Choices. OTA-BA-358. Washington, D.C.: U.S. Government Printing Office.

Van de Kamp, J. 1990. Letter to the editor. Los Angeles Times, March 29, p. B6, col. 4.

Voelker, R. 1990. Researcher suggests side effects of RU-486 may be underreported. American Medical News, October 26, p. 8.

Walsh, K. 1989. The Bush administration's modest plan to help pro-life backers. U.S. News & World Report 106(16):26.

Willke, J. 1990. The abortifacient RU 486: Gathering clouds? National Right to Life News, September 17, p. 3.

Yinger, N. 1990. Focus on maternal mortality. Population Today 18(May):6.

Commentary

William N. Hubbard

RU-486, used in sequence with a prostaglandin (PG), was developed collaboratively by Hoechst-Roussel in France and the World Health Organization (WHO). The latter has sponsored wide clinical trials with an emphasis on developing countries. Swedish data, and those from other developed countries, contributed to the research, which still continues. Although no commercial licenses are available from Hoechst-Roussel at this time, WHO has research contracts with a few academic institutions in the United States.

Although the Food and Drug Administration will accept well-developed data from other countries in reviewing an investigational new drug (IND) or new drug application (NDA), these are generally supplementary to, not a substitute for, data required from the sponsor. A recent Institute of Medicine publication, *Science and Babies* offers a short discussion of these issues. Because RU-486 is intended for convenience use by healthy young women rather than as a therapy for an incapacitating or life-threatening disease, the criteria for judging risks of use compared with demonstrable benefits may be expected to be relatively more demanding.

The fact that the drug is registered in France does not dilute the requirements for U.S. registration. The good laboratory practices and specific protocol

William N. Hubbard, currently retired, was formerly dean of the Medical School at the University of Michigan, and president of the Upjohn Company.

requirements for animal studies that must be completed before clinical registration studies can begin make it probable that two or more years of animal work would be needed before an IND would be approved.

Since RU-486 is not used alone because of its relatively low effective rate of 80 percent, but rather is used in sequential conjunction with a second unapproved drug—a member of the PG family—the designs of both animal and clinical protocols are complicated and nearly unprecedented. The result can reasonably be expected to include a longer period for development.

The usual standard of two well-controlled clinical trials demonstrating clinical endpoint differences at a 95 percent confidence level cannot be applied because neither a placebo group nor either single or double blinding would be ethical or feasible. These considerations suggest the probability that long-term follow-up of patients from the trials would be needed, and further, that a system of close monitoring of outcome of use after approval would be required. Absent the statistical analysis from randomized controlled clinical trials, it is reasonable that a relatively much larger number of patients would be required in order to make a reasonable "epidemiologic" judgment of safety and efficacy.

Conservatively, five to seven years would be required to recruit for two approved clinical trials, collect and analyze the data, and compile and submit a completed NDA. The review process is not predictable, but in light of poor experience with drugs in the nontherapeutic group used in healthy people for a significant part of the fertile years, it is prudent to expect an extensive and very critical review lasting at least three to five years. Ten years from beginning the registration protocol to final approval of the NDA is probably an optimistic estimate of the time required.

Legal liability and the costs of insurance against personal injury and punitive damages have been a major factor in limiting the availability of intrauterine devices and oral contraceptives as well as frustrating the recovery of costs of developmental research. In this case, the risks include failure to abort—now about 5 percent of cases—and putative causal relationship of treatment to any birth defect if a failed abortion is carried to term delivery. So great is this potential liability that it could effectively cripple if not bankrupt a large company. Such liability risks could be better managed by a small company funded by stock ownership at a distance, perhaps by a limited partnership. In this case the liability would not change, but the recoverability would be limited.

Because a few patients may have excessive bleeding after a completed abortion by RU-486/PG use, surgical resources for emergency dilatation and curettage *must* be available when this combination is used. Because there is a discrete rate of failure of complete abortion of approximately 1 out of every 20 patients, arrangements for surgical evacuation of the failed abortus *must* be available. Furthermore, the patient must be prepared in advance for this procedure because the degree to which the fetus has been compromised by the failed procedure cannot be known but may be extensive.

In estimating cost-benefit of RU-486 use, the costs of physician supervision and care as well as the standby costs of intervention for complications or failure must be included. The tort liability and insurance costs against damages will be a significant portion of the fee for physician services.

The total market is confined to the fertile years of women on the occasions of an unwanted pregnancy, limited to those areas where the surgical backup described above is available and where induced abortions by nonsurgical methods are legal (currently, for example, this excludes Japan—a major market). The exact number of users is not predictable, but it is not reasonable to assume that suction curettage would fail to continue as a method of choice for many women. In comparison with drugs affecting infectious diseases, cancer, heart disease, mental disorder, pain, arthritis, and metabolic disorders, the market is minuscule. Since unwanted pregnancy is unlikely to be termed a disease by the Congress of the United States, the so-called orphan drug act is unlikely to apply.

The role of boycott of the company providing abortifacients by those who oppose abortion products has been widely discussed. There are no data that would limit the freedom of opinion in this matter. It is banal to acknowledge that no company enjoys either this publicity or the loss of sales that is implied by a boycott. On the other hand, it is unlikely that an indicated medication will be withheld from a patient because of its source. There is no way to measure objectively the occurrence of sales that are not made.

Finally, in making a decision to undertake the development of RU-486/PG, a company must consider the lost value of opportunities for development of other drugs that were displaced. The irrevocable decision is the one *not* to develop an entity; the decision *to* develop is always conditional on progress. Drug candidates are more numerous by far than the number of products that can be developed. Future financial support of research depends on a choice of future products whose market will repay costs and provide for growth. Whether RU-486/PG will compete successfully for product development will depend on the number and quality of other product candidates, their therapeutic significance, the extent of need for the agent, and the time-cost of money needed for their development and distribution.

Commentary

Peter F. Carpenter

This case study is a factual, if biased, discussion of why RU-486 is not presently available in the United States. The conflict in this instance is between individuals who want access to a particular drug and some members of the broader society who feel that such access would be morally (rather than scientifically) wrong. It is difficult but still far easier to balance differences of scientific opinion than to balance differences of moral values. Most of the participants and constituencies involved in the RU-486 controversy appear to have defined the issue in terms of requiring a yes or no answer to the question "Should RU-486 be available in the United States?" That question is based on the hidden assumption that an appropriate decision-making process already exists, or that no such process is desired because the decision will be made on the basis of a moral, political, or economic point of view. There was little agreement as to a mutually accepted way of dealing with the issue.

The RU-486 decision was clearly *not* a stand-alone issue; it was deeply embedded in the larger abortion rights issue, and this greatly impeded and obscured the decision process.

The foreign events of this case are well documented. The domestic events are not so well documented, but that may be inevitable because many of

Peter F. Carpenter, a former pharmaceutical company (ALZA) and federal government (Office of Management and Budget) executive, is a visiting scholar at the Center for Biomedical Ethics at Stanford University.

those events were, in fact, "nonevents" (i.e., things that did not happen or negative decisions not [yet] subject to public analysis). Because the case dealt with nondecisions or non-public decisions regarding U.S. availability of RU-486, the actual decision-making process was difficult to describe; only limited information about this process was available to the author for presentation in the case study.

The formal French approval process was predetermined, but the subsequent decision by the French government to require product marketing was an ad hoc process. To the extent that there was a U.S. decision-making process, it was totally ad hoc. This ad hoc process was evolutionary, but without either a guiding principle or any attempt to construct a rational process to directly address the issue from multiple perspectives. This "decision-making process" consisted of well-organized public relations campaigns. The threat of boycotts supplanted reasoned scientific and political debates, and will probably become an inappropriate model for "deciding" difficult decisions that involve both biomedical innovation and moral questions.

The question about whether RU-486 should be available in the United States has evolved into a highly polarized debate between vocal and economically powerful constituencies on opposite sides of the issue with practically no participation by larger and more broadly based constituencies. The absence of a formalized decision-making process allowed the issue to be decided, albeit temporarily, without input from all of the affected constituencies and as a result the current (non)decision is unlikely either to be a stable decision or, absent new actors, to lead to a better process the next time around.

A gradual softening of Roussel's position not to make the product available for sale outside of France will eventually remove a significant obstacle to availability in the United States. However, at that point someone or some institution will need to take responsibility for creating a *process* whereby this issue can be properly addressed by all affected constituencies.

The Human Genome Project: The Formation of Federal Policies in the United States, 1986-1990

Robert Mullan Cook-Deegan

The human genome project began to take shape in 1985 and 1986 at various meetings and in the rumor mills of science. By the beginning of the federal government's fiscal year 1988, there were formal line items for genome research in the budgets of both the National Institutes of Health (NIH) and the Department of Energy (DOE). Genome research budgets have grown considerably in 1989 and 1990, and organizational structures have been in flux, but the allocation of funds through line-item budgets was a pivotal event, in this case signaling the rapid adoption of a science policy initiative. This paper focuses on how those dedicated budgets were created.

This case is not about the genome project itself, because that is still a nascent enterprise, but rather about the process by which it was conceived, formulated, and ratified at several levels in various federal science agencies. Describing this process is an exercise in contemporary history, retaining the advantages of direct access to the principal decision makers but necessarily suffering from a lack of perspective that only decades can bring. There are three main sources of information.

Robert M. Cook-Deegan is a physician, formerly with the congressional Office of Technology Assessment and the Biomedical Ethics Advisory Committee. In 1991 he joined the Institute of Medicine as Director of the Division of Biobehavioral Medicine and Mental Disorders.

First, I conducted interviews with the people involved. The first formal round of interviews occurred in January and February 1987, with most of them conducted during a two-month travel marathon spent visiting many western cities in the United States to gather facts for the congressional Office of Technology Assessment (OTA). Several more interviews took place later in 1987, principally in Boston, New York, and Washington, D.C. A second major round of interviews took place in July and August 1988. Since July 1986, I have also attended dozens of scientific symposia, administrative meetings, hearings, and other public events related to the genome project. At those events, I have spoken with the individuals cited in this paper, as well as several hundred more, many on a regular basis (once per quarter or more frequently).

The second source of information consists of planning documents, memos, letters, and other information gathered first for OTA and later in preparation for a book funded by the Alfred P. Sloan Foundation. Many of the people I interviewed opened their files to me, and I have copied material from OTA, the National Research Council, the University of California at Santa Cruz (UCSC), Cold Spring Harbor Laboratories, the DOE genome offices in Germantown, Maryland, the Office of the Director, NIH, and the National Center for Human Genome Research at NIH. This study has been an extraordinary opportunity to sift through the history of a science program in its infancy. Staff in the agencies were extremely generous with their time and free in allowing me access to documents. I have by no means gone through all the material in all these places; rather, I copied those documents identified as critical by those who made the decisions, or I filtered out pertinent material from large file collections. Finally, I systematically surveyed the science and lay literature for articles referring to the human genome project through mid-1988. Press accounts document the story, but they are also a part of it, as the channels of communication are themselves mechanisms for producing action.

The first section of the paper deals briefly with the origins of mapping and sequencing technologies. This topic is discussed because these technical capacities are the reason the genome project exists at all. Technical advances are not the focus of the paper but rather a backdrop to understand the ensuing story about policy formation; consequently, the technical background section is brief but dense, and it may be rough going for nonscientists or scientists outside molecular biology and genetics. If this is the case, the NRC or OTA reports on mapping and sequencing explain the technical background at greater length in lay language (National Research Council, 1988; U.S. Congress, OTA, 1988a).

The new technical means led to bureaucratic adaptations in the science agencies, and the paper's second section describes the history of the numerous individuals who originated different conceptions of systematic genome-scale research. It also tracks how the technical ideas were translated into science programs at DOE, NIH, and the Howard Hughes Medical Institute (HHMI). This history is mingled with the concomitant process by which these science programs were funded by Congress. Securing a budget for a new program is the first step that requires justification to a community beyond the science agencies, because the budget processes within the executive branch and the justification of budgets to the appropriations committees in Congress both entail considerable effort. Securing a budget requires convincing those with broad-ranging responsibilities well beyond a particular scientific community not only that something new is needed but that it is needed more than other items competing for funds in the federal budget. Programs must contend not only with other life science programs but also with broader national priorities within science and with any federal programs that entail annual appropriations.

In the case of the genome project, the legislative and bureaucratic developments hinged on arguments, made principally by scientists themselves, about the merits of the enterprise. Some of the principal arguments and issues raised in the process of persuasion are teased apart in the final section of this paper. The justifications proffered for public funding of the genome project generated a set of obligations that the project will have to meet, and I briefly note these and discuss whether keeping such promises matters. Four brief appendices elaborate on certain specific issues mentioned only briefly in the text.

The future of the genome project remains in doubt. Public fears of how genetic information might be handled, discomfiture with the power of such intimate knowledge, and democratic distrust of powerful elites are all elements that could disrupt the working consensus that currently favors public support. Opposition to a new style of biology and research management has been intense since the beginning and shows little sign of abating. There is no disease-oriented constituency supporting the program, and so the genome program is largely a creature of the molecular biologists and human geneticists who conceived it and supported it in its early stages. The human genome project is thus, more than many other areas of biomedical research, under pressure to produce results, and it is likely to be held to greater standards of accountability than other projects for the initial promises made on its behalf. Whether the genome project is judged a social benefit is contingent on how its results are used, and there will be considerable uncertainty about this for several years at least.

The genesis of the human genome project highlights the complex interplay between people and the institutions in which they work, illuminating how much difference a few individuals can make but also demonstrating how constrained those individuals are, how persistent they have to be, and how little power any one person has in the great march of science. A few individuals independently conceived a large-scale genome project, a much larger number of scientists reformulated the initial plans in a way that commanded greater support within the scientific community, and policymakers ratified the judgments made by scientists, thus providing resources to begin work. The genome project is now poised to begin in earnest, and its results over the next few years, and the uses to which those results are put, will determine the success or failure of the endeavor.

TECHNICAL AND SCIENTIFIC BACKGROUND

The genome project coalesced from a number of independent developments. Historical strands can be traced to evolutionary and population genetics, medical genetics, molecular biology, detection of mutations, advances in instrumentation, and computational biology. The principal factor was a meeting of the fields of human genetics and molecular biology. One field has long been largely clinical and descriptive; the other has been highly reductionist and focused on mechanics. As these two worlds came together in the 1970s and 1980s, each was fundamentally transformed, a process that continues today. The human genome project is a result of this collision.

Human gene mapping began in 1911, when researchers deduced that, because of its pattern of inheritance, color blindness lay on the X chromosome. For five decades thereafter, study of the odd inheritance patterns of X-linked disease was the only reliable mapping method. In the late 1960s, two technical developments occurred. First, somatic cell hybridization became a mapping strategy. This method mixed chromosomes by fusing together cells from humans and other organisms. The mixed chromosomes fragment and reorganize into metastable cell lines that retain various amounts of human deoxyribonucleic acid (DNA). It turned out that rodent-human cell lines, after a few generations, generally retained mainly rodent and only a small amount of human DNA and were relatively stable over time. By assembling large numbers of such cell lines, and devising clever ways to select only those cells that contained functional genes of interest, it became possible to map genes. During this period, it also became possible to differentiate the 24 distinct human chromosomes under the light microscope by staining them with DNA-binding dyes, producing a karyotype (normally 22 pairs of autosomes and either a pair of Xs, in females, or an X and Y, in males). In a photograph of the nucleus of a cell, the chromosomes could be directly seen and large-scale deletions, rearrangements, and duplications detected. Somatic cell hybridization and karyotyping launched human geneticists on their quest for a complete gene map (McKusick, 1988).

In the mid-1970s, restriction enzymes, recombinant DNA techniques, and the enormous variety of molecular biological techniques for selectively cutting and copying DNA ushered in a new era in gene mapping. Recombinant DNA led to the isolation and cloning of hundreds of human genes, but there was another significant spinoff: mapping by linkage to DNA markers. The idea was to find landmarks along the human chromosomes that would allow geneticists to determine which parts of which chromosomes were inherited from which parent. Once located, the markers could be used to trace the inheritance of bits of chromosomes through families, so that the inheritance of markers could be compared with the inheritance of diseases or other traits.

There are, very roughly, 3 million differences in DNA sequence "spelling" between any two people. Most of these differences have no detectable effect on the individuals, but they can be measured by direct analysis of DNA. If there are enough markers and enough people in a family to do the statistics, one can "link" the inheritance of a genetic character (a disease or trait) to the inheritance of a chromosomal marker. The closer a gene is physically to the marker being studied, the less often it will be separated in the process of producing sperm and egg cells, and the greater the statistical linkage to the marker. Because the marker's chromosomal location is known, at least approximately, this information locates the gene nearby.

Kan and Dozy first used linkage to a sequence difference to detect different variants of hemoglobin in 1978 (Kan and Dozy, 1978). The first published suggestion that a systematic collection of such markers be made occurred in 1979 (Solomon and Bodmer, 1979). A landmark paper published a few months later (Botstein, 1980) elaborated the idea in considerably more detail, initiating an explosion of genetic linkage mapping in the 1980s.

Methods of studying the inheritance of markers and genetic characters harken back to the mathematical genetics developed late in the last century and early in this one. The scientific approach is fundamentally classical genetics—the study of the inheritance of observable differences among individuals—supplemented by clinical observation to define the genetic characters under study and augmented by the modern tools of molecular marking. The process relies on the mathematics of probabilities to make correlations. The communities that studied evolutionary and population genetics immediately understood the significance of genetic linkage mapping. They were joined by a few medical geneticists who were comfortable with the statistical techniques of linkage. When the method yielded success in locating the gene responsible for Huntington's disease in 1983 (Gusella et al., 1983) and the gene responsible for polycystic kidney disease in 1985 (Reeders et al., 1985), clinical genetic research quickly adopted it.

By the mid-1980s, genetic linkage mapping was part of the mainstream of human genetics. *Newsweek* magazine quipped in late 1987 that there was a disease a week being mapped by genetic linkage (Begley et al., 1987). Technical advances further extended the ability to work backwards from an approximate gene location, determined by linkage to a marker, to find the gene itself and identify its product (in most cases, a protein). The first successful search for a gene starting from its chromosomal location ended in 1987, with the cloning of a gene that causes the rare condition chronic granulomatous disease (Royer et al., 1987). This achievement was soon followed by location of the Duchenne's muscular dystrophy gene (Koenig et al., 1987) and retinoblastoma (Friend et al., 1986; Lee et al., 1987). In these cases, however, the location was known from patterns of inheritance (on the X chromosome for Duchenne's muscular dystrophy and on chromosome 13 for retinoblastoma), or from human-hamster hybrids, and the study of individual patients who had lost specific portions of the X chromosome.

The process of going from chromosomal location to isolated gene is slow, tedious, unreliable, and often frustrating. (Intensive work over seven years failed to produce the Huntington's disease gene, for example.) But many prevalent disease-causing genes have been isolated in this way, most notably the gene that causes cystic fibrosis (Kerem et al., 1989; Riordan et al., 1989; Rommens et al., 1989). Cystic fibrosis was the first case in which the gene was mapped initially by genetic linkage; then the regional DNA was studied until a gene was found and its product identified, a membrane protein thought to be involved in the regulatory flow of chloride ions into cells. The idea that mapping can be the critical first step in understanding genetic disease has thus been confirmed in principle and in practice, but there is a long way to go before the more than 4,000 known disorders have been correlated with genes and gene products. The late 1980s were the period that saw human genetics, and with it the study of genetic diseases, joined with molecular biology in happy matrimony.

Molecular biology is largely a post-World War II phenomenon. Its two seminal events are Avery, MacLeod, and McCarty's discovery in late 1943 of DNA as the "transforming principle," conferring heritable traits (Avery et al., 1944), and Watson and Crick's revelation in 1953 of the double helical structure of DNA (Watson and Crick, 1953). These are, indeed, two of the high points in twentieth-century science and culture.

The distinctive signature of molecular biology is its approach to understanding function through the study of molecular structure. The double helical structure of DNA is the touchstone of this approach, explaining at once how information can be transmitted from generation to generation or from cell to cell during development, and also how information can be decoded into cellular processes through DNA-directed synthesis of proteins and ribonucleic acid molecules. One tenet of molecular biology is to study simple systems of living things, and early work in molecular biology, Delbrück and Luria's "phage" group in particular, focused on the simplest—viruses that infect bacteria (Judson, 1979). Beginning in the 1960s, however, molecular biology invaded field after field, applying its increasingly powerful tools to questions of greater complexity. By the mid- to late 1970s, molecular genetics was applied with astonishing success to the study of cancer and resulted in the discovery of oncogenes.

The first disease characterized at the molecular level was sickle cell anemia. In 1949, genetic studies by Neel showed that it was a recessive genetic disease, and biochemical studies by Pauling and colleagues (1949) indicated that it was caused by a chemical change in the structure of hemoglobin. In the mid-1950s, Ingram identified the difference between sickle and normal hemoglobin by breaking the protein into small fragments and looking for differences. He was able to establish that in the sickle cells a single glutamine amino acid had been replaced by valine in one of the two pairs of protein chains that make up hemoglobin (Ingram, 1957). This difference suggested a mutation in the DNA encoding of the beta chain of hemoglobin. Until the past few years, most of the tools of molecular biology were applied following this paradigm, that is, studying individual genes, one at a time, by biochemical analysis. Application of molecular techniques to chromosome mapping came from pushing molecular biological techniques at both ends—on the one hand, forcing chromosomal mapping to higher resolution, ultimately enabling direct decoding of the DNA base pair sequence, and on the other hand, developing techniques to separate and clone larger and larger fragments of DNA, culminating in reproduction of megabase stretches of DNA.

Before the development of these techniques, the handling of large fragments of DNA was difficult for several reasons. First, the manipulations involved in preparing it for analysis often sheared the long, fragile strands. Second, the widely used analytical techniques could only separate fragments of up to thousands of base pairs in length. Finally, because of the modified viruses and plasmid vectors used, the length of DNA that could be cloned was also limited to a range of from several thousand to a few tens of thousands of base pairs. During the early to mid-1980s, it became possible to handle long strands of DNA without breaking them by manipulating them in gels rather than in solutions. It also became possible to separate DNA molecules of up to several million base pairs in length using pulsed-field gel electrophoresis, first developed by Schwartz and Cantor, who pioneered several innovations in electrophoretic separation methods (Schwartz and Cantor, 1984). Moreover, cloning vectors that could consistently contain 30,000 to 40,000 base pairs became standard fare through incremental improvements in dozens of laboratories. With these concomitant advances, it became possible to take DNA from chromosomes, clone it, and analyze it to reconstruct the order of cloned DNA fragments, so that eventually a complete map of the original DNA could be assembled. This kind of map had the enormous advantage that the chromosomal DNA would be not only mapped but also cloned and stored in the freezer for further analysis. If such a tool had been available for the tip of chromosome 4, for example, those searching for the Huntington's gene in that region could have studied the DNA directly as soon as they located the gene. Having the DNA cloned would make the search for closer markers and candidate genes much simpler and faster. The DNA sequence would be another leap forward. Work on both fronts is now proceeding.

Two groups began independently to apply the cloning and ordering strategy to make ordered maps of yeast, in Olson's laboratory at Washington University, and of nematodes, in Sulston and Coulson's laboratory in Cambridge, U.K., and Waterston's at Washington University. Work began in the early 1980s and began to show promising results by 1986 (Coulson et al., 1986; Olson et al., 1986). The genome of the nematode is roughly the same size—100 megabases—as a small human chromosome, and it thus became conceivable to map the human genome by extension of the nematode method. Such an extension followed a tradition in molecular biology to focus on a new problem an order of magnitude greater than one that has been solved before. (The exact size of the leap was open to discussion, but the principle was widely accepted.)

DNA sequencing was developed by groups located in both Cambridges, more or less simultaneously, using entirely different approaches. Sanger's group in Cambridge, U.K., developed DNA sequencing after a dedicated and deliberate effort that started with protein sequencing, progressed to the sequencing of ribonucleic acid, and culminated in DNA sequencing. Sanger presented a partial sequence of a virus to an awestruck audience in May 1975 (Judson, 1987) and published a modified, simpler method in 1977 (Sanger et al., 1977). Maxam and Gilbert, working in Cambridge, Massachusetts, developed DNA sequencing from their attempts to study directly the regulation of gene expression in bacteria. Gilbert's group had been early pioneers in the field. They isolated their first DNA segment and deduced their first DNA sequence during 1972-1974. This first sequence consisted of 24 base pairs and took two highly competent investigators two years to achieve (W. Gilbert, Harvard University, personal communication, July 1988). The next step was to use chemical modifications of DNA bases to study directly the DNA protein-bound segments that regulate gene expression. Maxam and Gilbert realized they had come upon an approach that, with some further work, would permit direct DNA sequencing (Kolata, 1980). By August 1976, they were ready to distribute the chemical recipes used in their sequencing reactions at a Gordon conference (one of many small, closed gatherings of scientists held in New Hampshire colleges each summer). They also published their method of DNA sequencing in 1977 (Maxam and Gilbert, 1977).

Molecular biology thus generated a cornucopia of technological tricks that allowed scientists to think seriously about constructing physical maps of chromosomes and determining their DNA sequence. Some human geneticists were quick to apply the developing techniques to study diseases, but with a few exceptions, molecular biology was a separate field from human genetics. Nonetheless, the two disciplines were rapidly converging, as molecular biology worked its way into yet another field ripe for the picking.

The early to mid-1980s also saw two other important technological developments: diffusion of the personal computer and automation of microchemical manipulation. The computer revolution was imported from other areas but quickly adapted to the needs of biologists. It was important because it put personal computers in thousands of laboratories that were unacquainted with them. It permitted more analysis of raw data, and there was a natural harmony with the digital analysis of linear DNA sequence information. As information processing became faster and cheaper by orders of magnitude every few years, biologists, including molecular biologists, began to use computers more and more.

Automation of microchemical processes made possible experiments that were too tedious to do by hand. Automation was successfully cultivated at only a few university centers and in companies that either were already selling instruments to biologists or had been newly formed to do so. Instruments were devised first to sequence and synthesize proteins for analysis of their amino acid building blocks. Analysis of DNA was the next step. Serious efforts to synthesize short segments of DNA, a capability essential to developing highly sensitive probes for analyzing genetic experiments, began in the late 1970s; they had by 1980-1981 proved successful.

Automation of DNA sequencing began around this time in both Japan and the United States. In the United States, the first efforts leading to the current generation of DNA sequenators began in 1980 at the California Institute of Technology, or Caltech, under a five-year grant from the Weingart Institute. The first government support, through the National Science Foundation (NSF), came only in 1984 after a successful prototype was developed. In Japan, the Science and Technology Agency in 1981 began to support a project to automate DNA sequencing that involved several corporate sponsors (Fuji Photo, Seiko, and Matsui Knowledge Industries). The automation effort at the European Molecular Biology Laboratory in Heidelberg began several years later, supported by several European governments.

All of these technological developments surged during 1980-1985. In their wake came ideas for a concerted genome project, and several farsighted people independently brought them forth.

ORIGINS OF DEDICATED GENOME RESEARCH PROGRAMS

The idea of a systematic gene map of human chromosomes was not new. Human geneticists had talked of it for decades. The notion of large-scale sequencing was also discussed soon after sequencing techniques became widespread in 1977. Several groups talked of sequencing the HLA region involved in immune regulation and the regions encoding antibody protein genes. The European Molecular Biology Laboratory seriously discussed a dedicated project to sequence *Escherichia coli* in 1980-1981. Solomon and Bodmer (1979) mentioned the benefits of finding DNA markers throughout the chromosomes, and Botstein and colleagues analyzed in detail the significance of a systematic effort in this area (Botstein, 1980) in a landmark 1980 paper. Yet none of these ideas for a collective effort took hold within the federal government. DNA sequencing was widely used, but it remained the province of thousands of small laboratories focused on small regions. The Cambridge, U.K., group, under Sanger and then Barrell, were almost alone in sequencing the entire genomes of progressively larger organisms.

The key idea in genome projects was a dedicated effort to map and sequence whole organisms or significant parts of their genomes (e.g., an entire chromosome or chromosomal region). Government support for such technically focused efforts was slow to develop. Several attempts to entice NIH to construct a genetic linkage map were rebuffed, in part because the logical mechanism was a service contract or other nongrant mechanism. These were considered highly suspect because, in part, they had been used to support cancer research of only marginal usefulness. One corporation, Collaborative Research, Inc., and a private philanthropy, the Howard Hughes Medical Institute, stepped in to fund laboratories dedicated to generating DNA markers. These two laboratories, under the direction of Helen Donis-Keller (Collaborative Research) and Ray White (HHMI, Utah), contributed more than half the DNA markers that existed on the human genetic map in 1987 (Donis-Keller et al., 1987). The idea of focused mapping received some support when it fit into the format of a small scientific project, as in the case of physically mapping yeast, but several proposals to apply these methods to human chromosomes were rejected by scientific review groups in the mid-1980s.

In 1985 and 1986, however, several groups began to buck the tide. The first discussion of a large dedicated genome project came at a workshop convened at the University of California at Santa Cruz in June 1985. In the fall of the same year, Norman and Leigh Anderson proposed that sequencing the genome and cataloging all known genes should be a concerted national effort, but the idea was recorded in a relatively obscure journal and never caught fire (Anderson and Anderson, 1985).

By a curious twist, the history of the genome project is connected to the Keck telescope that now graces Mauna Kea, joining the cluster of other large telescopes on a Hawaiian mountaintop. The story behind this connection merits a digression because it is a classic example of how the quest for funds breeds scientific entrepreneurship and how thinking about Big Science infiltrated the field of biology.

Robert Sinsheimer was chancellor of UCSC in the fall of 1984. He was a biologist who wanted to leave a mark on his institution. In his own words, he "wanted to put Santa Cruz on the map in biology." He was also faced with a problem: he knew about a pot of money but had no way to spend it.

The events leading to this development were initially tied not to biology but to astronomy. The UCSC astronomy department had become extremely enthusiastic about building the largest optical telescope in the world. (UCSC had an excellent international reputation in astronomy, which was a great source of pride for the university.) One problem, however, was the prohibitive cost of producing the mirror for such a telescope. This problem was solved in principle by packing together 36 small hexagonal mirrors, rather than producing a single large mirror, which lowered the estimated costs from $500 million to $70 million. With this development, UCSC decided to seek funding for a telescope from private donors. A story was run in the San Jose *Mercury*, and the university received a call from a person familiar with the newly formed Hoffman Foundation, created after the death of Max Hoffman, the U.S. importer of Volkswagen and BMW automobiles. After further inquiry, the foundation indicated that Hoffman's wife might be interested in contributing $36 million to help finance the world's largest telescope. David Gardner, president of the University of California system, was contacted, and the money was accepted. It was the largest single contribution to the University of California in its history. Mrs. Hoffman died the next day.

The university continued to search for funds, but it began to have difficulty securing the additional donations, in part because it was a state university largely supported with taxpayer dollars and in part because the agreement with the Hoffman Foundation included naming the telescope for Max Hoffman. Caltech was approached to explore the possibility of a joint effort, assuming it could help raise the requisite funds. Caltech secured an additional $15 million from among its trustees, and then it contacted the W. M. Keck Foundation, established with monies from Superior Oil. The Keck Foundation was willing to help but wanted to fund the entire effort and have the telescope named after Keck. According to this plan, the $36 million from the Hoffman Foundation and other prior donations could be used as operating capital. When the Hoffman trustees were approached with the idea as well as another proposal to build twin telescopes, however, both overtures were rejected. The University of California returned the check for $36 million. The Keck telescope saw first light in December 1990 managed by the California Association for Research in Astronomy, the University of California-Caltech group established for the project.

To return to the genome thread of the story, Sinsheimer's problem late in 1984 was what he might do to recoup the Hoffman funds. He decided to develop a proposal for a big, attractive project. He began by considering what opportunities might be lost in biology because of an exclusive focus on projects that could be done by small groups without special facilities. After rejecting a number of possibilities, he hit upon the idea of sequencing the human genome. He called in UCSC biologists Robert Edgar, Harry Noller, and Robert Ludwig to discuss setting up an institute at UCSC for this purpose. At first the three were stunned by the idea, thinking it ludicrous in its audacity, but after some discussion they felt it was worth further consideration. Edgar and Noller then prepared a position paper, dated Halloween 1984, that described the genome sequencing institute as

a noble and inspiring enterprise. In some respects, like the journeys to the moon, it is simply a "tour de force;" it is not at all clear that knowledge of the nucleotide sequence of the human genome will, initially, provide deep insights into the physical nature of man. Nevertheless, we are confident that this project will provide an integrating focus for all efforts to use DNA cloning techniques in the study of human genetics. The ordered library of cloned DNA that must be produced to allow the genome to be sequenced will itself be of great value to all human genetics researchers. The project will also provide an impetus for improvements in techniques . . . that have already revolutionized the nature of biological research . . .

As the next step in the project, the UCSC group decided to call a meeting of experts from around the world. Noller wrote to Frederick Sanger, the two-time Nobel laureate whose DNA sequencing methods were described above, and with whom Noller had worked early in his career. Sanger wrote back: "It seems to me to be the ultimate in sequencing and will probably need to be done eventually, so why not start on it now? It's difficult to be certain, but I think the time is ripe."

The meeting was held on May 24 and 25, 1985. The group assembled included those pushing the limits of DNA sequencing (Bart Barrell, Leroy Hood, and George Church), some originators and practitioners of genetic linkage mapping (David Botstein, Ronald Davis, and Helen Donis-Keller), large-scale physical mappers (John Sulston and Robert Waterston), mavens of large DNA fragment analysis (Leonard Lerner and David Schwartz), and a mathematician concerned with analysis of DNA sequence (Michael Waterman). An important addition, however, was made at the last minute.

While the meeting was being organized, Walter Gilbert, co-inventor of the chemical modification DNA sequencing method and one of the most highly respected minds in molecular biology, was off in the Pacific after having resigned as chief executive officer of Biogen, Inc. The Santa Cruz group strongly wanted his blessing, and after some effort Edgar finally reached him in late March. Gilbert was in transition back to his faculty position at Harvard, and he agreed to come. His presence became central to the unfolding genome story.

After the meeting, Sinsheimer summarized its conclusions, which Steven Hall later reported, capturing the modesty of the meeting in "Genesis, the Sequel" (Hall, 1988). The group agreed that it made sense to pursue systematic development of a genetic linkage map, a physical map of ordered clones, and the capacity for large-scale DNA sequencing (Sinsheimer, 1989). The sequencing effort early on should focus on automation and development of faster, cheaper techniques. This summary was sent to several potential funding sources, including HHMI and the Arnold and Mabel Beckman Foundation, but there was no response. Donald Fredrickson, then president of HHMI, was at that time also hearing ideas about a different variety of genome project from Charles Scriver, then a member of the HHMI medical advisory board. HHMI decided to investigate further but did not agree to fund the Santa Cruz proposal.

Gilbert was an extraordinarily articulate science visionary. In a memo to Sinsheimer two days after the workshop, he translated the Santa Cruz group's ideas into specific operating plans and became the torchbearer for the effort to generate enthusiasm, taking the ideas generated at the workshop into the power centers of molecular biology. He gave informal presentations on sequencing the genome at a Gordon conference and at the first international conference on genes and computers in August 1985. Gilbert was extremely well connected and infected several of his colleagues with his enthusiasm. (Two of them in particular—Paul Berg and James Watson—figure later in the story. Both Nobel laureates like Gilbert himself, they were counted among the most respected and powerful figures in molecular biology.) Gilbert also gave the genome project much greater notice than it would otherwise have achieved, earning feature stories on his role in it from *U.S. News and World Report* (McAuliffe, 1987), *Newsweek* (Begley et al., 1987), *Boston* magazine (del Guercio, 1987), *Business Week* (Beam and Hamilton, 1987), *Insight* (Holzman, 1987), and the *New York Times Magazine* (Kanigel, 1987). In addition, he and Leroy Hood wrote supporting articles for a special section in *Issues in Science and Technology* published by the National Academy of Sciences (Gilbert, 1987; Hood and Smith, 1987), and he and Walter Bodmer wrote editorials for *The Scientist* (Gilbert, 1986; Bodmer, 1986b). Gilbert thus kept the steam up in the genome project engine, even as Sinsheimer's attempts locally at UCSC were meeting bureaucratic resistance from the University of California system.

Sinsheimer, however, was also sounding out his colleagues about the idea of a genome sequencing institute. He spoke to James Wyngaarden, director of NIH, at a meeting in Washington, D.C., sometime in late February or early March 1985. His personal note about this conversation stated that Wyngaarden was quite supportive and urged Sinsheimer to put together a proposal to the National Institute of General Medical Sciences (NIGMS) after the May workshop. Wyngaarden judged that "it would not be too difficult to get congressional funding for the project, through NIGMS," according to Sinsheimer. Two years later, Wyngaarden recalled this conversation only vaguely but agreed that he would probably have said something like what Sinsheimer reported.

It would have been logical to seek funding from NIH, but such a course presented several problems. The cost estimates from the Santa Cruz meeting—$25 to $40 million to build an institute, with an annual budget of roughly $10 million—were far too high for a grant or standard research program. The project would require a special appropriation, which raised the difficulties of approaching Congress. This step also required the approval of the president of the University of California system. Sinsheimer judged that the university system's support was contingent on getting a large private donation to start things off and proposed that he approach the Hoffman Foundation with his new idea. The president's office, however, stalled for several months on the proposal, perhaps because it did not accord the genome institute a high priority or because it was concerned about conflict among the various campuses in the system, many of which could argue that they were better positioned to house a genome institute. Whatever the reason, the approach was never made, and the initial impetus for the sequencing idea—the potential availability of funding from Hoffman—proved a dead end. Moreover, no other private donor ever materialized. Sinsheimer later lamented, "I thought the extraordinary significance of the project would be more self-evident to some of the prospective donors than proved to be the case" (R. Sinsheimer, personal communication, September 1988). In the end, without the needed private support, the idea of a genome institute at UCSC died a slow, quiet death.

THE DEPARTMENT OF ENERGY PLAN

A more successful seed was planted in December 1984, when DOE sponsored a meeting at Alta, Utah, to discuss how to measure heritable mutations in humans (Cook-Deegan, 1989). Ray White of the University of Utah organized the meeting at the behest of Mortimer Mendelsohn of Lawrence Livermore National Laboratory and David Smith of DOE. The specific question to be addressed was whether new DNA-based methods were sensitive enough to detect any increase in mutations among survivors of the Hiroshima and Nagasaki atomic bomb blasts. A group of scientists engaged in developing new DNA analytical techniques were invited to participate. The conclusion of the meeting was that the methods could not yield an answer with the scale of effort that was currently feasible, but the workshop had a more lasting effect as a result of the coincidence of several events. The workshop was in progress just as Schwartz and Cantor were producing the first data using pulsed-field gel electrophoresis for mapping, as George Church was beginning to think of new approaches to DNA sequencing directly from DNA in the native genome of an organism, and as Maynard Olson's physical mapping efforts in yeast were beginning to bear fruit. Its timing was propitious.

OTA staff were preparing a report on technologies to measure heritable mutations in humans because the issues of exposure to Agent Orange, environmental toxins, and radiation were beginning to come before congressional committees (U.S. Congress, OTA, 1986). Mike Gough, the OTA project director, was present at the meeting and discussed the various technologies in a draft report that was sent to DOE for review. Charles DeLisi, as newly appointed head of DOE's Office of Health and Environmental Research, reviewed the draft and recalled looking up from its pages with the idea for a dedicated project focused on DNA sequencing and computation (DeLisi, 1988).

DeLisi and David Smith of DOE moved quickly on many fronts in the December lull of 1985. They asked the biology group at Los Alamos National Laboratory for its comments on DeLisi's idea, and just before Christmas the group responded with a dense, somewhat scattered, but extremely enthusiastic five-page memo. The principal author was physician Mark Bitensky. The memo concerned sequencing the entire human genome and barely mentioned physical or genetic mapping. It provided estimated costs, noted that such a project could become a "DNA-centered mechanism for international cooperation and reduction in tension," and extolled the potential technical and human health benefits. The Los Alamos group even persuaded Frank Ruddle to agree to testify before Congress. With this initial feedback, Smith and DeLisi began to pull the bureaucratic levers in Washington.

In a note to Smith, DeLisi outlined an approach to garner support from the scientific community, from his superiors at DOE, and from Congress. In a return note to DeLisi dated December 30, 1985, Smith mentioned previous discussions of sequencing the human genome at a Gordon conference and at a meeting at the University of California the previous summer but said he did not know what had come of these efforts. He also anticipated the criticisms that would plague the DOE proposal for some time to come: that it was not science but technical drudgery, that directed research was less efficient than letting small groups decide what was important and then do it, and that effort should be concentrated on genes of interest rather than global sequencing. In a reply the next day, DeLisi contended that "regarding the grind, grind, grind argument . . . there will be some grind; what we are discussing is whether the grinding should be spread out over 30 years or compressed into 10." He presciently noted that "we are talking about $100-150 million per year spread out over somewhat more than a decade . . . " and further asserted that such a project would certainly rate as more important than the lower 1 percent of grants that funding of this magnitude would displace. He suggested that the political effort should focus not on whether it would displace other work but instead on how to gain support for new funding.

In January 1986, DeLisi discussed the idea with his superior, Alvin Trivelpiece, who as director of the Office of Energy Research reported directly to the secretary of energy (then Herrington). Trivelpiece supported the project and charged the DOE biological sciences advisory committee (the Health and Environmental Research Advisory Committee, or HERAC) to report back to him about the idea. This action by Trivelpiece followed several discussions with DeLisi about the possibility of doing a genome project in DOE. The two men had discussed why the agency did not have the same high stature in biology that it had in high-energy physics, and both aspired to change that situation by providing a project that would propel DOE to the forefront of biology. As part of the outreach to the scientific community, Los Alamos was asked to convene a workshop (1) to find out if there was consensus that the project was feasible and should be started, (2) to delineate medical and scientific benefits and to outline a scientific strategy, and (3) to discuss international cooperation, especially with the Soviet Union.

During 1986, the wheels continued to turn. A workshop was held at Santa Fe on March 3 and 4, with "a rare and impassioned esprit," according to Bitensky's memo that summarized it. Discussions at the workshop resulted in a clear emphasis on physical mapping by ordering clone libraries as a crucial first step (collected papers from 1986 Santa Fe Workshop, DOE, not published; Bitensky, 1986). In letters back to the conference organizer, Mark Bitensky, there was consensus on the importance of a new project, a fair degree of agreement on what should be done next, and a wide range of opinions about how to organize the effort. Anthony Carrano and Elbert Branscomb from Lawrence Livermore National Laboratory stressed the importance of clone maps and warned that "a program whose announced purpose was simply to 'sequence the human genome' might unnecessarily and incorrectly arouse fears of territorial and financial usurpation in the biomedical research community." They were certainly right in that regard. In contrast, David Comings was rather far off the mark when he averred that the whole physical mapping component might be funded "without any stirring up of any congressmen or other related creatures." The creatures were not so docile; indeed, they proved downright ornery.

By May, DeLisi had produced an internal planning memo to carry the request for a line-item budget. The memo was transmitted to Trivelpiece and from there up through the DOE bureaucracy. By the time the memo was prepared, the project had been broken into two phases. Phase I had three components. The first, physical mapping of the human chromosomes, to last five or six years, took up much of the first phase. The other two components in Phase I were development of high-speed automated DNA sequencing and a research program to improve computer analysis of sequence information. DeLisi's background in computational biology came to the fore here. Phase II, which was contingent on success in Phase I, entailed sequencing the banks of DNA clones put together in a physical map of the chromosomes.

In his memo to Trivelpiece dated May 6, DeLisi spoke of a project analogous to a space program, but requiring the efforts of many agencies and a more distributed work structure, with "one agency playing the lead, managerial role . . . DOE is a natural organization to play the lead management role." In a separate memo DeLisi requested a budget of $5, $10, $19, $22, $22, and $22 million dollars for fiscal years 1987-1992. The plans survived internal DOE review, and a series of meetings were scheduled in late 1986 with Judy Bostock, the DOE life sciences budget officer in the White House Office of Management and Budget (OMB), in conjunction with planning for fiscal year 1988 and beyond. Bostock was a physicist from the Massachusetts Institute of Technology, with a strong interest in biology, especially in improving the speed and efficiency of biological research. The budget briefing documents for DeLisi's Office of Health and Environmental Research/OMB meetings included a budget projection for fiscal years 1987-1990 of $5.64, $11.55, $18, and $22 million. In the DOE copy "$22 million" for 1990 is scratched out and replaced with "$23.5," and there is a handwritten note that the changes resulted from discussions with OMB. The document's cover sheet specifies a four-year project beginning October 1, 1987, extending to September 30, 1991, and costing $95 million. By simple arithmetic, this suggests there was an agreement for a fiscal year 1991 budget of $40 to $45 million. Decisions about a Phase II budget were to be made in 1990 and 1991. Bostock confirmed that there had been minor revisions, but essentially the proposal worked out by DOE and OMB in fall 1986 became the basis for a multiyear program agreement.

The DOE HERAC endorsed the plan for a DOE genome initiative in a report from its special ad hoc subcommittee. The subcommittee was composed of 14 scientists, only one of whom was from a national laboratory. It was a blue-ribbon scientific group chaired by Ignacio Tinoco, a highly respected chemist from the University of California at Berkeley (then on sabbatical for a year at the University of Colorado in Boulder). The report urged a budget of $200 million per year, and made a case for DOE leadership of the effort. A few observations must be made about this advisory process, however. First, the subcommittee's budget projections were not at all connected to the multiyear DOE-OMB budget agreement discussed above. The subcommittee first considered budget projections on February 5 and 6, 1987, at a meeting in the Denver Stouffer's Hotel (see the discussion of costs below). The DOE-OMB agreement is dated one and a half months earlier, December 18, 1986. DeLisi had briefed OMB earlier, on September 5, and received tentative agreement (Hall, 1988). Clearly, DeLisi was willing to listen to the subcommittee's advice, but it is equally clear that the commitment to go ahead with a project, including a multiyear budget, was made long before DeLisi knew what the subcommittee would say. Second, at its final meeting to draft the report, the subcommittee did not discuss which agency should lead the effort. This deficit was pointed out to HERAC when it met to consider the subcommittee's report in March; by April, when the report was released, Tinoco as subcommittee chairman and Mort Mendelsohn, a member of the subcommittee and chairman of HERAC, had canvassed members to gain support for language in favor of DOE leadership. Later interviews with members of the subcommittee revealed that at least 7 of the 14 had reservations about giving DOE a blank check; they agreed to the suggested language, however, because they perceived a lack of action on the part of NIH and thought the project so important that it should be done no matter which agency did it.

In the waning days of 1985, DeLisi and Smith forged a plan that propelled the human genome project onto the public agenda. It is clear from memos and personal notes that they did this deliberately and with the purpose of establishing a new mission for the DOE-supported laboratories centered on sequencing the human genome. The process for obtaining funding included successful transit of the DOE bureaucracy and agreement from a highly involved OMB budget officer.

Yet despite the go-ahead from the bureaucracy, the job was not complete: now came the two-step congressional process. Here DeLisi was less adept, although he managed it. Any new action of the federal government requires congressional authorization and appropriation. These twin processes are interdependent but distinct. Authorization falls to a pair of committees, one each in the House and Senate. Which of the authorization committees handles a particular science agency is determined by an intricate set of jurisdictional rules negotiated over the years by the committees. The authorizing committee structure is not exactly parallel between the House and the Senate because the two houses have different boundaries, drawn in part to accommodate the individual interests of past and current committee chairmen. The appropriations process, in contrast, is a parallel process with a relatively stable annual routine.

The President's budget proposal is submitted in January each year and then goes to the appropriations committees. Except in unusual circumstances (as occurred once during the Reagan years, violating the spirit, if not the letter, of the Constitution), the House takes action first, and the Senate works from the House figures. If there are new programs under consideration, appropriations are theoretically, and in most cases actually, contingent on prior passage of an authorization statute. The appropriations committees are not to legislate but rather to fund activities under rules set forth by other committees. The interpretation of this proviso can be liberal or strict, depending on the circumstances.

To get the genome program started, DeLisi took $4.5 million in funds from the preexisting fiscal year 1987 budget and reallocated them to the genome effort. Such limited "reprogramming" is common practice, permitted by the appropriation and authorization committees within reasonable limits with written justification. For 1988 and later budgets, however, DOE needed support from its authorization committees and funding from the appropriations committees. DeLisi had noted the need for congressional action in his December 1985 note to David Smith, and he had held some meetings with congressional staff in 1986. There was little problem in the Senate, as DOE had the strong support of Senator Pete Domenici and tacit approval of Senator Wendell Ford, the key figures on the authorization committee. Domenici also sat on the appropriations and budget committees and could be counted on for support there. The problem was in the House.

Staff of the relevant DOE authorization subcommittee in the House were getting mixed signals about the DOE genome initiative. They had read the generally negative response to it in *Science* magazine, and a few calls to contacts in the molecular biology field elicited both support and opposition. Eileen Lee was the committee's resident biologist, and was understandably uncertain about the tack the committee should take. The problem was further complicated by the politics of DeLisi's other biology programs. The committee staff of the majority party were generally disposed to support initiatives coming from DOE staff, who were, after all, paid to do just such planning, but DeLisi's relations with the committee were problematic and it was unclear to the staff whether they should expend the political capital to defend him on the genome initiative. Claudine Schneider, ranking Republican on the committee, was dissatisfied with DOE's record on research into environmental health hazards, and her staff director, Eric Erdheim, was rumored to have called the Delegation for Biomedical Research to ask James Watson to testify against the DOE genome program. (Erdheim did, indeed, speak with Bradie Metheny, lobbyist for the delegation, but nothing came of it; Erdheim was not so much opposed to the genome project as suspicious of any new proposal coming from DeLisi. Watson stated in an interview a few months later that he was never asked to testify. DeLisi had a backup if he ran into trouble in the subcommittee, however, because Manuel Lujan, ranking Republican on the full committee, came from New Mexico and was well known as a national laboratory supporter. If Schneider had wanted to change DOE's direction, she would at least have had to notify him.)

Eileen Lee arranged for Leroy Hood to testify before the committee, after calling OTA and several other contacts for suggestions. Hood agreed, oblivious to the political maelstrom swirling around him, and on

March 17, 1987, projected a passionate vision of the genome project (U.S. Congress, House, 1987a). Hood strongly supported a new genome initiative and proposed a role for DOE, NIH, and NSF, thus deftly ducking the troublesome question of which agency should hold the reins. Schneider's latent distrust broke the surface in a series of questions about DOE reports on health effects of radiation on submarine workers, Hiroshima and Nagasaki survivors, and nuclear plant workers and reports on least-cost energy, but the genome program glided through the hearings unscathed. The appropriations process was less troublesome than authorization and presented no major obstacles once the genome project had OMB approval.

The DOE budget process for fiscal years 1988 and 1989 held true to the initial agreement with OMB—the agency sought $12 million and $18 million, respectively, for the two years. It exceeded the initial agreement only in 1990, when it sought $28 million instead of $22 million.

The seeds that Charles DeLisi planted found fertile soil in the U.S. Senate, but for very different reasons. Senator Pete Domenici was a staunch supporter of the national laboratories in New Mexico, although he had long believed that they produced far fewer long-term benefits for the local economy of his state than they should. He convened a panel to discuss the future of the national laboratories one Saturday morning, May 2, 1987, in the U.S. Capitol. Domenici's staff brought together an impressive group of people, including former Senator Barber Conable, now head of the World Bank; Donald Fredrickson, former director of NIH; Ed Zschau, former California congressman and successful entrepreneur; and the directors of several national laboratories. In the middle of the meeting, Domenici posed the question, "What happens if peace breaks out?" This question was of great concern because the vast bulk of work supported at the two laboratories in New Mexico was focused on nuclear weapons production and defense-related research and development. Domenici wanted to know how the immense research resources of the national laboratories could be better integrated into local economies. He also sought a new mission for the labs that did not depend on cold war rhetoric and that might move them into the growth areas of science, which clearly included biology. There was no way that Domenici could have foreseen the events of late 1989 and the transformation of Eastern Europe, but it did seem likely that sooner or later the Reagan defense spending juggernaut would lose steam.

Donald Fredrickson, then president of HHMI, suggested that the national laboratories might play a role in the human genome project. Jack McConnell, director of advanced technologies for Johnson & Johnson, took hold of the ideas discussed at the meeting and worked with

Domenici's staff to draft legislation that resulted in Senate Bill No. 1480, giving DOE the mandate to mount a genome project. (The bill also legislated issues relating to technology transfer in semiconductors and military research and included some patent policy directives.) By that time, Los Alamos was already in the thick of beginning its genome program, but this show of strong support from the Senate secured its future at a time of potential vulnerability.

It was clear from the outset that the DOE initiative would include national laboratory centers for genome research. Taking advantage of national laboratory resources was one of two principal justifications for DOE assuring the lead role in the project (the other being the areas of related research that were part of the DOE mission, particularly mutation detection). It was also clear that Los Alamos National Laboratory would be one such center, because it housed groups working on the cloning techniques, was the site for GenBank (the DNA sequence data base), and was in Domenici's home state (Domenici sat on both the authorization and appropriations committees for DOE and was also a ranking member of the budget committee). Most people assumed that Lawrence Livermore also would be designated a center, because it housed the other group engaged in large-scale cloning and DNA library-ordering efforts.

There were several problems, however. First, both Los Alamos and Livermore were weapons laboratories. This fact placed them in a different administrative category in DOE and made them somewhat less subject to direction by the Office of Energy Research, and the Office of Health and Environmental Research within it, because the laboratories answer to those parts of DOE concerned with national security policies. This administrative aspect also makes technology transfer issues (e.g., negotiation of patent agreements and personnel exchanges) more difficult because such transfers are covered by a different set of contracts with the University of California. (DOE-funded laboratories are operated by contractors. The University of California operates Los Alamos, Livermore, and Berkeley.) Finally, Livermore is sited on a flat, dry, windswept California plain whereas its sister laboratory, Lawrence Berkeley, nestles among the eucalyptus groves in the foothills overlooking beautiful San Francisco Bay. It would be much easier to recruit new researchers to a beautiful spot near one of the world's most prestigious universities than to an isolated steppe known best for the birth of the fusion bomb.

Early in the DOE initiative, the various national laboratories were invited to submit proposals for review, and many did so, including both Berkeley and Livermore. The Berkeley proposal was initially rejected by DOE staff, which did not surprise those who had worked on the proposal in Berkeley, who knew it was in serious trouble. But in September 1987, press reports of an American Association for the Advancement of Science meeting announced that Berkeley had been designated a center. This decision was apparently the result of discussions between DeLisi, Bostock, and other DOE and OMB higher-ups. Livermore, on the other hand, retained its project to map chromosome 19 and several other ongoing efforts, but was not given center status for several years.

The Berkeley center began with a first-year budget of roughly $3 million but without an approved proposal or a site visit. The designation was made with the expectation that Charles Cantor would become the center's director, but negotiations with him were still going on when the announcement was made. Clearly, Berkeley's designation as a center was a judgment—which required the agreement of upper management at DOE and OMB that establishing a new resource center at Berkeley was a better course of action than having to solve all the bureaucratic problems associated with supporting the ongoing work at Livermore.

DeLisi and Smith's anticipation of some arguments that would be made for and against the program was excellent. But what was missing from their thoughts proved to be just as important—competition with NIH and acceptance among molecular biologists and human geneticists. DeLisi remarked later that "moving unilaterally was not my preference, nor did I consider it optimal." One source of great enthusiasm was Vincent DeVita, director of the National Cancer Institute, where DeLisi had worked before. The problem, from DeLisi's perspective, was that the National Institute of General Medical Sciences supported the fields of science most relevant to the genome project. DeLisi saw a hole, put his head down, and ran. He put the genome project on the public agenda, but not without getting tackled.

The well-known NIGMS response was that if it were to be done, they should do it, but it should not be done . . . One of my choices was to use the NIH style of cautious consensus building. At times, perhaps most of the time, that is the best procedure; but in my judgment, this was not such a time. I made a deliberate decision to move vigorously forward with the best scientific advice we could muster (HERAC). I am quite willing to take the criticism, rational or not, that such movement provokes . . . . I would have been far more timid about subjecting myself to . . . criticisms . . . if I saw my future career path confined to government. (C. DeLisi, personal communication, March 1990)

Several technical elements are also remarkable by their absence from early consideration. The DOE proposals for the project contain very little discussion of genetic linkage mapping—the first and arguably the most important step in making the project useful to the research community—and scant attention to the study of nonhuman organisms as either pilot projects or even scientifically important topics. One could argue that these areas were outside the range of biology research at DOE, but this is straining the argument because genetic linkage mapping is highly mathematical, requires systematic repetitive searches for DNA markers, and thus presents a great opportunity for just the sort of large group effort advocated by DOE. The omissions were undoubtedly in part also premised on a tacit understanding that the requisite work would of course get done. The omissions were, however, noted by biologists.

DOE strongly emphasized bacterial genetics immediately after World War II, and continued to support many groups working on nonhuman biology. Whatever the justifications, the neglect of genetic linkage mapping and nonhuman genetics drove a wedge between DOE and much of the biomedical research community. The enthusiasm driving the DOE human genome proposal proved sufficient to keep it going, but it was a rough ride.

On March 7, 1986, as many of the Santa Fe workshop participants were returning to their laboratories, *Science* magazine published an article by Renato Dulbecco (1986). Dulbecco, a Nobel laureate and president of the Salk Institute, was highly respected for his quiet demeanor and careful approach to science. The article thus brought wide attention and generated a wave of discussion in the laboratories of universities and research centers throughout the world. Dulbecco argued that the early emphasis in cancer had been on exogenous factors—viruses, chemical mutagens, and their mechanisms of action. Cancer research was at a turning point, he said, so "if we wish to learn more about cancer, we must now concentrate on the cellular genome." The nature of the connection to research specifically on cancer was imprecise; but scientists took note of the proposal, coming as it did from a scientist of Dulbecco's stature. Like Sinsheimer, Dulbecco came to the idea of the genome project deliberately thinking big. He had been preparing a review paper on the genetic approach to cancer. Although cancer clearly is not a purely genetic disease except in rare cases, it is equally clear that the steps leading to uncontrolled cellular growth involve changes in DNA.

Dulbecco further explained his rationale in a January 1987 interview. His argument for sequencing was that genetic techniques were among the most powerful in biology and extensive sequencing information would be a tool of immense utility in the study of cancer. He saw the sequence as a reference standard against which to measure the changes in DNA that take place in cancer. He argued that some such standard was needed because of human genetic variation. In other species, such as the mouse, for which there are some 150 well-characterized, genetically homogeneous strains, controlled breeding is possible; in humans it is not. He saw the human gene sequence information as itself generating new biological hypotheses for experimental testing. Dulbecco believed that sequence information would be an intimate part of understanding some of the most fundamental problems of biology—cancer, chronic disease, evolution, and development. He noted the need for biology to encompass some collective enterprises of use to all, in addition to its extremely successful agenda of mounting small, narrowly focused inquiries. When asked what he thought about big science in biology, he smiled and said perhaps that would take care of itself over time.

THE SCIENTIFIC COMMUNITY RESPONDS

By the summer of 1986, the rumor networks of molecular biology were abuzz with talk of the DOE human genome proposal. News of the Santa Fe workshop had been disseminated by the participants and those in the mainstream of molecular biology were beginning to take the idea seriously. As is so often the case, Cold Spring Harbor Laboratory became the focal point of the debate. In June 1986 the lab sponsored a large meeting titled "The Molecular Biology of *Homo sapiens*." The symposium brought together the giants of human genetics and molecular biology, with 123 speakers and an audience of 311 (Watson, 1986). The genome project was the hottest topic of discussion. Walter Bodmer, a British human geneticist familiar with both molecular methods and mathematical analysis, was the keynote speaker. Well known for his broad view of the field, he emphasized the importance of gene maps and the advantages of a DNA reference dictionary. Bodmer argued that the project was "enormously worthwhile, has no defense implications, and generates no case for competition between laboratories and nations." Moreover, it was better than big science in physics or space because it was "no good getting a man a third or a quarter of the way to Mars . . . . However, a quarter or a third . . . of the total human genome sequence . . . could already provide a most valuable yield of applications" (Bodmer, 1986a). He concluded his talk by urging a commitment to systematic mapping and sequencing, as "a revolutionary step forward."

Victor McKusick, dean of human genetics and keeper of Mendelian Inheritance in Man, the gold standard human genetic disease data base, was the next speaker. He summarized the status of the gene map and finished his talk by urging a dedicated effort to genomic mapping and sequencing (McKusick, 1986). He argued that "complete mapping of the human genome and complete sequencing are one and the same thing," and explained the intricate interdependence of genetic linkage maps, physical maps, and DNA sequence data. He urged the audience to get on with the work and pointed to the future importance of managing the massive flood of data to come from human genetics.

The issue came to a head at an evening session not originally on the program. Paul Berg was unaware of the discussions in DOE and Santa Cruz but he had read Dulbecco's article and suggested to Watson that it might be useful to have an informal discussion of a genome sequencing effort at the Cold Spring Harbor meeting (P. Berg, personal communication, March 1990). Watson called Gilbert to find out if he would chair such a session with Berg (W. Gilbert and J. Watson, personal communication, June 1989). Berg thus arrived at the symposium to find that Watson had scheduled the session and that he and Gilbert would chair it.

The purpose of the session was to discuss the proposals for a genome project. Berg led off by trying to have the symposium participants discuss the scientific merits of mapping and sequencing and what technical approaches might make the effort feasible. Gilbert then got up and briefly described the Santa Cruz and Santa Fe meetings, following with the essentials covered in his earlier letter to Sinsheimer. He noted that the DNA sequence was accumulating at the rate of 2 million base pairs per year, in which case there would be no reference sequence for the genome for a thousand years. Gilbert thought that figure could be reduced to 100 years with no special effort but that a dedicated effort involving 30,000 person-years, on the scale of the space shuttle project, would produce a dramatic acceleration with enormous benefits. He began to write down numbers—large numbers that evoked great interest from the audience. The numbers on costs, however, provoked the most vigorous reaction. Gilbert estimated that, at $1 per base pair, there could be a reference sequence for approximately $3 billion dollars.

Berg called for discussion about whether it would be worthwhile to have the DNA sequence of the human genome. David Botstein rose to the podium and asked that scientists "not go forward under the flag of Asilomar," meaning presumably that they should be aware of the political elements of their endeavor from the outset. He noted that if Lewis and Clark had followed a similar approach to mapping the American West, a millimeter at a time, they would still be somewhere in North Dakota; he also cautioned that scientists were amateur politicians and should be wary of making grand political proposals. Botstein voiced concern that researchers would become "indentured" to a mindless sequencing project and closed by pleading that molecular biologists "maybe accept the goal, but not give away our ability to decide what is important because we have decided on the space shuttle" (D. Botstein, remarks recorded by C. Thomas Caskey). This speech set loose the dammed-up energy of the assembly, and infectious applause spread through the audience. Several speakers followed, including Maxine Singer, Leonard Lerman, Peter Pearson, and Giorgio Bernardi, as well as other well-known molecular biologists. Many reiterated Botstein's sentiments; others supported the notion of an appealing proposal that could attract public support but were ambivalent about its impact on science. David Smith of DOE spoke midway through the session on the focused nature of the DOE proposal, but he was clearly on the defensive, even admitting in response to one question that perhaps DOE should not lead such an effort. His comments were largely lost in the wash. (Smith noted later, however, that many people in the audience had come forward privately to indicate their support.) Berg struggled from time to time to refocus the meeting on the technical and scientific aspects of the proposals, but his cause was lost. As the session ended, it was clear that molecular biologists were not enthused by the DOE human genome project, perceiving it as a misguided bureaucratic initiative and, more important, as a direct threat to their own research funding.

The dispute was covered by Roger Lewin of *Science* magazine, and his news articles were the first signals of the coming debate that encompassed many in science and government (Lewin, 1986a,b). The first step, however, was to shift the scene of the action from the quiet scientific mecca of Cold Spring Harbor to Washington, D.C.

A gala event held on the NIH campus, July 23, 1986, was sponsored by HHMI. Donald Fredrickson, former director of NIH and then president of HHMI, introduced and closed the meeting chaired by Walter Bodmer, which became something of a celebration for a redefined genome project. There were several brief presentations about the technologies and about what was going on in U.S. agencies and in other parts of the world. Mainly, however, it was a show of power—a battleship summit for molecular biology.

The HHMI interest can be traced along several paths. HHMI staff credit Ray Gesteland and Charles Scriver as the people principally responsible for interesting the institute in gene mapping. Gesteland was a student in the Watson laboratory in the mid-1960s and became a Hughes Investigator at the University of Utah. He suggested to George Cahill, HHMI vice president for scientific training and development, that HHMI support research on some ideas for systematic genetic mapping proposed by a group in Massachusetts, in particular, Ray White. Cahill recruited White to go to Utah, a feat accomplished in part by the attraction of the incredibly rich and detailed Mormon pedigrees kept by the university that might be useful for clinical genetic studies. (It also helped that White liked to ski.) Thus, in November 1980, White began to construct a genetic linkage map.

Charles Scriver, a Canadian and human geneticist of international reputation, had served on the HHMI Medical Advisory Board from the late 1970s to the mid-1980s. (During this period the institute's annual funding for biomedical research increased from just over $10 million to more than $200 million, following the death of Howard Hughes in 1976.) Scriver was fascinated by the prospect of a human genome project, thinking primarily of the immense impact systematic mapping could have on clinical genetics and the patients he saw each day in his Montreal genetics clinic. Yet he called the decision to fund genetic linkage mapping, for which he became a champion on the Medical Advisory Board, "a close thing" on the part of HHMI.

Scriver became convinced, mainly through conversations with Francis Ruddle and later with White, that support of genetics data bases was essential, and he worked to persuade the other members of the Medical Advisory Board. As a result, HHMI began to support human gene mapping workshops held every two years, the Human Gene Mapping Library at its facility near Yale University, and the computerized version of McKusick's Mendelian Inheritance in Man data base (Pines, 1986).

A special meeting to discuss the HHMI human genetic resources effort was convened in Coconut Grove, Florida, on February 15, 1986. The meeting focused on how to manage the massive increase in information about genetic marker maps, locations determined by somatic cell genetics, and new DNA probes. It took place two weeks before the DOE meeting in Santa Fe on sequencing the genome but covered a completely different set of issues that only later took refuge under the umbrella of the human genome project. Watson met with Fredrickson on April 1 to indicate his strong support for an HHMI presence in genome research.

A July meeting at NIH was scheduled to gain information for a meeting of the Hughes trustees in August. In the wake of Cold Spring Harbor, the focus on data bases converged with the dispute about the DOE proposal to generate a tension surrounding the HHMI forum at NIH. The forum thus became another turning point in the debate, but the new direction was not entirely clear. Roger Lewin opened his report of the meeting in *Science* with the observation, "The drive to initiate a Big Science project to sequence the entire human genome is running out of steam" (Lewin, 1986c). Hood, whose views on sequencing were taken quite seriously, asserted that massive sequencing was premature and that the focus instead should be on improving the technologies. But the meeting was far from an outright rejection of the genome project—it merely rechanneled its energies.

Those attending the meeting agreed that the time was ripe to mount a special initiative in gene mapping. Bodmer could not contain himself when David Smith presented an outline of the DOE genome initiative, and Bodmer interjected that the proposal did not acknowledge the importance of genetic mapping. While Smith continued, Sydney Brenner, seated at the meeting table, conspicuously passed a note to Gilbert and Watson that was read by those around them: "This is a retreat." DOE was on hostile turf there in the NIH homeland, and the meeting was another event in a several-year period of tension between NIH and DOE regarding management strategies. Indeed, which agency would lead the effort became the dominant topic of discussion surrounding the genome project until well into 1988. The importance of the HHMI forum, however, lay in the fact that the question had imperceptibly shifted from whether to start a genome project to what it encompassed, how best to do it, and who should lead it.

HHMI was presumed to be a neutral party in the dispute, a philanthropy with international reach and a commitment to shared informational resources in human genetics. The institute was seen as a small partner to the federal agencies, rapidly responding when federal agencies could not, and filling in niches left vacant by the NIH behemoth. The shape of the HHMI program was becoming clear. A special presentation on the genome project was scheduled for the HHMI trustees in August. Maya Pines, a highly respected science writer, was commissioned to write a background piece on gene mapping and sequencing as background for deciding on continued support of basic genetics and a multiyear funding initiative for genomic data bases (Pines, 1986). The proposal was approved, with George Cahill (later, Max Cowan) and Diane Hinton of HHMI assigned principal administrative responsibility.

Before and after the Cold Spring Harbor meeting, James Watson was busy behind the scenes, trying to put together the pieces of a project that would be to his liking. Watson had been a power broker in molecular biology, since soon after he and Francis Crick discovered the double helical structure of DNA, and he had a well-deserved reputation for speaking his mind. Within the scientific community, many found him distasteful, but almost every molecular biologist learned to respect his biological intuition, his ability to frame important questions, and his talent for creating an environment in which bright people could contend with the best in the world. First at Harvard and later at Cold Spring Harbor Laboratory, he was an impresario of topnotch molecular biology, and he used his status as "the father of DNA" to get what he thought was needed.

He thought the nation needed a genome project—but not the one offered by DOE. Consequently, he enticed Berg and Gilbert to hold the

Cold Spring Harbor rump session on the genome project, and he began to agitate for involvement of the National Academy of Sciences (NAS), supporting its efforts to mount a study quickly. His position was quite simple, and he stated it publicly at the HHMI meeting: "I am for the project, although everyone I talk to at Cold Spring Harbor is against it." He was following his intuition, again, against the stream.

CALLS FOR EVALUATION

NAS was a logical place to go for an assessment of research strategy. Devising a national plan for mapping and sequencing clearly involved substantial scientific and technical issues, for which the National Research Council (NRC) at the Academy was created. Furthermore, the Academy process ensured a systematic assessment often absent from open-ended debate, and its reports carried special weight in Congress and in the executive agencies. Convening a panel on the genome project was a considerable risk to genome supporters at the time, however, because sentiments were largely against the DOE proposal, which had dominated discussion to that point. An Academy report that equivocated or came out against a genome project would likely kill the idea for several years at least. A positive report would not guarantee its success, particularly if it required extra funding, but a negative report would be an almost insurmountable obstacle.

Plans to involve NAS were hatched around the time of the Cold Spring Harbor meeting in June 1986. On July 3, John Burris, executive director of the Academy's Board on Basic Biology, wrote a short proposal to fund a small group meeting to discuss the genome project in August. A discussion of the options was placed on the agenda of the board's meeting in Woods Hole, Massachusetts, on August 5. The meeting included DeLisi, Wyngaarden, Watson, Cantor, Gilbert, Hood, White, Ruddle, Kingsbury, Ruth Kirschstein (director of NIGMS), Frank Press (president of the Academy), and several Academy staff. The board noted its support for physical mapping and expressly withheld its support from a massive sequencing program. It suggested that the NRC might wish to organize a study to formulate whether any special project made technical sense and if so, what its goals should be. A proposal was prepared, and Watson directed Burris to Michael Witunsky of the James S. McDonnell Foundation for funding of the study. Within a week, McDonnell had sent a check to the Academy. Bruce Alberts, known to be generally opposed to large targeted research efforts in biology because of an editorial he had written for *Cell* (Alberts, 1985), was selected to chair the project because he would be seen as neutral. Furthermore, his experience in writing a major textbook gave him the tools to make sure a report was written quickly and well. The original hope was to complete the study in six months, or at least by mid-summer 1987.

Several people identified as skeptics were appointed to the panel, notably Botstein and Shirley Tilghman. The committee was also peppered with Nobel laureates: Gilbert, Watson, and Daniel Nathans from Johns Hopkins. Sydney Brenner was invited to represent the views of British mappers and sequencers, and John Tooze from the European Molecular Biology Organization was asked to speak for the Europeans as a group. An effort to secure a Japanese scientist was unsuccessful, although at least one was invited. Cantor, Hood, and Ruddle represented different technical backgrounds, and McKusick, Leon Rosenberg (dean of Yale Medical School), and Stuart Orkin (whose laboratory had done seminal work on chronic granulomatous disease and many other conditions) represented the field of human genetics.

Alberts and Burris hatched a strategy intended to build consensus slowly, if that proved possible. The first meeting on December 5, 1986, was intended to give the committee a sense of the general lay of the land, with presentations from the U.S. organizations with special genome-related activities (NIH, DOE, NSF, HHMI, and OTA) followed by a survey of activities in Europe. The remainder of the day centered on deciding what a final report should cover and what information needed to be gathered for it. The committee elected to focus early meetings almost exclusively on technical background and to postpone discussion of policy options and funding until the technical stakes were clear. To that end, they brought in individuals with "hands-on" experience in the fields under discussion. A January meeting had three technical sessions: (1) genetic linkage mapping, somatic cell hybrid mapping, and physical mapping; (2) large-scale sequencing; and (3) data bases related to protein and DNA structure.

In the meantime, the dynamics of the committee took an interesting turn. Walter Gilbert announced plans to form the Genome Corporation to map and sequence the genome as a private company and consequently he resigned from the NRC committee when he did so to avoid a conflict of interest. Gilbert had been a strong proponent of a fast-track genome project. Several committee members felt he was such a strong champion that it was becoming difficult to reach any consensus because his assertiveness elicited a backlash from several other members. His resignation paradoxically made it possible for those who were highly skeptical of the project to gracefully redefine it and shift to its support.

The next meeting, in March, began with a discussion of genetic linkage mapping in greater detail, with Donis-Keller, Gusella, and White all making presentations. The afternoon was an attempt to assess the political context, with presentations from OTA and Wyngaarden. Gilbert's slot had been filled by Maynard Olson, whose work in physical mapping and large DNA fragment cloning was in the thick of the technologies under discussion. Indeed, Bruce Alberts viewed "my major contribution to the NRC as the appointment of Maynard Olson to replace Gilbert" (personal communication, October 12, 1990). Olson also brought a philosophical approach well suited to forging consensus. It was he who noted the importance of having enough genetic linkage markers to assemble a physical map, thus cementing the "marriage" of those twin objectives, and he also clearly articulated the distinctive feature of genome research that would set it apart from other genetic studies: a focus on projects of increasing scale (size of DNA to be handled or mapped, degree of map resolution, speed, cost, accuracy, or other factors). He argued that support should be given to those projects that promised to increase these scale factors by three-to tenfold. The second day of the March meeting opened with Cahill describing the HHMI interests. The rest of the day was devoted to trying to sort through the first drafts of several technical background chapters and beginning the process of deciding what would be said about policy. It became clear that the skeptics had been converted by the project's redefinition.

In effect, the NRC panel was a microcosm of biomedical research. Its deliberations for the first time systematically assessed the arguments for and against a dedicated genome project and surveyed the various technical components necessary to bring it together. Alberts called the NRC committee "the most fun of any committee I have worked on" because of the talented people on it, the rapid learning process it entailed, the uncertainty of its outcome, and its direct impact on policy (personal communication, August 18, 1988). The NRC report succeeded to a remarkable degree in setting a scientific agenda—the critical missing element from 1986 to early 1988.

The report, however, had one critical weakness—its recommendations about how the project should be organized. The scientists on the committee made little attempt to survey what the agencies were doing, and there was a great deal of activity going on in NIH, in DOE, and in Congress. The committee commissioned only one paper, by Eric Juengst and Albert Jonsen, on the ethical implications of the research. The committee members had some informal contacts, principally with NIH, but there was no systematic attempt to gather information critical to making a policy recommendation. The federal bureaucracies are highly complex, and the political process is unpredictable; having an impact requires extensive knowledge about the backgrounds of large bureaucracies, jurisdictional boundaries in Congress, and the histories of pivotal figures. Such knowledge is necessary to make credible recommendations, or at least formulate options, that do not seem naive or counterproductive. One of the reviewers who received the penultimate draft of the NRC report had great familiarity with the organization of science agencies and was appalled by the organizational options. This response and others provoked a rewrite of the section and many last-minute changes. It is clear from subsequent interviews that the committee did not have enough data on which to base a recommendation but felt it had to do so anyway to fulfill its responsibility. There had been no meeting to discuss this topic, and the phone calls that were conducted in its stead did not permit a solid consensus to form.

The report was released recommending that there be one lead agency but failing to specify which one (NRC, 1988). The option preferred by the NRC required Congress to decide whether NIH or DOE should lead the genome project. Clearly, the preferable organizational structure would have been to develop a program de novo from within one agency, but this was historically not how it happened. It was too late to make the program fit the ideal. The NRC committee ignored the fact that by 1988 each agency had multimillion-dollar budgets, advisory committees, planning documents, and, just as important, expectant constituencies and congressional patrons. In addition, it was not clear what was meant by a "lead agency." If it meant that one agency should have a formal mandate, with funding coming from several sources, then it would have been politically feasible but effectively meaningless. How would NIH as "lead" agency decide how DOE should spend its funds? If it meant all the funding should come from one place, then it required a dismantling of either the NIH or the DOE programs, a politically hopeless task, particularly when congressional interests were taken into account. The main reason for fumbling the administrative recommendation was ambivalence about both NIH and DOE. NRC committee members were disappointed by what they saw as a faint-hearted commitment from Wyngaarden and near hostility from Kirschstein. Yet DOE undermined its credibility by asserting it wanted to do the project to detect mutations and monitor human exposure to radiation and environmental toxins. This was seen as asking to buy a sledgehammer to put in thumbtacks. There was also suspicion of DOE peer review, fomented by the process by which the genome center had been established at Lawrence Berkeley Laboratory.

Congress was following the debate and independently taking steps to gather the information needed to make policy choices. McKusick presented the arguments for mapping the human genome at a 1986 meeting of a biotechnology advisory panel at OTA, at the invitation of OTA staff Gary Ellis and Kathi Hanna. When the news from Cold Spring Harbor was reported, it attracted the attention of several Hill staff. I wrote a memo in mid-July to OTA upper management urging that the agency undertake a study because the issues were highly technical and complex and because DOE and NIH were on a collision course. A short discussion with Lesley Russell, science advisor to John Dingell, chairman of the Energy and Commerce Committee, led to a request for a proposal from Dingell to which OTA responded. By pure happenstance, the OTA and the NAS projects were approved in the same hour on September 30, 1986.

With separate governmental departments (in the form of NIH and DOE) vying for position, there were only two places to resolve the issue—in the White House or in Congress. Science policy in the Reagan administration was largely dictated by the budget process. Until the final year of the administration the ritual was to propose unrealistically low NIH budgets, leaving room for increased funding in other areas. NIH was one of the most popular executive agencies in Congress because of its medical research mission and a reputation for being well run and "clean," if a bit stodgy and paranoid. For the first seven years under Reagan, Congress increased the NIH budget far above the requested amount, a course of action that effectively gave power over the NIH budget, especially new budget items, to the appropriations committees in the House and Senate. This process contrasted starkly with that of the DOE budget, for which the President's request was much more likely to be cut than augmented. For DOE, the "inside game" that DeLisi played, going through formal budget review in DOE and OMB, was much more important than for NIH. NIH's budget, on the other hand, was an "outside game," played in the public arena of congressional politics—hearings, press reports, and Capitol Hill meetings.

Tracking the policy aspects of the genome project was left to OTA. Patricia Hoben kept abreast of technical developments and wrote a clear, well-illustrated introduction to the technologies. Jacqueline Courteau gathered information about data bases and repositories and sought information about foreign genome plans. Other staff collected information about what U.S. agencies and research institutions were doing in the field of genome research. Papers on Japan and Europe were commissioned, as was this history of the biology and of analogous periods of development in physics. OTA commissioned two papers to assess the ethical implications of the project, and several papers were commissioned and dozens of letters sent to gain technical background (a process unnecessary for the NRC committee). The OTA process was relatively open, with four panel meetings and workshops, each of which was attended by more than 100 people. The drafts were circulated to roughly 200 people, and served as an informal communication link among those following genome activities.

In contrast to the NRC report, which lays out a clear scientific strategy, OTA had virtually no role in setting the scientific agenda because it was not positioned to render a scientific judgment. Yet consensus on the strategy was a necessary precondition for the political decision about how to fund a program; thus, the NRC and OTA reports complemented one another. NRC performed the most important function, namely, articulating a scientific program that captured the insights of those who saw the need for collective resources and focused efforts. OTA systematically gathered information about government programs and acted as a well-informed but neutral observer, expert in science policy but not about the science itself. It fell to OTA to propose the options for coordinating the NIH and DOE efforts.

The OTA report was used mainly in two hearings on the NIH and DOE programs, held in April and June 1988. Senator Lawton Chiles (D-Fla.) had introduced a bill, when the Domenici legislation met with resistance, to create an interagency task force to tackle the genome. The new bill was passed by the Senate by a margin of 88-1 and sent to the House. NIH and DOE were faced with two options: conspicuous cooperation or a strong likelihood of legislation mandating a specific framework not entirely to their liking. They opted to sign a memorandum of understanding in hopes of staving off House action on the bill, having reached a tacit agreement with staff from both the Science, Space, and Technology and the Energy and Commerce committees. The content of the memorandum was immaterial, but the process was important for each agency in facing the reality that they would both have genome programs for the foreseeable future and that Congress would be quite sensitive to interagency bickering.

Until the release of the NRC and OTA reports, and, indeed, for a few months afterward, staff from both agencies appeared to believe that Congress would somehow designate their agency the lead organization. They expressed disappointment that NRC and OTA had not made a tough call, but in fact there was no call to make. The existence of twin genome programs was in the cards as soon as DOE pushed its first formal authorization and appropriation through Congress. The only strategy that could have prevented the birth of two programs was either the death of both in a fit of internecine warfare or a preemptive strike by NIH in spring or summer 1987. DOE could not have stopped NIH from mounting an effort once leaders at NIH concurred and the NRC committee reached a consensus, and NIH could have stopped DOE only before it cleared its authorization hurdles for the 1988 budget.

THE NATIONAL INSTITUTES OF HEALTH AND CONGRESS RESPOND

The critical figure in the effort to secure funding for an NIH genome program was James Wyngaarden. From Duke University Medical School, where he had been chairman of its largest department, medicine, for 15 years, Wyngaarden became the director of NIH after being nominated by President Reagan in spring 1982. He was highly respected as a clinician and human geneticist, and he accepted the job with some reluctance, stating this openly. In his confirmation hearings before the Senate, he noted, "I did not actively seek the post . . . my acceptance of that honor is out of a sense of obligation based on an awareness of the vital role of NIH in biomedical research . . . " and went on to emphasize the importance of basic biomedical research as the best long-term strategy to solve the nation's health needs (U.S. Congress, Senate, 1982). In a 1988 interview, he said he accepted the position because of considerable worry about what might happen to NIH if a caretaker were nominated instead of a person thoroughly familiar with the biomedical research process.

Wyngaarden first heard about the genome project in London at a meeting of the European Medical Research Council in June 1986, when someone asked him what he thought about a DOE plan to spend $3.5 billion sequencing the human genome. Shocked, Wyngaarden said this idea seemed to him "like the National Bureau of Standards proposing to build the B-2 bomber." At this same time, Ruth Kirschstein, director of NIGMS, began to get feedback from the March workshop in Santa Fe.

DeLisi of DOE had invited an NIH representative to the Santa Fe meeting in March, but the invitation got lost in the deluge of mail that enters the NIH director's office. He had sent background materials about the meeting afterward, as preparation for a meeting of himself, Wyngaarden, and Norman Anderson. When he returned from London, Wyngaarden asked Ruth Kirschstein to bring together an NIH panel to decide what might be done in response to the DOE foray. Kirschstein summarized the June 27 meeting of that group in a memo dated July 2 to Wyngaarden, noting that "first and foremost, while it is clear that the Department of Energy has taken, and will continue to have, the lead role in this endeavor, the NIH must and should play an important part." The group recommended that Wyngaarden focus the upcoming Director's Advisory Committee meeting in October on the genome project, in time to make plans for the fiscal year 1988 budget. They also noted the need for increased support of GenBank, the data base that stored DNA sequence information.

The October 16-17, 1986, meeting of the Director's Advisory Committee had another all-star cast that included Nobel lights and Nobel aspirants. The meeting was more structured than the HHMI forum of several months before, and the policy issues were becoming more evident. The meeting's main conclusions were that (1) NIH should eschew "big science" or a crash program, (2) the study of nonhuman organisms was just as important as the study of humans, (3) it would soon be feasible to sequence the human genome, and (4) information handling was already a problem. An NIH working group was appointed after this meeting, to be chaired by Wyngaarden and including Kirschstein, Duane Alexander (director of the National Institute of Child Health and Human Development), Betty Pickett (director of the Division of Research Resources), Donald Lindberg (director of the National Library of Medicine), and Jay Moskowitz (Program Planning and Evaluation), with George Palade (Nobel laureate from Yale) as the lone outsider. Rachel Levinson was named executive secretary. The working group met in November and December and produced recommendations for enhanced support of data bases as well as two new research program announcements.

Wyngaarden's early concern was to ensure that NIH had a major role in any large genome program that went forward but without making any long-term commitments. He was in favor of the concept of the genome project "from the very start," but resisted the impetus to go too far out on a limb when there was so much dissension among NIH-supported researchers. In a revealing analogy, he likened his position on the genome project to Lincoln's waiting for success at Antietam to announce the Emancipation Proclamation, so as not to lose Union support from Europe. His second analogy was to Roosevelt's delay in pushing the Lend-Lease Act until public sentiment supported the course he had already chosen. However, Wyngaarden did support the genome project, and strongly, where it counted the most—in the appropriations process.

In his summary statement to the House and Senate appropriation committees for fiscal year 1988 (in February and March 1987), Wyngaarden gave gene mapping a high profile. He mentioned NIH's centennial and the urgency of acquired immune deficiency syndrome (AIDS) research, and then flagged the genome project. A straight reading of his text would suggest it had second priority to AIDS. The NIH appropriation for genome research did not require a special authorization, as such research clearly fell within the bounds of NIH's biomedical research mission. Unless someone in Congress objected, much could be done through appropriations alone. Fiscal year 1988 was one of the years in which the NIH budget dance was played by ignoring the administration proposals, and Congressman David Obey said as much. Because the NIH director is part of the administration, Wyngaarden had to toe the administration line in supporting budget requests to Congress. Any testimony before legislative or appropriations committees is reviewed by officials in the Department of Health and Human Services and in the Office of Management and Budget. But the bureaucracy cannot interfere with Congress's authority to ask whatever questions it likes, and interfering with honest answers is a violation of federal whistleblowing laws. The appropriations committees thus had a simple way to ascertain NIH's true priorities, as opposed to those in the administration's fictitious request. Each year, they merely asked the NIH director what he would do with sums of money in addition to those requested, in $100 million increments.

In the House appropriations hearing, Congressman David Obey, who had read an article in the *Washington Post* about the genome project, tapped into what had become the major issue related to genome research by asking several questions about gene mapping. He wanted to know why DOE was proposing to lead such a project. Wyngaarden replied that the agency had legitimate interests in detecting mutations but that NIH was outspending DOE by a hundred to one in the relevant fields and so NIH should— He was about to finish his policy recommendation when Obey interrupted, asking for further clarification of DOE's interest. Wyngaarden never finished his recommendation but said to *Nature* magazine several weeks later that he thought it was presumptuous of DOE to claim leadership when it was spending less than $10 million a year in the area (Palca, 1987). Again he was not pressed on what NIH should do about it. Leslie Roberts of *Science* magazine opened the "Research News" section of the September 18 issue with a depiction of interagency squabbling (Roberts, 1987) that captured the confused positions of scientists and administrators during this formative period.

David Kingsbury of NSF, who emerged as one of the mediating forces, attempted to channel the conflict, first through the Biotechnology Science Coordinating Committee (formed principally by the White House Office of Science and Technology Policy to deal with interagency disagreements over the release of genetically altered organisms into the environment) and then the Domestic Policy Council (a cabinet-level group). Kingsbury's decision to mediate meant that NSF had to stay out of the competition, and NSF's policy position was quite clear for several years— it had no genome program per se, although its support for instrumentation and nonhuman biology was directly relevant. (This was clearly a position crafted in that bureaucratic netherworld where truth wears gray.)

Kingsbury's political situation deteriorated quickly, however, when he was implicated in a conflict-of-interest investigation related to his financial connections with Porton, a company that grew out of the chemical warfare establishment in England and that had aspirations in biotechnology. NSF thus was removed from contention for several years, reentering only in 1989 with its instrumentation centers and proposals for a plant genome program focused on *Arabidopsis thaliana*, a weed with a conveniently small genome.

Interagency disagreements at the strategic policy level had little material impact on those individuals who were administering grants and sponsoring activities in NIH and DOE, or among those researchers receiving grants from the agencies. If anything, there were special efforts to work jointly because of the intense public scrutiny, at least among readers of *Science* and *Nature*. Indeed, the degree of disruptive battling between NIH and DOE was less than for other high-stakes turf disputes *within* the Public Health Service—for example, among the National Institute on Aging, the National Institute of Neurological and Communicative Disorders and Stroke, and the National Institute of Mental Health regarding Alzheimer's disease funding in the late 1970s to mid-1980s; or among the National Cancer Institute, the National Institute of Allergy and Infectious Diseases, and the Centers for Disease Control over AIDS research beginning in the mid-1980s.

Squabbling over the genome nonetheless reached directly into Congress in the form of legislation. Senator Pete Domenici introduced S. 1480 early in 1987, the bill crafted by Jack McConnell and Domenici's staff to promote technology transfer from DOE-funded national laboratories. A section was devoted to the genome project. Domenici's bill gave a mandate to the secretary of energy to map the human genome and directed the secretary to establish and head a consortium dedicated to this purpose. Coordination of research from other agencies was to occur through a National Policy Board on the Human Genome, chaired by the secretary and including the NIH director, the NSF director, the secretary of agriculture, and other officials. Domenici attempted to add the bill as an amendment to the trade bill under active consideration in spring 1987, and his staff began to call other Senate and House committees with jurisdiction. Key to this effort were Senator Chiles, chairman of the NIH appropriations subcommittee and of the entire Budget Committee and generally accepting of NIH initiatives in biotechnology, and Senator Edward Kennedy, chairman of the NIH authorization committee.

By an irony typical of congressional politics, the genome project was linked to orange groves in Florida. Chiles's interest in biotechnology stemmed from a 1982 or 1983 meeting with one of his constituents, Francis Aloysius Wood, dean of the School of Agriculture at the University of Florida. Wood caught the senator's attention by describing how gene manipulation could move the frost belt 60 miles north, which meant more land could be devoted to cultivating a large crop plant of immense importance to Florida. Wood had found a graphic way to explain how the use of so-called ice-minus bacteria might delete some of the genes that cause ice crystals to form on fruit, thus lowering the temperature at which the fruit sustained damage. Changing the temperature at which fruit becomes damaged would reduce the annual worries of Florida's orange growers and effectively expand the territory acceptable for planting.

When the Senate became Democratic in the 1986 election, Chiles became the chairman of the appropriations subcommittee for NIH. His interests at NIH focused on biotechnology policy. The genome project became linked to biotechnology through Domenici's bill and through the language used by scientists to justify the project. When Domenici's bill first came to his attention, Chiles spoke with his legislative aide Rand Snell in a brief conversation en route from the Senate floor after a vote. The DOE element didn't seem quite right; it didn't seem fair to NIH. Later, Patricia Hoben from OTA happened to be meeting with Snell from Senator Chiles's staff on another matter, the competitiveness of U.S. biotechnology. When she heard about the proposal, she asked whether there had been outside consultation with university researchers. 'She suggested that Snell call Bruce Alberts, chairman of the NRC study committee. Alberts was noncommittal but indicated that there was, indeed, ambivalence about DOE leadership and a strong feeling among some on the committee that NIH should be the lead agency. Chiles refused to bite on Domenici's bill and thus began a long process of negotiation that led to a Chiles-Kennedy-Domenici bill, S. 1966, which included a genome project provision modified from Domenici's to give NIH and DOE joint leadership.

Kennedy's staff also called their contacts. During the week, a storm of protest calls came into the offices of Domenici, Chiles, and Kennedy, and the idea of passing the Domenici bill as an amendment to the trade bill was dropped. The Industrial Biotechnology Association, a trade association for the larger biotechnology companies, began a survey of its members in response to the Domenici bill. The survey showed a strong consensus in favor of funding a genome project, but only under the aegis of NIH.

Domenici held a workshop in Santa Fe on August 31, 1987, to determine what should be done about the genome project. It was Charles DeLisi's last day on the job at DOE: he was leaving to head a department of mathematical biology at Mt. Sinai Medical Center in New York City. Domenici urged his strong support for a DOE role in genome research. Norman Anderson pulled out all the stops in a moment of zeal:

I think so far as the man in the street is concerned ... to say that here is the possibility at one shot of finding the cause of some 2,500 human diseases is really stunning. ... A century from now, as history books are written, the big projects that were important in this century are the genome project, and after it possibly space and then the atomic bomb (the order of those, I don't know). But the man who first proposes to do the genome project in the United States Congress is in history. (U.S. Congress, Senate, 1987b)

It was a good way to get Domenici's attention.

Back in Washington at hearings on Domenici's bill on September 17, 1987, Wyngaarden articulated his desire for what one might paraphrase "the mission and the money, but not the management." This came during an interchange with Domenici in the question-and-answer session following Wyngaarden's testimony:

Domenici: *If you were assured that it was not the intention of the legislation to in any way denigrate or detract from your ongoing activities, would you recommend that the United States of America have a policy of mapping the human genome as expeditiously as possible?*

Wyngaarden: *Yes, sir. Unequivocally, yes.*

Domenici *(several exchanges later): If Congress wants to do it, how do we do it? Just give the NIH more money under their existing program and give DOE some more money ...*

Wyngaarden: *I think that is a very good way to do it.*

Domenici: *And would it get done?*

Wyngaarden: *Yes.*

Domenici: *Without any changes in the law?*

Wyngaarden: *I think so.*

James Decker, representing DOE, concurred with Wyngaarden.

Domenici *went on: I love you both and I think you are great. But I absolutely do not believe you. I believe it would get done. But I am quite sure that it would not get done in the most expeditious manner, because I do not think you would be charged with doing that. I do not think you would send up any requests of a priority nature with reference to it, because you do not have enough money to do what you are doing. And if you tried to send up the request, it would be thrown in the waste basket at OMB ... (U.S. Congress, Senate, 1987a)*

Wyngaarden and Domenici locked horns for several minutes more over definitions of what the other had meant, but it was clear that the basic issue was the mutual distrust between the legislative and executive branches of government. Congress, in the person of Domenici, did not trust the agencies to act quickly, and the agencies, principally in the person of Wyngaarden, did not want to have Congress tying internal priority-setting and budgeting processes in knots. Neither side could score a decisive win, and the policy process in this case was typical in that it unfolded over many months of thrusts and parries.

Within NIH, and among the power brokers in molecular biology, there was a division of opinion about the NIH role. Kirschstein articulated one position strongly. She was particularly concerned that the genome project not become a political juggernaut that could endanger small-group pursuit of basic genetic knowledge, for which NIGMS was the largest source of funding in the world. NIGMS issued two new announcements for grants in mapping and computation in May 1987, to demonstrate a special willingness to support such work, but did not formally commit dedicated funds for this purpose. These two grant announcements were the main product of the genome working group set up after the NIH Director's Advisory Committee the previous October.

Earlier, Kirschstein had canvassed all the NIH institutes to find out how much was being spent on grants that involved gene mapping or DNA sequencing and had produced a figure of $313 million in fiscal year 1987, of which $90 million was for work on humans. The grant officers of her own institute spent several days poring over their portfolios to come up with the figures, revealing the energy with which Kirschstein worked to support her position that NIH was already acting aggressively. Kirschstein argued that the NIGMS announcements were "not exactly business as usual, but not highly targeted either." Rachel Levinson, a member of Wyngaarden's staff who worked on the genome policies, agreed with this viewpoint and maintained that there was no need "for a concerted effort because it is not new. Every institute has work related to mapping and sequencing" (Roberts, 1987). This position was no doubt intended to assuage fears of a major shift in policy that could threaten investigator-initiated research, but it backfired. The message heard by the opinion leaders in molecular biology, including many Kirschstein supporters, was that NIH thought it was doing all it needed to do.

Many scientists, however, saw this contention as failure to appreciate the collective and dedicated efforts needed to finish maps and develop new technologies. NIH's neglect of dedicated genetic linkage mapping and DNA sequencing instrumentation was cited as symptomatic of a deficiency in NIH's resource planning. In interviews with dozens of molecular biologists, including Berg, David Baltimore, Botstein, Watson,

Gilbert, Hood, and others, NIH's official position was decried for missing the point of the genome project—to fill a need for concerted and focused efforts to create common resources. Whether Kirschstein took this position because she saw it as essential, or whether she was attempting to placate those worried about the genome project's impact on other basic genetic research and defend NIH against incursions from DOE, cannot be determined now, but it set the NIH genome program on a course that made separation from NIGMS inevitable.

NIH's first dedicated funding for genome research—$17.2 million—came in December 1987, when President Reagan signed the 1988 appropriations law (two months into the fiscal year). To determine how to allocate the funds, Wyngaarden convened an ad hoc advisory committee on February 29 and March 1, 1988, in Reston, Virginia, only a few weeks after release of the NRC study, which recommended a vigorous $200 million annual genome effort. The committee was chaired by David Baltimore, a Nobel laureate who had written against the Big Science genome project approach (Baltimore, 1987). The ad hoc committee made recommendations that closely followed those contained in the NRC report. Watson urged that an esteemed scientist be appointed director of the NIH genome efforts. Later, he stated, "I did not realize that I could be perceived as arguing for my own subsequent appointment" (Watson, 1990).

Whether Watson's arguments contributed to his subsequent appointment is unclear; nevertheless Wyngaarden named Watson director of a new genome office in October 1988. Watson then hired Elke Jordan, former associate director under Kirschstein and erstwhile resident of Matthew Meselson's laboratory when it was down the hall from Watson's in the 1960s. He also hired Mark Guyer, a bacterial geneticist who had worked at Genex Corporation before joining the NIGMS staff. Several people who were interviewed for this history thought Watson's ascension to the position of genome director was due to sexism or power seeking. Watson did, indeed, want power—enough to get the genome project moving. It seems clear, however, that he did not initially contemplate running the project himself.

One pointed exchange took place between Kirschstein and Watson in August 1987 at an OTA workshop on the costs of the genome project. The meeting was chaired by Berg and was intended to ferret out strategies for genome mapping and sequencing by forcing a discussion of budget items that would be of concern to Congress. At one point, the discussion digressed to management issues. Kirschstein and Watson clashed over the need for assertive planning by NIH. Watson wanted powerful direction; Kirschstein argued for the wisdom of the investigator-initiated grant mechanism. Watson was interviewed after the

OTA meeting and asked if he were willing to be the "czar" that he thought necessary. He said no, saying "I can't think of a job I'd like less" (Roberts, 1987). He later called several other people to find someone willing to take the job, but none of those who were able were also willing.

In his actions regarding the genome project, Wyngaarden made a tough call between the advice provided by Watson and others in his camp and the advice offered by Kirschstein and others in hers. In the end, the NIH director decided a question of policy directly. To her credit, Kirschstein supported the project publicly even after it was moved away from NIGMS, calling it "an important part of what the Public Health Service is all about in the next century," although allowing that it had politically "taken on a life of its own" (Jenks, 1989). Certainly, no one could doubt that.

THE PROJECT IS FUNDED

Wyngaarden was successful on another front—obtaining a genome budget at NIH. In his replies to the House Appropriations Committee for fiscal year 1988, he asked for $30 million in genome research funds in his fifth increment of $100 million above the administration request, and another $15 million in the eleventh increment (the penultimate of 12 such increments) (U.S. Congress, House, 1987b). After Wyngaarden testified in early spring 1987, David Baltimore and Watson met to brief members and staff of the House and Senate appropriations committees. They were invited to speak informally as part of a series of occasional meetings put together by Bradie Metheny on behalf of the Delegation for Basic Biomedical Research. Baltimore and Watson met briefly just before the session on May 1 to go over their remarks. The meeting included Congressmen William Natcher and Silvio Conte, chairman and ranking Republican of the NIH appropriations subcommittee, and also Congressman Joseph Early, a subcommittee member and staunch NIH supporter of many years. Senator Lowell Weicker, then chairman of the Senate appropriations subcommittee for NIH, was also present. The principal aim of the meeting was to promote funding for AIDS research. Watson, however, also supported adding $30 million to NIH's budget for genome research (Watson, 1990).

The House responded to Wyngaarden by appropriating $30 million for genome research. The Senate was less enthusiastic, inserting only $6 million. Maureen Byrnes, staff to Senator Weicker, recalled that he was not as enthusiastic about the genome project as the House delegation; other senators, such as Tom Harkin, were more enthusiastic but were also more junior and thus were unable to influence decisions as strongly. The House and Senate bills went to a conference committee for resolution of differences. The usual response in such cases was to split the difference unless one house could convince the other. In this case, the arithmetic mean of $18 million emerged from the House-Senate conference, passed, and became law. Because of Gramm-Rudman-Hollings rescissions, NIH had a final appropriation of $17.2 million for genome research at NIGMS that year. In private conversations, NIGMS staff estimated that $5 million of this was diverted from existing funds and the rest was "new" money.

An additional $3.85 million found its way to NIH's coffers in the 1988 to fund a National Center for Biotechnology Information. The regents of the National Library of Medicine (NLM) identified molecular biology as an important area in which the NLM's emerging expertise in electronic data basing would become increasingly important. An outside support organization, the Friends of the National Library of Medicine, took up the cause and drafted a bill for Congressman Claude Pepper to introduce. Pepper was an old friend of Fran Howard, who was a long-time NLM supporter—later an employee—as well as the sister of the late Hubert Humphrey and the widow of a prominent academic physician at Johns Hopkins. The bill was to establish an information management center to support biomedical research and biotechnology efforts in the United States, with annual budget authority rising to $10 million. Pepper held a moving hearing on the bill on March 6, 1987, but the hearing was under the auspices of his subcommittee on the Select Committee on Aging, which has no legislative authority. Pepper called members of the legislative committees, but the news did not reach staff of the Energy and Commerce Committee, which had legislative jurisdiction. (Staff for those committees learned of the hearing through OTA and NIH.) NIH, unlike many other agencies, is authorized for three-year intervals as a rule, and 1987 was not one of the years when such a bill was in Congress. There was thus no logical vehicle to which the NLM bill could be attached, and so it stood as a freestanding act. These factors delayed action on it, and eventually it was folded into the NIH authorization passed a year and a half later. However, the appropriations committee acted before then, appropriating $3.85 million for fiscal year 1988 with Pepper's full support, with the understanding that it was to be spent for the purposes specified in the languishing Pepper bill.

NIH appropriations for fiscal year 1989 were more or less routine, with NIGMS requesting $28 million for genome research in this, the final year of the Reagan administration. Congress and the President had agreed on a two-year budget plan the previous fall, in the wake of the October 1987 stock market crash, and the President's budget request held to this agreement. In fact, this was the one year under Reagan when the NIH request was taken seriously by the appropriations committees, and the requested amount was granted. There was one added feature by then, in that the NRC genome report had been made available for the appropriations hearing cycle. Representative Natcher led off his questioning of Wyngaarden by asking how the $28 million budget request from NIH fit with the $200 million recommended by the NRC committee. This gave Wyngaarden an opening to explain that there would be higher budget requests in future years.

Natcher also asked which agency should assume the leadership of the project. Wyngaarden was unequivocal and direct in his answer: "I think NIH is the appropriate agency" (U.S. Congress, House, 1988). The congressional hearing took place within weeks of the NIH ad hoc advisory committee meeting in Reston, Virginia. Wyngaarden's strong support for NIH leadership on the human genome project in Reston and now before the appropriations committee were the clear statements of purpose that had been eagerly awaited by opinion leaders in molecular biology. The NIH program began to pick up steam.

What led to Wyngaarden's assertion of leadership is instructive. He was beset by disagreement about the proper style for promoting genome research, with Kirschstein and Watson articulating incompatible options. He had to choose. To aid his decision, he scheduled the ad hoc planning meeting in Reston, and he had already met with Watson and Baltimore on December 17, 1987, to discuss AIDS research and the human genome. Watson expressed his views about how NIH had missed the boat on the genome project and was clear in his opposition to Kirschstein's approach. With the backing of an NRC report presenting a coherent approach and advocating a focused effort with a $200 million annual budget, Wyngaarden chose the high road.

NIH's appropriations for 1990 involved several complications. NIH forwarded a budget request to the Department of Health and Human Services that went on to OMB, with a final request of $62 million as the result. When the President's budget request came out, it asked for $100 million for genome research at NIH. (The $62 million apparently had been increased to $100 million by dividing up some excess monies left from the removal of other programs during OMB review [John Barry, free-lance writer, personal communication, May 1990].) The increase surprised NIH and signaled support for the NIH genome project high in OMB or elsewhere in the White House; but in the end it did not matter, as the appropriations committee staff used the initial request level from NIH as the basis for their deliberations. The final 1990 appropriation was $59.5 million after last-minute adjustments.

Now that the genome budget had become sufficiently large, Wyngaarden discussed with the appropriations committee staff the need to create a separate administrative center for the project for the 1990 fiscal year. The House agreed to allocate the 1990 budget request to a new center that the department would create by administrative fiat. The Senate, however, was looking for ways to fund new initiatives in health and human services, and, as a result, the 1990 NIH genome budget was subject to last-minute negotiations. One eleventh-hour proposal reduced the genome budget from $62 million to $50 million, with the $12 million added to funds taken from elsewhere in NIH to fund programs for the homeless. In the end, however, the Senate agreed to roughly the same budget figure as the House but left the funds in NIGMS. In conference, the report followed the House, creating a new center.

This process illustrates the twofold vulnerability of new programs at NIH. Activities that show a rapid percentage rise in funding from year to year are highlighted by the procedures used by appropriations staff to track budgets, and NIH takes up an increasingly high fraction of the discretionary funding in the Department of Health and Human Services. The department disburses more than $300 billion in funds each year, but the vast bulk goes to entitlement programs—Social Security, Medicare, and Medicaid—that are not subject to congressional appropriations or direct agency control. This makes NIH's $8 billion budget loom large as a potential source of funding "offsets" to support new initiatives for health and social services.

The budget history also illustrates the illusory dichotomy between "new" and "existing" monies. One of the most divisive debates within the biomedical research community has been miscast in these terms, with supporters of investigator-initiated small grants contending that the genome project was carved from their province, while staunch defenders of the genome project argue that the political attractiveness of the project has increased the size of the pie without in any way cutting into other efforts.

There is scant evidence for pure versions of either view. Would the $87 million 1990 genome budgets at NIH and DOE have been appropriated elsewhere for biomedical research if there had been no genome proposal? Only those who actually made the decisions for the appropriations committees could answer such a question, but they simply did not make the decisions on these terms—nor should they. The NRC report and the rhetoric supporting the genome initiative leaned heavily on the principle that the new initiative should come from "new" funds, but this kind of money did not exist. The genome budget was not given a great deal of attention in the appropriations process, and it was merely one of thousands of such decisions; in interviews with appropriations committee staff, it was clear that this was not a highly contentious part of the budget deliberations and did not generate enough controversy to leave strong memory traces.

There are hints that substantial pressures are being felt to reduce the overall NIH budget to leave more room for other health and social service spending, as in the case of the homeless funding. If this were the case, it would lend support to the contention that, without the dedicated genome line item and the new NIH administrative center, there would have been a lower overall NIH budget, and that the genome project provided a new justification for a budget increment. But the budget history makes clear that it was largely left to NIH, specifically Wyngaarden, to indicate internal NIH priorities, and the funds given to the genome project would probably have gone to NIH in any case. The argument thus is not truly about new or existing funding but about NIH priorities. Initial funding in 1988 was just under 2 percent of a budget supplement appropriated to NIH beyond the presidential request (amounting to 0.2 percent of the overall budget). Was Wyngaarden right in his decision to dedicate the funds to the genome project? The answer hinges on whether the genome project filled an unmet need. The NRC committee and leaders of the biomedical research community certainly identified a weakness in the pattern of NIH funding—a neglect of genome-scale mapping efforts, inattention to development of new technologies, and insufficient funding of data bases and shared resources.

The real question is whether addressing these needs merits just under 1 percent of the NIH budget now and up to 2 or so percent of the budget in the future. Is this field more important than the several hundred grants that could be funded for other biomedical research? The answer depends on whether one believes that society will benefit more from funding an additional 3 to 4 percent of investigator-initiated grants or from devoting attention to developing maps and technologies useful to all of molecular genetics. The debate is not about a funding *mechanism*—the funds will be dispersed by the same mechanisms used throughout NIH, although differently from tradition in basic genetics, which has been undirected research. The decision is analogous to deciding when a new territory is crowded enough to want to build roads and make rules about land and water use. The genome is largely virgin territory, but molecular biologists have begun to stake claims. When is it time to devote resources to planning and constructing projects for the common good?

Wyngaarden and Kirschstein placed the genome project on the NIH agenda, principally through the appropriations process. Kirschstein's reputation among appropriations committee staff as a solid administrator of great integrity was a necessary element. Wyngaarden first created the line item in response to a ritual question from Congress and then shepherded the budget request through its labyrinthine appropriations process. The process of securing an NIH budget was much messier and more public than securing funds for DOE, a process that required input from a dozen or so individuals but the direct approval of only a handful. The NIH process did not take much longer, but it involved input from hundreds to thousands of individuals and the direct approval of scores of them.

The DOE process was initiated by a few individuals who sensed an opportunity; the NIH process entailed a cacophonous but productive discussion that redefined the project and flagged the policy issues it would raise. Because of its conspicuousness, the NIH process was also much harder on, but more exciting for, the individuals involved. During 1987 and well into 1989, there was an article almost every month in the news pages of *Science* or *Nature*, or both. The genome project was a way for one's name to become widely known—but not always with the "spin" one might want. The extensive coverage also meant that Wyngaarden, Kirschstein, DeLisi, Watson, Gilbert, and others often learned of personal criticisms first by reading about them, an injury that always leaves scars.

SOCIAL ISSUES EMERGE

The debate about the genome project changed substantially in 1989, moving from the question of which agency should lead it to issues of international scientific cooperation, economic competition, and concern about social implications of the research. These issues had always been in the background, but with successful joint planning by NIH and DOE and little controversy about budget levels, attention turned to them. In Europe, concern about the history of eugenics delayed by a year the approval of a 15 million ECU (European currency unit, slightly over a dollar in value) genome project. In the United States, there were two congressional hearings, one by Ralph Hall's international scientific cooperation subcommittee in the House and the other by Senator Albert Gore's science subcommittee. International and ethical issues were foremost in both hearings. On October 19, Hall summarized his concern about equitable sharing of the research burden: "If you want to ride on the train, you've got to buy a ticket" (U.S. Congress, House of Representatives, 1989). Watson, testifying before him, concurred. George Cahill, representing the Human Genome Organization, acknowledged the problem but pointed to the destructive impact on science of imposing any unilateral restrictions on data flow. This issue arises from the two faces of science—at once the pursuit of pure knowledge, conforming to moral values that transcend national borders, and also an investment in the future of national economies, expected to produce technological capacities that will yield new products, new jobs, and new wealth. As the rate of growth of the U.S. national economy lagged far behind that of Japan in the late 1970s and through the 1980s, and as Japan captured selected high-technology markets once the sole province of U.S. corporations, members of Congress became concerned that Japan was commercially exploiting the basic research results paid for by U.S. taxpayers. Economic competitiveness became the buzzword of the day; although there were few concrete policy options to address the concern, it would clearly persist as an issue for the genome project for years to come.

The Gore hearing, held November 9, 1989, touched on international data sharing but concentrated even more on the social implications of the project (U.S. Congress, Senate, 1989). These were not entirely new, having been raised by other work in human genetics, but the highly public debate about the genome project brought these issues to the fore. The project would clearly result in much greater knowledge about human genes and would produce technologies to make genetic tests faster, cheaper, and more accurate, as well as applicable to many more diseases. The issues of genetic discrimination in employment or insurance, and the prospects of backdoor racism through genetic screening and testing, were thus more urgent because of the genome project. Indeed, just as the genome project was being formulated, a run of books began on issues related to genetic screening, genetic testing and counseling, and related issues (Holtzman, 1989; Nelkin and Tancredi, 1989; Rothstein, 1989; U.S. Congress, OTA, 1988b). These issues bespoke a renewed public concern about how genetic tests would be used.

Watson saw the need to confront these issues early in the project and stated at the press conference announcing his appointment as associate director of NIH, head of a new Office of Human Genome Research, in October 1988, that he thought the NIH genome program should spend some money to discuss the ethical implications of the work. He elaborated these ideas further at a speech at UCLA in December 1988. Watson foresaw the importance of educating the public through courses, books, and public meetings, and of devising new means to think through the consequences of genome research and anticipate public policy needs. His argument was that, although the genome project was "completely correct" in pursuing gene maps and DNA sequence data as fast as possible, it was essential to be completely candid about how such information could be abused and to suggest laws to prevent such abuse, because, as he said "we certainly don't want to mislead Congress" (Watson, 1988).

As one of the next speakers, I first had to recover from my surprise. This was not the Watson I expected from reading *The Double Helix*.

Watson's commitment to the consideration of the ethical implications of the project was clarified at several subsequent meetings, and the NIH advisory committee agreed to devote 3 percent of the NIH genome budget to fund the activities of a working group chaired by Nancy Wexler of Columbia University's College of Physicians and Surgeons, and to support a research program.

This commitment was noted in Watson's opening statement before Senator Gore, and Gore commented on it favorably in his opening remarks and again after Watson spoke. Robert Wood, acting director of DOE's Office of Health and Environmental Research, spoke after Watson. As Wood was reading his prepared statement into the microphone, Gore turned to his staff and me, seated behind him, and asked if DOE had made a similar commitment of funds to study the ethical and social implications of the genome project. We were not sure but could not remember seeing any budget commitment in the prepared statement. Gore interrupted Wood to ask. Wood began a reply to the effect that he believed that the NIH effort would address the necessary issues and that DOE was quite concerned about them. Gore responded by asking specifically whether DOE had made a commitment similar to NIH's. Wood said no, and Gore stepped up to the plate. He suggested quite strongly that they do so and noted that there would be future hearings on the genome project at which this issue would come up. Gore's position was reiterated by Senator John Kerry. It was as clear a congressional signal as can be made (U.S. Congress, Senate, 1989).

Gore's interest in the implications of human genetics dated from the early 1980s, when he held a series of hearings on human gene therapy, in vitro fertilization, and biotechnology. In talks with constituents he had found that genetics was especially worrisome to the general public, and he shared some concerns. It was not an antiscience bias but rather an inchoate discomfiture with the prospects of meddling in something as fundamental as a person's genes. Gore had introduced legislation in 1983 that eventually led to the ill-fated Biomedical Ethics Advisory Committee (which quietly died in September 1989 without issuing a report), and his interests in the topic had continued unabated.

Gore was not alone among senators in these concerns. Edwin Froelich was a physician and staff person for Senator Orrin Hatch, ranking Republican on the Senate committee that authorizes NIH activities. Froelich called DeLisi to his office late in 1986, soon after he learned of the DOE plans for a genome project. He expressed grave concern about the project and urged that the research be scrutinized for its broader impact, particularly whether it would lead to more prenatal diagnosis and abortion. He likewise called Ruth Kirschstein when he heard of the NIH plans in 1987. Kirschstein and W. French Anderson then met with him to reassure him that NIH was, indeed, concerned about these matters. (Froelich wanted some assurance that there would be explicit attention to such matters, or the program would be in jeopardy.) In several meetings late in 1988, Barbara Mikulski, the brusque senator from Maryland, also expressed concern to me and others about "go-go" science that potentially might race far in advance of the policies developed to contain its adverse impacts on individuals and society. More pointedly, Congressman David Obey raised serious questions about how insurers and employers might use genetic information to discriminate unfairly against certain individuals. He urged strongly in the House appropriations hearings for the 1991 budget (held early in 1990) that NIH come up with a systematic plan to deal with such issues.

Human genetics was of special concern for several reasons. First, it appeared threatening because it studies the very stuff of life—not directly who we are but the "recipe book" that makes each of us possible. Second, human genetics offered technological options that were not available before. Before genetic testing was developed, individuals at risk for Huntington's disease or anxious about whether they were carriers of sickle cell or Tay-Sachs disease did not have to worry about such tests. Technology brought choice, sometimes agonizing choice. This situation was not different in principle from other medical advances, but it seemed to hit especially hard in the case of genetic disease, which is caused by factors utterly beyond the control of the person carrying the genes. Finally, genetics had been used as a tool for political abuse in the past.

Human genetics research labored in the shadow of eugenics and racial hygiene. A new spate of scholarship detailed the role of scientists and physicians in promoting the racist agenda of those movements in the first half of this century (Kevles, 1985; Lifton, 1986; Muller-Hill, 1988; Proctor, 1988; Reilly, 1977). The medical model of nondirective genetic counseling explicitly rejected the tenets of eugenics and racial hygiene, but the magnitude of the abuses left a strong legacy of distrust. Nonscientists were not about to give this trust automatically; scientists would have to earn it.

Several observers, both scientists and nonscientists, predicted that the research program and other activities to investigate the ethical, legal, and social implications of human genetics would be an important legacy of the genome project, perhaps even its most substantial one. Concomitantly with the National Center for Nursing Research at NIH, the National Center for Human Genome Research did, indeed, become a pioneer in offering NIH support for such work. Although bioethics had been supported intermittently by NIH in the past, it had not had the support of any ongoing program and lacked a dedicated budget.

The commitment to fund such work was a dramatic departure from past practices, an innovation in NIH policy that was likely to have deep and long-lasting impacts on NIH well beyond the genome center.

STILL, ORGANIZATIONAL ISSUES

The organization of the genome project remained in flux. Under threat of legislation, NIH and DOE signed a memorandum of understanding in fall 1988, choosing a joint agreement rather than a structure imposed by the Chiles-Kennedy-Domenici bill. The agreement ratified an existing informal arrangement but grew into substantially more, as bona fide cooperation began to seem advantageous to both agencies. Throughout 1989, staff from NIH and DOE met to discuss how to carry out the terms of the memorandum. They finally settled on a joint NIH-DOE advisory group, composed of members of the advisory panels for each agency's outside advisory group.

Watson was insistent on having a "serious" planning document. Rand Snell and Michael Hall, of Senator Chile's staff, inserted language into the 1989 appropriations conference report, a document that accompanied the bill to explain congressional intent, expressing concern about interagency coordination and stipulating that NIH and DOE develop "the optimal strategy for mapping and sequencing the human genome" in time for the 1991 budget cycle (U.S. Congress, Senate, 1988). The research was given a big boost at a joint NIH-DOE planning retreat held at the Banbury Center, Cold Spring Harbor Laboratory, in late August 1989.

For many months, there had been an informal coordinating committee: Diane Hinton of HHMI, Mark Guyer of the genome office, Irene Eckstrand of NIGMS, John Wooley of NSF, and Ben Barnhart of DOE. Others attended occasionally. The loosely coordinated plans formed by that group began to gel when combined in a retreat setting with the powerhouses of genome research at Banbury. The advisory committees for both DOE and NIH were present, as well as invited experts from other laboratories engaged in genome research.

Going into the meeting, NIH and DOE staff were expecting to prepare a five-year plan. DOE's Barnhart and Norton Zinder, of Rockefeller University, thought that no specific planning draft would emerge from the retreat (Palca, 1989), but they proved themselves wrong. Zinder organized the discussion into task areas, and a format of specifying goals and the means of achieving them developed naturally out of this discussion. Much of the meeting focused on how to construct physical maps, sets of ordered, overlapping cloned DNA fragments. Maynard Olson and others mentioned the idea of using short stretches of DNA sequence as unique "tags" that would serve as landmarks on the chromosomes that could be used by laboratories using different methods. The suggestion was seized upon quickly, and a group agreed to author a paper for *Science* (Olson et al., 1989; Roberts, 1989). Thus, the shape of the plan that the staff had hoped to develop became considerably clearer after the retreat; NIH and DOE staff agreed that the report on the five-year plan should follow the goal-oriented format (NIH/DOE, 1990).

The human genome project began to come of age in late 1989 and 1990. Secretary of Health and Human Services Louis Sullivan created the National Center for Human Genome Research in October 1989, giving the project administrative authority to spend federal funds, pending approval of an advisory council. Much staff time went into organizing chromosome-specific meetings, workshops on cloning large DNA inserts, DNA sequencing, informatics, and other topics. Upper management, particularly Elke Jordan and Mark Guyer at NIH and Ben Barnhart at DOE, focused heavily on preparing a joint five-year plan to present to Congress. The two oversight hearings in October and November 1989 gave way to appropriations hearings in both houses of Congress in spring 1990. The process for reviewing grants began to become more routine for the genome proposals, although there continued to be disagreement about the specific goals and scope of the project among grant reviewers. Steps were taken to establish standing review panels for genome grants in mid-1990, and the advisory council charter was approved. Watson declared that, because the first few years had been dedicated to getting organized, the genome project should officially begin with fiscal year 1991. And so it began.

CONCLUSIONS

The history of the genome project makes it clear that scientists played a crucial role in starting it, and they were the sources to which policymakers turned for advice along the way. The NRC was particularly influential, but there were many independent mechanisms as well. Hundreds of scientists attended the meetings that hatched the genome scheme. Scientists were also called upon as independent witnesses in hearings in addition to NRC and OTA staff. There were no disease constituencies who rose to champion the project, in contrast to cancer, heart disease, Alzheimer's disease, or AIDS. There was strong support from the Alliance for Aging Research and a few other groups in 1989; these sources did not constitute a wellspring of public sentiment but rather the support of organization members in leadership positions. Indeed, aside from scattered press reports, the public remained largely ignorant of the project even after it had been under way for three years.

Public policy on the genome project was formed in the cruel daylight of productive conflict, and key actors in federal agencies responsible for conducting research did most of the political spadework. It is impossible to judge now whether the genome project would have happened without DeLisi's efforts, but it certainly would not have happened as fast. Probably, there would have been considerable discussion about sequencing, about data bases, about genetic linkage maps, about physical mapping, and about computational biology, but these "abouts" could conceivably have remained segregated in their scientific communities of origin. The human genome project need not have emerged so quickly from the collision of human genetics and molecular biology, and it need not have been projected as a major new initiative meriting serious high-level political attention. Large-scale mapping and sequencing efforts might well have emerged piecemeal and been resolved incrementally, but the proposals would have met substantial resistance within the scientific disciplines. The genome project provided a vehicle for biological projects on a larger scale with a greater focus on technological improvement per se.

The science agencies did not have to discover the human genome project as a way to package the road-building work of human genetics. Indeed, given the bureaucratic tendencies toward caution and narrow definitions of mission, they might well have resisted any new initiative but for the prodigious efforts of a few champions. DeLisi put the genome project on the public agenda. Once it was there, it provoked competition between DOE and NIH and forced the issue to the surface of science policy. Wyngaarden rose to the challenge, and Congress then had to make several decisions about budgets and agency leadership. Watson channeled his prodigious energies into the project, and gave it scientific credences it desperately needed.

Without strong impetus from DOE, NIH almost certainly would not have reacted as strongly, as quickly, or as systematically as it did. Without these agencies vying for leadership, neither might have fought quite so hard to assess its options, secure its budget, or influence the opinions of the scientific community. The extraordinary number of meetings on the genome project testify to the fact that, once the idea of the project was aired, it was immediately perceived as exciting and important. Norton Zinder noted the consistency with which the genome project was first greeted with skepticism and then accepted as inevitable (N. L. Zinder, Rockefeller University, personal communication, March 1990). Sinsheimer, Dulbecco, and DeLisi were the first to sense the importance of a new push for human genetics. But in science policy as in science, being first matters more than being absolutely right.

A few pivotal scientific figures—the scientists who took the trouble to learn about the policy process and to interact with it—clearly had enormous influence. Watson was preeminent among these, but Hood, Gilbert, Bodmer, Baltimore, Berg, Dulbecco, Alberts, Cantor, Olson, and others had major effects at critical junctures. Many scientists from the national laboratories played decisive voices in steering DOE policies. Still, not every contribution was totally positive. Some scientific input was naive and some almost destructive. Scientists were rather poor at making the policy issues clear and were often quick to form opinions without fully informing themselves of the political consequences. The NRC recommendation of a lead agency was one such mistake.

Sometimes there were remarks that fanned the flames without focusing the heat. Robert Weinberg, for example, was quoted in *New Scientist* as saying, "I'm surprised consenting adults have been caught in public talking about it . . . it makes no sense" (Joyce, 1987). This may well have been the case of a wayward pronoun, a loose "it" floating freely in that dangerous space between a reporter and his source. The context of this remark made it unclear whether Weinberg referred to the entire project or to the prospect of sequencing it alone. He later recalled referring to the latter (personal communication, December 12, 1990) and disavowed opposition to a concerted mapping effort, but at the time, the remark was cited by staff on Capitol Hill as opposition to the project as a whole. Even apart from losing whatever nuances surrounded the original arguments, politicians are well able to filter such isolated judgments. Politics is, after all, waged as a war of words, and politicians are accustomed to the rhetorical excesses of interest groups anxious to support a position.

Most of the policy statements made by scientists had little impact because those in Congress who were making decisions were insulated from them. Most members of Congress had a few regular sources of scientific information on which they relied, and they also listened to committee staff, the NRC, and OTA. Scientists, for their part, talked mainly to one another. Few took the time to visit with policymakers or to write for an audience outside science journals and science news publications. There was remarkably little effort to build a broad public constituency, a strategy that would instinctively have appeared important to an elected official. When reporters came, many scientists were eager to be quoted, but there were remarkably few attempts to articulate a broader vision of why the general public should support a genome project at taxpayer expense. Most of the debate was a narrow one regarding the unanswerable question of whose ox would be gored if the monies for the genome project were not actually "new."

Gilbert, Watson, Hood, Cantor, and a few others were unusual in the degree to which they took public communication seriously. Ironically, this sensitivity cost them support within the scientific community, which saw these efforts as grandstanding. The issue recurs time and again in connection with public support of science, falling in the gray border zone between selling to and educating the public. Every politician knows that one needs support to get things done, and deliberately maintaining a high profile is a necessary component of policy formation in the world of modern media. DOE recognized this early on and sponsored a science writers' workshop at Brookhaven National Laboratories, which led to several articles. The Alliance for Aging Research, the American Medical Association, and DuPont sponsored a national conference with general media coverage in mind. A cover feature appeared in *Time* magazine a few weeks before the conference (Elmer-DeWitt et al., 1989; Jaroff et al., 1989), and there was a wave of articles afterward. The many national scientific meetings also generated press coverage. These activities, however, were hardly broad public education, relying as they did on snapshots of scientific opinion. There was no systematic assessment of what the public was worried about until the project was well along—it clearly *was* worried—and little attempt to identify issues of which the public was as yet unaware. The task of public education was largely left for the future.

Now, the future of the genome project depends on several factors: (1) whether it produces scientifically useful data, in particular, whether the systematic approach is quickly shown to be useful as a way to understand major diseases and illuminate fundamental biological questions; (2) whether it broadens its base of support among scientists and in the general public; and (3) whether it successfully confronts the broader social implications that emerge as human genetics advances.

APPENDIX A

Where Was OSTP?

The job of the White House's Office of Science and Technology Policy (OSTP) is to help make science policy. Its director is the President's science advisor. OSTP's purpose and position make it the logical place to resolve disputes such as those that arose between NIH and DOE during 1987 and 1988. Why, then, was it ineffective? The question cannot be answered completely, but a few observations are relevant. First, OSTP is severely limited by staff constraints. For most of the period in question, there were only two life scientists in OSTP, left to attend to AIDS, environmental issues, international science agreements, and the ceremonial and diplomatic duties inherent in any White House office. It was quite easy for urgent issues to displace those that were merely important when there were so few staff covering broad expanses of federal policy.

Second, OSTP was not trusted by the agencies or OMB. If OSTP had been better staffed it might have been effective. But life sciences were given short shrift at an agency regarded as marginally effective even in its area of greatest expertise—military research. OSTP eventually began to hold monthly meetings about the genome project that included representatives from the Department of Agriculture, NIH, DOE, NSF, and HHMI, but the agency staff attending them, without exception, found them to be nonproductive.

OSTP has enormous power to convene high-level meetings, but for such meetings to succeed, either OSTP staff must have the power to enforce decisions—giving agencies a strong incentive to prepare their positions carefully—or they must know the issues and agencies' interests well and have the agencies' respect and an expectation of fair judgment. Because OSTP was irrelevant to the budget process, interagency science policy decisions were made elsewhere, that is, by OMB and Congress.

OSTP did have some effect in one area regarding the genome project: it nearly ruined an opportunity to create a platform for U.S.-Japanese cooperation on the program. OSTP was given principal responsibility for negotiating a U.S.-Japan science and technology agreement and participated in discussions about life sciences in Tokyo in April 1989. The United States came to the table with five proposals, most of them involving forestry and fermentation, areas of Japanese strength. Japan came with nine areas, two of which were related to genetics and another that was specifically focused on the human genome project. The OSTP representative dismissed the Japanese genome proposals as not showing promise for U.S.-Japan collaboration under the agreement because the United States was seen as so far ahead in these areas. This perception was true, in fact, but an opportunity was missed to leverage the Japanese government into much greater support for genome research, which might have avoided at least some of the controversy that later ensued over data sharing by U.S. and Japanese genome investigators.

The Japanese Ministry of Education (Monbusho, which supported most university-based research) had just received a report supporting a major commitment to genome research. Japan's Science and Technology Agency had translated into English another report that reached more or less the same conclusion. Apparently, Monbusho and the Science and Technology Agency were counting on U.S. support to approach their own Ministry of Finance to ask for substantial budget increases, but the OSTP statement in April scuttled this strategy. The cabinet-level Japanese science council issued a report supporting genome research in May, but the damage was done. Monbusho and the Science and

Technology Agency succeeded in each gaining two-year programs, but funding for them fell considerably short of their aspirations. It set them back until well into 1990.

In June 1989 a controversy with the United States over the level of research support in Japan began to heat up at an international genome meeting in Moscow and erupted publicly in October. The controversy had the effect of focusing renewed attention on the genome project in Japan, and scientists there became optimistic that more support might be forthcoming. As this volume goes to press, U.S. negotiations with Japan about the genome project are pending.

APPENDIX B

Can the Genome Project Keep Its Promises?

The genome project was "sold" on four main points: (1) it would create tools to combat human disease by expediting the process of biomedical research; (2) it would stimulate domestic economic development by keeping the United States in the lead in biotechnology; (3) it would enhance national prestige; and (4) it would stand as a cultural achievement to be hailed for centuries. Of these, the promise to promote understanding of health and disease seems secure. Because the main products of the genome project will be information (maps and sequence data) and methods of broad applicability (cloning, detecting, sequencing, and analyzing DNA), the genome project will certainly help elucidate the mechanisms of disease, and even when elucidation does not lead to cure, it may suggest means of prevention or amelioration.

Sickle cell anemia is a case in point. It has often been cited as an example of how molecular knowledge can fail to have clinical impact, but persuasive arguments can also be made for exactly the opposite position. Knowledge of a molecular defect in hemoglobin in this condition has been available since 1949, but this has not led to a cure. Morbidity and mortality rates for sickle cell anemia, however, are severalfold lower than four decades ago. Has molecular knowledge made a difference? Knowing which gene is involved has not led to direct gene therapy—at least not yet—but knowing the mechanism of disease *has* directed the development of new treatment strategies that have improved management of the disease by small increments over the years, and has provided a means for monitoring the effects of various treatments.

Noting that genome research will help in the study of disease does not answer the question about the optimal balance between the collective, concerted effort to map and sequence the genome and more decentralized, undirected research, or that done in pursuit of particular diseases. It does mean that the money spent on the genome will not be wasted. If in 10 years researchers and policymakers generally agree that the money was spent wisely, then this efficiency criterion will also have been met. The continuing debate about whether the genome project is displacing better science hinges on three points, none of which is susceptible to rigorous analysis: (1) whether the genome project displaced other biomedical research, that is, whether the increase in NIH funding associated with the genome project would have gone to NIH in any event; (2) if such displacement occurred, whether the displaced science was of equal or greater merit (a notoriously difficult issue to judge); and (3) whether biomedical research was the best use of funds that might otherwise have been used to house the homeless or provide other social services (an equally impossible question).

The other three promises are more difficult to assess. The relationship of the genome project to biotechnology is murky and confused. Genome research will clearly push the limits of DNA-based methods, and these advances will have broad applicability, not only in research but also in medical diagnosis and treatment, agriculture, pharmaceutical development, and other industrial sectors. Even more important, those who learn genome research will be at the cutting edge of techniques, and this training is the most effective means of technology transfer.

If economic development were the principal goal of policy, however, rather than acceleration of biomedical research, would the genome project be the most direct route? The genome project is more likely than most other research to have industrial spinoffs, but direct funding of instrumentation, methods development, fermentation technologies, protein engineering, structural chemistry, and other targets is arguably at least as important because it would be focused on choke points of industrial development, as opposed to pure research. Industrial development of new technologies is widely acknowledged as the weakest point of U.S. technology policy, while basic science is its greatest strength (U.S. Congress, OTA, 1984). The genome project is one step in the direction of technological development because three- to fivefold increases in speed, scale, or cost reduction are explicit goals of its technology development component. Nevertheless, technologies more directly related to commercial application might be even more efficient in improving economic returns on public biotechnology investments. Several other countries are pursuing such commercially targeted policies; thus, time will tell whether the U.S. genome project was, as some scientists asserted, the best way to retain biotechnological supremacy.

The arguments regarding national prestige and cultural endowment are undecidable. If the United States has the largest program and the program is judged successful, then it will add to our national prestige. So do Olympic gold medals, but the U.S. government does not fund the efforts leading to them. Further, arguing that a science program adds to prestige would have to satisfy the condition that it does so more quickly, surely, and cheaply than alternatives to the same end. This condition seems a heavy burden for long-term scientific or technical projects to carry. Such an argument may have worked for the Apollo project in the 1960s, when the U.S. economy was overwhelmingly the healthiest on the planet, but it is unlikely to carry the day in the 1990s. National prestige is a tenuous basis on which to form any policy, and it is especially risky as a foundation for science and technology funding.

If the genome project is as successful, and has as few adverse social side effects, as the optimists predict, it will undoubtedly be hailed as a major cultural advance. If the project fails technically, or if the information derived from it and the methods developed as part of it are transformed into tools for genetic discrimination or racism, then it will be judged a disaster. The degree to which scientists and health professionals take responsibility for seeing that the fruits of their labor are used to promote freedom, rather than circumscribe it, will be critical to the ultimate judgment about the benefits of the human genome project. Enthusiastic pronouncements, such as those voiced by Norman Anderson in Santa Fe, fill the pages of history books—sometimes as examples of prescient insight and other times as examples of egregious folly. History's verdict on such predictions is harsh and depends entirely on whether they are right.

APPENDIX C

Is Cost Wobble a Serious Problem?

There were many attempts to formulate budgets for the human genome project. The earliest were performed in conjunction with the Santa Cruz meeting, at the first Santa Fe meeting, and at meetings held thereafter. There were many different strategic approaches with diverse component parts that yielded wildly different projections. The early estimates are chronicled in Appendix B of the OTA report (U.S. Congress, OTA, 1988a). The generation of cost figures played a pivotal role in forcing consideration of the technical options. Cost figures also became a focus of policymaking, as those funding the project wanted to know how much they would be expected to spend. Scientists who were engaged in the genome debate quickly became aware of this expectation, and the cost projections of the three advisory committees were remarkably similar. The reasons for this concurrence are instructive.

Since DOE was the first federal program to start, it was also the first to begin discussion of budget projections. This took place at two levels, within the DOE bureaucracy and among scientists promoting the genome project from the outside. Charles DeLisi's internal process is noted in the text. The external process began at the first Santa Fe conference in March 1986, where the budget numbers were extremely diverse and generally focused only on one or two components. By the second Santa Fe conference in January 1987, planning had become more serious. Several of the invited participants met over lunch at that conference to discuss what the budget should be. David Padwa, who had previously been involved with founding the agricultural biotechnology company Agrigenetics, noted the political constraints on the budget. It had to be large enough to command congressional attention, so it would have to be at least $50 million to $100 million per year, but it could not be so large that it threatened other research interests.

The budget discussions continued a month later, at a meeting of the scientific advisory committee assembled to render advice on DOE's genome project. The DOE HERAC subcommittee met to discuss costs on February 5 and 6, 1987, a month before its report was to be considered by the full committee. The subcommittee met for an afternoon session, during which there was some discussion of costs, but generating cost estimates had been delegated to Lee Hood, who was not scheduled to appear until the next morning. The meeting started at 9 a.m. on the 6th, but Hood's plane had been delayed, so the group began to discuss what could be done within the range of budgets it was thought reasonable for the Office of Health and Environmental Research to request. There was some discussion of how much physical mapping and sequencing could be done with $20 million to $40 million, the maximum the subcommittee considered politically feasible. Hood entered the meeting at 10 a.m., armed with some handwritten notes that included a menu of necessary technologies and attached costs. The proposal included technology development, physical mapping of the human genome, mapping and sequencing of model organisms (yeast and bacteria), and regional sequencing of interesting chromosomal regions (e.g., those packed with genes). Hood's estimates were $200 to $300 million per year for a full program. A shocked silence settled over the room. Someone asked if that was at all possible, being a full order of magnitude higher than what had been discussed before. Hood did not wait for or provide an answer but instead asked passionately whether the budget would drive the vision or the vision drive the budget. Swept away, the group niggled over technical details of how to make the projections and settled on a figure of $200 million, thus exceeding Padwa's threshold. Those present at the Santa Fe discussion, including Charles Cantor, then endorsed the importance of having the budget reflect what was needed to begin a realistic scientific program, and not to let perceived budget ceilings force the group into making promises they could not keep.

The NRC committee process for setting a budget was somewhat different. A subgroup was tasked to produce cost options. Botstein spearheaded this effort and came up with three options that would enable various amounts of genetic linkage mapping, physical mapping, sequencing, and other activities. He suggested annual budgets of $50 million, $100 million, and $200 million, with completion dates sooner for the higher figures (the year 2000 for $200 million versus 2025 for $50 million). The estimates were based in part on previous technical presentations on mapping and sequencing methods but mainly on how many people in how many laboratories could be funded at the different budget levels. Watson objected to the range of options, noting that it would naturally incline the committee members to seem reasonable by choosing the middle option. He therefore suggested a $500 million-per-year crash program as a fourth option. (Because Botstein had already deemed his top option the crash program, Watson's was variously dubbed the crash-crash or crash-boom.)

Comments began on Botstein's right and went counterclockwise around the table. One by one, the members supported some special effort, although there was no convergence on any one figure until a second go round the table. Then, there seemed to be a general acceptance of something near the $200 million figure, with Botstein responsible for reviewing the figures again after the discussion. The committee ultimately projected a need for $200 million a year for 15 years: $60 million for 10 centers, $60 million for grants and technology development, $55 million per year in early years for construction and capital costs, and $25 million per year for administration, a stock center, a data management center, quality control, and peer review (NRC, 1988).

The OTA budget projections were based on a two-stage process. A workshop was convened in August 1987, chaired by Paul Berg. The participants included representatives from the major funding agencies and scientific groups engaged in mapping and sequencing, as well as others familiar with quality control, data bases, and costs of materials distribution and handling. After some discussion, the panel agreed on cost figures for genetic linkage mapping and physical mapping. When the discussion turned to sequencing, however, it became contentious, lapsing into several disagreements about what strategy should be followed, how much reagents would cost, and how much automation could save. Subsequent estimates of the costs of storing DNA clones were shockingly high, and the last hour of the meeting was dominated by debate about how the project should be managed and which agency should lead it.

Beyond genetic linkage and physical mapping estimates, the exercise failed to produce a cost table. The process did force the alternative strategies to the surface, however, and these were sent along with alternative cost estimates to all the participants and an additional 30 or 40 people with technical or science administrative background. This procedure yielded estimates in a much narrower range, which were summarized in an appendix to the OTA report. One clear decision was made at OTA: attempting to project more than a five-year budget was impossible because of technical uncertainties, and even estimates beyond two years were highly suspect. OTA estimated costs beginning at $47 million the first year and increasing to $228 million over five years.

How did all the estimates fall into such a narrow range? There are two explanations. First, there was really only one way to project costs—to estimate how many people could be productively engaged in the various component tasks. With genetic linkage mapping, the wobble came from disagreement about how high the resolution needed to be. The costs per marker were fairly certain because there were several years of experience in finding markers and mapping them. In the case of physical mapping, there was some experience with nematodes and yeast and a sense that new methods to clone larger fragments would reduce costs. For the other components, the wobble overwhelmed the axis of rotation. At bottom, all of these estimates were highly subjective intuitions of what would be needed.

The question of estimates based on intuition raises the second factor ensuring some convergence. The group of people making these estimates was fairly small, and they talked to one another frequently, if nowhere else than at that week's genome meeting. Hood, for example, was on all three advisory committees, for DOE, NRC, and OTA.

A policy problem is thus apparent in placing the authority to make budget projections, clearly one of the most important considerations in genome project planning, in the hands of such a limited number of people. Yet there are few alternatives when dealing with cutting-edge technologies. The group of people consulted was small because the number of experts who ran relevant programs was small, and there was no way to avoid this problem. Further, the process was not as narrow as it might seem from the discussion above: at least the OTA cost workshop was well attended (by more than 100 observers, in addition to the participants) and covered prominently by science journals (including a feature piece in *Science* [Roberts, 1987]), which elicited unsolicited comments from many quarters. Nevertheless, the fact remains that the basic cost estimates came from the handful of scientists who had direct experience with the technologies.

APPENDIX D

What Is "Technically Feasible" in the Policy Context?

When discussions about the genome project began in 1985, scientists claimed that only recently had it become technically feasible to sequence the entire human genome. It is not clear what was meant by this statement, but this and similar language cropped up in dozens of letters, articles, meetings, and private discussions. It is not technically feasible to sequence the human genome in 1990, despite a half decade of impressive gains in power, speed, and simplicity of component steps (e.g., cloning larger DNA fragments, ordering clone libraries, DNA sequencing, and analyzing map and sequence data). Many scientists might more accurately have said that the sort of problems posed by the project were of a kind that seemed likely to be solved without conceptual breakthroughs or revolutionary technological innovations. Carefully qualified statements, however, fit poorly into media sound bites and can be as inimical to communication with policymakers as deliberate obfuscation.

This type of communication is a problem endemic to any scientific enterprise requiring long-term federal support. It is an artifact of the time-scale mismatch between policy formulation and scientific or technical achievement, and the communication style mismatch between science and science policy. The medium of science is written, usually in the passive voice, carefully qualified, and driven by data. Communication about policy is verbal, oriented toward action, and driven by issues. Arguments must be made in favor of a scientific agenda many years before that agenda can be met, in order to ensure that the budget and infrastructure are in place so work can go forward if the intervening technical obstacles are overcome. Visionary scientists leap over considerable technical obstacles because they assume obstacles can be overcome; the money has to be ready and waiting when the science arrives. This process is related to the issue of promise keeping noted above, except that it is focused on how the technical objectives of a project can be met, rather than on whether those objectives relate to a larger mission such as promoting health, combating disease, or generating wealth through biotechnology.

Science has a healthy skepticism about glib pronouncements of what will be possible—but then so do politicians. Skepticism about claims is a natural reflex, without which no politician can long remain in office. Contending with interest groups is the very stuff of political life, but in crafting science policy, scientists have conflicting roles as objective observers and stakeholders.

The predictions made in 1987 that there would be a complete physical map of the human genome in a "few years" and that DNA sequencing would cost "only a few pennies a base" were clearly wrong. On the other hand, some parts of the X chromosome spanning more than 2 million base pairs are contained in ordered clone libraries; more than 10 million base pairs of the nematode genome have been contiguously mapped by overlapping clones. And although the longest continuous sequence to date is still only 200,000 base pairs, the *hprt* gene region on chromosome X has been sequenced, and large expanses of chromosome 4 and the T-cell receptor region are now being sequenced—projects unthinkable even in 1987.

There are no easy answers here. It does not seem that Congress has been seriously misled about the technical feasibility of mapping the genome. The current five-year plan stipulates specific goals and presents these openly to Congress, a remarkably forthright strategy. By producing this document, NIH and DOE have provided Congress and OMB with the tools by which to measure their progress in future years. Success or failure of the effort will thus be much easier to assess. It is a bold strategy: if a technical obstacle suddenly appears, support for the entire enterprise might evaporate, although this is unlikely. In the worst-case scenario technically (leaving aside for the moment the possible social abuses of genetic information), there will be a great deal of useful sequence data even if only 5 percent or so of the genome is sequenced, because investigators will attack the most clearly interesting regions first. Genetic and physical maps will be useful no matter how incomplete, but the value of the genome project depends on their completeness. The current NIH-DOE joint planning strategy is critically dependent on setting the right goals, requiring a stretch but not a break, and marshaling the resources necessary to meet them.

REFERENCES

Alberts, B. M. 1985. Limits to growth: In biology, small science is good science. Cell 41:337-338.

Anderson, N. G., and N. L. Anderson. 1985. A policy and program for biotechnology. American Biotechnology Laboratory September/October:1-3.

Avery, O. T., C. M. MacLeod, and M. McCarty. 1944. Induction of transformation by a deoxyribonucleic acid fraction isolated from Pneumococcus Type III. Journal of Experimental Medicine 79:137-158.

Baltimore, D. 1987. Genome sequencing: A small-scale approach. Issues in Science and Technology 3:48-50.

Beam, A., and J. O'C. Hamilton. 1987. A grand plan to map the gene code. Business Week April 27:116-117.

Begley, S., with S. E. Katz and L. Drew. 1987. The genome initiative. Newsweek August 31:58-60.

Bitensky, M. 1986. Sequencing the Human Genome. Santa Fe, N.M.: Office of Health and Environmental Research, U.S. Department of Energy (published by the University of California under contract W 7405-ENG-36, Los Alamos National Laboratory, N.M.).

Bodmer, W. F. 1986a. Human genetics: The molecular challenge. Pp. 1-3 in Molecular Biology of Homo sapiens. Cold Spring Harbor Symposia on Quantitative Biology, Vol. 51. Cold Spring Harbor, N.Y.: Cold Spring Harbor Laboratory.

Bodmer, W. F. 1986b. Two cheers for genome sequencing. The Scientist October 20:11-12.

Botstein, D. 1980. Construction of a genetic linkage map in man using restriction fragment length polymorphisms. American Journal of Human Genetics 32:314-331.

Cook-Deegan, R. M. 1989. The Alta summit, December 1984. Genomics 5:661-663.

Coulson, A., J. Sulston, S. Brenner, et al. 1986. Toward a physical map of the genome of the nematode *Caenorhabditis elegans*. Proceedings of the National Academy of Sciences (USA) 83:7821-7825.

del Guercio, G. 1987. Designer genes. Boston Magazine August:79-87.

DeLisi, C. 1988. The human genome project. American Scientist 76:488-493.

Donis-Keller, H., P. Green, C. Helms, S. Cartinhour, B. Weiffenbach, K. Stephens, T. P. Keith, D. W. Bowden, D. R. Smith, E. S. Lander, et al. 1987. A genetic linkage map of the human genome. Cell 51:319-337.

Dulbecco, R. 1986. A turning point in cancer research: Sequencing the human genome. Science 231:1055-1056.

Elmer-DeWitt, P., with A. Dorfman and J. M. Nash. 1989. The perils of treading on heredity. Time March 20:70-71.

Friend, S. H., R. Bernards, S. Rogelj, R. A. Weinberg, J. M. Rapaport, D. M. Albert, and T. P. Dryja. 1986. A human DNA segment with properties of the gene that predisposes to retinoblastoma and osteosarcoma. Nature 323:643-646.

Gilbert, W. 1986. Two cheers for human gene sequencing. The Scientist October 20:11.

Gilbert, W. 1987. Genome sequencing: Creating a new biology for the twenty-first century. Issues in Science and Technology 3:26-35.

Gusella, J. F., N. S. Wexler, P. M. Conneally, S. L. Naylor, M. A. Anderson, R. E. Tanzi, P. C. Watkind, K. Ottina, M. R. Wallace, A. Y. Sakaguchi, A. M. Young, I. Shoulson, E. Bonilla, and J. B. Martin. 1983. A polymorphic DNA marker genetically linked to Huntington's disease. Nature 306:234-238.

Hall, S. S. 1988. Genesis: The sequel. California (July):62-69.

Holtzman, N. A. 1989. Proceed with Caution. Baltimore, Md.: Johns Hopkins University Press.

Holzman, D. 1987. Mapping the genes, inside and out. Insight May 11:52-54.

Hood, L., and L. Smith. 1987. Genome sequencing: How to proceed. Issues in Science and Technology 3:36-46.

Ingram, V. M. 1957. Gene mutation in human haemoglobin: The chemical difference between normal and sickle cell haemoglobin. Nature 180:326-328.

Jaroff, L., with J. M. Nash and D. Thompson. 1989. The gene hunt. Time March 20:62-67.

Jenks, S. 1989. Gene map budget given a boost. Medical World News February 13:94.

Joyce, C. 1987. The race to map the human genome. New Scientist March 5:35-40.

Judson, H. F. 1979. The Eighth Day of Creation: The Makers of the Revolution in Biology. New York: Simon and Schuster.

Judson, H. F. 1987. Mapping the Human Genome: Historical Background (Mapping Our Genes contractor reports, Vol. 1, NTIS Order No. PB 88-160-783/AS). Office of Technology Assessment, U.S. Congress.

Kan, Y. W., and A. M. Dozy. 1978. Polymorphism of DNA sequence adjacent to human beta-globin structural gene: Relationship to sickle mutation. Proceedings of the National Academy of Sciences (USA) 75:5631-5635.

Kanigel, R. 1987. The genome project. New York Times Magazine December 13:44, 98-101, 106.

Kerem, B.-S., J. M. Rommens, J. A. Buchanan, D. Markiewicz, T. K. Cox, A. Chakravarti, M. Buchwald, and L.-C. Tsui. 1989. Identification of the cystic fibrosis gene: Genetic analysis. Science 245:1073-1080.

Kevles, D. J. 1985. In the Name of Eugenics. Berkeley, Calif.: University of California Press.

Koenig, M., E. P. Hoffman, C. J. Bertelson, A. P. Monaco, C. Feener, and L. M. Kunkel. 1987. Complete cloning of the Duchenne muscular dystrophy (DMD) cDNA and preliminary genomic organization of the DMD gene in normal and affected individuals. Cell 50:509-517.

Kolata, G. B. 1980. The 1980 Nobel prize in chemistry. Science 210:887-889.

Lee, W. H., R. Bookstein, F. Hong, L. J. Young, J. Y. Shew, and E. Y. Lee. 1987. Human retinoblastoma gene: Cloning, identification, and sequence. Science 235:1394-1399.

Lewin, R. 1986a. Molecular biology of Homo sapiens. Science 233 July 11:157-160.

Lewin, R. 1986b. Proposal to sequence the human genome stirs debate. Science 232:1598-1600.

Lewin, R. 1986c. Shifting sentiments over sequencing the human genome. Science 233:620-621.

Lifton, R. J. 1986. The Nazi Doctors. New York: Basic Books.

Maxam, A. M., and W. Gilbert. 1977. A new method for sequencing DNA. Proceedings of the National Academy of Sciences (USA) 74:560-564.

McAuliffe, K. 1987. Reading the human blueprint. U.S. News and World Report (December 28, 1987/January 4, 1988):92-93.

McKusick, V. A. 1986. The gene map of Homo sapiens: Status and prospectus. Pp. 15-27 in Molecular Biology of Homo sapiens. Cold Spring Harbor Symposia on Quantitative Biology, Vol. 51. Cold Spring Harbor, N.Y.: Cold Spring Harbor Laboratory.

McKusick, V. A. 1988. The morbid anatomy of the human genome: A review of gene mapping in clinical medicine. Bethesda, Md.: Howard Hughes Medical Institute.

Muller-Hill, B. 1988. Murderous Science. New York: Oxford University Press.

National Institutes of Health and Department of Energy. 1990. Understanding Our Genetic Inheritance. The US Human Genome Project: The First Five Years, FY 1991-1995. Document DOE/ER-0452P. Washington, D.C.: National Institutes of Health, U.S. Department of Health and Human Services; and U.S. Department of Energy.

National Research Council, Committee on Mapping and Sequencing The Human Genome. 1988. Mapping and Sequencing the Human Genome. Washington, D.C.: National Academy Press.

Neel, J. W. 1949. The inheritance of sickle cell anemia. Science 110:64-66.

Nelkin, D., and L. Tancredi. 1989. Dangerous Diagnostics: The Social Power of Biological Information. New York: Basic Books.

Olson, M. V., J. E. Dutchik, and M. Y. Graham. 1986. Random-clone strategy for genomic restriction mapping in yeast. Proceedings of the National Academy of Sciences (USA) 83:7826-7830.

Olson, M. V., L. Hood, C. Cantor, and D. Botstein. 1989. A common language for physical mapping of the human genome. Science 245:1434-1435.

Palca, J. 1987. Human genome sequencing plan wins unanimous approval in US. Nature 326:429.

Palca, J. 1989. Gene mappers meet on strategy. Science 245:1036.

Pauling, L., H. A. Itano, S. J. Singer, and I. C. Wells. 1949. Sickle cell anemia: A molecular disease. Science 110:543-548.

Pines, M. 1986. Shall We Grasp the Opportunity to Map and Sequence All Human Genes and Create a 'Human Gene Dictionary.' Bethesda, Md.: Howard Hughes Medical Institute.

Proctor, R. 1988. Racial Hygiene. Cambridge, Mass.: Harvard University Press.

Reeders, S. T., M. H. Breunig, K. E. Davies, R. D. Nicholls, A. P. Jarman, D. R. Higgs, P. C. Pearson, and D. J. Weatherall. 1985. A highly polymorphic DNA marker linked to adult polycystic kidney disease on chromosome 16. Nature 317:542-544.

Reilly, P. 1977. Genetics, Law, and Social Policy. Cambridge, Mass.: Harvard University Press.

Riordan, J. R., J. M. Rommens, B.-S. Kerem, N. Alon, R. Rozmahel, Z. Grzelczak, J. Zielenski, S. Lok, N. Plavsic, J.-L. Chou, M. L. Drumm, M. C. Iannuzzi, F. S. Collins, and L.-C. Tsui. 1989. Identification of the cystic fibrosis gene: Cloning and characterization of complementary DNA. Science 245:1066-1072.

Roberts, L. 1987. Human genome: Questions of cost. Science 237:1411-1412.

Roberts, L. 1989. New game plan for genome mapping. Science 245:1438-1440.

Rommens, J. M., M. C. Iannuzzi, B.-S. Kerem, M. L. Drumm, G. Melmer, M. Dean, R. Rozmahel, J. L. Cole, D. Kennedy, H. Hidaka, M. Zsiga, M. Buchwald, J. R. Riordan, L.-C. Tsui, and F. S. Collins. 1989. Identification of the cystic fibrosis gene: Chromosome walking and jumping. Science 245:1059-1065.

Rothstein, M. A. 1989. Medical screening and the employee health cost crisis. Washington, D.C.: Bureau of National Affairs.

Royer, B., L. Kunkel, A. Monaco, S. Goff, P. Newburger, R. Baehner, F. Cole, J. Curnutte, and S. Orkin. 1987. Cloning the gene for an inherited human disorder—chronic granulomatous disease—on the basis of its chromosomal location. Nature 322:32-38.

Sanger, F., S. Nicklen, and A. R. Coulson. 1977. DNA sequencing with chain-terminating inhibitors. Proceedings of the National Academy of Sciences (USA) 74:5463-5468.

Schwartz, D. C., and C. R. Cantor. 1984. Separation of yeast chromosome-sized DNAs by pulsed field gel electrophoresis. Cell 37:67-75.

Sinsheimer, R. 1989. The Santa Cruz workshop, May 1985. Genomics 5:954-956.

Solomon, E., and W. F. Bodmer. 1979. Evolution of sickle cell variant gene [letter]. Lancet 1:923.

U.S. Congress, House. 1987a. Fiscal Year 1988 DOE Budget Authorization: Environmental Research and Development (No. 58). Subcommittee on Natural Resources, Agriculture Research, and Environment of the Committee on Science, Space and Technology, U.S. House of Representatives.

U.S. Congress, House. 1987b. Departments of Labor, Health and Human Services, Education, and Related Agencies Appropriations for 1987 (Part 4A). Subcommittee of the Committee on Appropriations, U.S. House of Representatives.

U.S. Congress, House. 1988. Departments of Labor, Health and Human Services, Education, and Related Agencies Appropriations for 1989 (Part 4A). Subcommittee of the Committee on Appropriations, U.S. House of Representatives.

U.S. Congress, House. 1989. Hearing on International Cooperation in Mapping the Human Genome. October 19, 1989, 2325 Rayburn House Office Building. Subcommittee on International Scientific Cooperation, Committee on Science, Space, and Technology.

U.S. Congress, Office of Technology Assessment. 1984. Commercial Biotechnology: An International Analysis. OTA-BA-218. Washington, D.C.: U.S. Government Printing Office.

U.S. Congress, Office of Technology Assessment. 1986. Technologies for Detecting Heritable Mutations in Human Beings. Washington, D.C.: U.S. Government Printing Office.

U.S. Congress, Office of Technology Assessment. 1988a. Mapping Our Genes—Genome Projects: How Big? How Fast? OTA-BA-373, Washington, D.C.: U.S. Government Printing Office.

U.S. Congress, Office of Technology Assessment. 1988b. Medical Testing and Health Insurance. Washington, D.C.: U.S. Government Printing Office.

U.S. Congress, Senate. 1982. Nominations. Committee on Labor and Human Resources.

U.S. Congress, Senate. 1987a. Department of Energy National Laboratory Cooperative Research Initiatives Act (S. Hrg. 100-602, Pt. 1). Subcommittee on Energy Research and Development of the Committee on Energy and Natural Resources. Washington, D.C.: U.S. Government Printing Office.

U.S. Congress, Senate. 1987b. Workshop on Human Gene Mapping (100-71). Committee on Energy and Natural Resources. Washington, D.C.: U.S. Government Printing Office.

U.S. Congress, Senate. 1988. Departments of Labor, Health and Human Services, and Education and Related Agencies Appropriation Bill, 1989, Report (Report 100-399, pp. 83-84). Senate Committee on Appropriations.

U.S. Congress, Senate. 1989. The Human Genome Project and the Future of Biotechnology. Subcommittee on Science, Technology, and Space, Committee on Commerce, Science, and Transportation. (S. Hrg. 101-528). Senate Committee on Commerce, Science and Transportation. Washington, D.C.: U.S. Government Printing Office.

Watson, J. D. 1986. Foreword. Pp. xv-xvi in Molecular Biology of Homo sapiens. Cold Spring Harbor Symposia on Quantitative Biology, Vol. 51. Cold Spring Harbor, N.Y.: Cold Spring Harbor Laboratory.

Watson, J. D. 1988. The NIH Genome Initiative. Los Angeles: Molecular Biology Institute, University of California.

Watson, J. D. 1990. The human genome project: Past, present, and future. Science 248:44-49.

Watson, J. D., and F. H. C. Crick. 1953. Genetical implications of the structure of deoxyribonucleic acid. Nature 171:737-738.

Commentary

Paul Berg

This case study abounds with interesting opportunities for both retrospective and prospective analyses of science policymaking. Moreover, the study's chronicle of the personalities, events, and decisions that led to the creation of the genome project provides a valuable record for evaluating the wisdom and effectiveness of the actions taken. Cook-Deegan's analysis also points out those policy decisions whose validity will have to be judged by events yet to come. Thus, this case study fulfills the purpose for which it was commissioned. It provides a record that is worth scrutinizing to determine how the policy and funding decisions were made and whether there are general and applicable lessons to be learned for advancing other biomedical programs.

Any new initiative in science funding needs a highly visible, easily understandable goal, and champions who can articulate that goal persuasively in the offices of influence and power. By almost anyone's criteria, mapping and solving the human genome's sequence was viewed as a bold and exceedingly ambitious scientific and technical challenge, but one that would very likely be expensive in terms of resources, personnel, and funding. Aside from its initial influential group of proponents—Sinsheimer, DeLisi, Gilbert, Dulbecco, Hood, and Cantor—the plan to sequence the entire human genome, when it

Paul Berg is the Willson Professor of Biochemistry and Director of the Stanford University Medical School's Beckman Center for Molecular and Genetic Medicine.

became known, was met with considerable consternation and resistance. After some vacillation, Watson emerged as the genome project's chief advocate and proceeded to orchestrate support from several practicing and committed scientists. Concomitantly, DeLisi and Wyngaarden managed the legislative and budgetary complexities characteristic of governmental bodies. Senator Domenici, concerned for his DOE and state constituencies, and Senator Chiles, protective of the NIH, dominated the congressional debate and its outcome.

Another influential participant was the NRC Committee on Mapping and Sequencing the Human Genome. Their report expressing unanimous support (including that of previously skeptical or opposing members) carried a great deal of weight with the scientific community and helped persuade Wyngaarden, the OMB, and the congressional bodies dealing with the proposal. The report prepared by OTA *(Mapping Our Genes—Genome Projects: How Big? How Fast?*; 1988a) also helped move the genome proposal toward acceptance by supporting its feasibility and emphasizing the wisdom of a phased program. The report also provided a more reasoned estimate of its costs and the ways they could be apportioned. However, the NRC and OTA reports diverged in their recommendations as to who should manage the project. The NRC chose not to express a preference for the managing agency, while OTA preferred a joint NIH-DOE management structure—a solution that may become a stumbling block in later stages of the project. However, the recently published NIH-DOE combined plan for the first five years of the project, harbors well for a cooperative collaborative research effort. This arrangement should also alleviate the often-voiced suspicions about the quality of DOE research and its peer review systems. But competition for funding and recognition between DOE's national laboratories and NIH-sponsored genome centers could threaten the presently well intentioned cooperation. Mutual understanding of research activities and a strong spirit of team play will be important ingredients of that partnership.

A puzzling feature of the discussions concerning management of the genome project is why the NSF never emerged as a contender, especially as the project is indisputably science and technology based. Was this because of NSF's lack of interest or lack of competence to manage such a project? Or was it because of the project's decidedly biomedical slant?

One aspect of the scientific debate is worth noting. As initially conceived, the human genome project's goal was to obtain the sequence of the 3 billion base pairs comprising the haploid genetic complement. But the debate among scientists broadened the scope of the project in several significant ways. One was to include a moderate resolution map of linked restriction fragment length polymorphism (RFLP) markers for use in locating disease genes. A second modification was to obtain a physical map of cloned DNA segments spanning the entire genome. Moreover, it soon became apparent that the sequencing efforts would have to await the completion of the first two objectives, as well as the development of faster, more accurate, and far less expensive sequencing technologies. Such a reformulation of the project was inevitable once fine scientific minds turned to developing a coherent and workable strategy.

Another major modification of the original plan was to increase the number of genomes to be included in the project. This modification was not intended to add funds to an already large project, but was a result of the recognition of the close correspondence in genetic structures and functions between even distantly related organisms. Furthermore, it was evident that such relatedness would inform and speed the work on the human genome. Additionally, research with yeast, *Drosophila*, nematode, and mouse genomes provides experimental models with which hypotheses and technologies can be tested without resorting to human experimentation.

Cook-Deegan points up several innovations in government-supported science. Besides the somewhat novel joint and coordinated sponsorship of genome research by NIH and DOE, there is the acknowledgment that ethical and cultural values need to be reconciled with the program's objectives and applications. Including public education in that function would be helpful because one of the ingredients lacking from the debate so far has been any evidence of significant public awareness of the human genome initiative's costs and implications. The amount of funding for education and ethical studies is not as important as the fact that an ethics panel exists and that congressional support is contingent on attention to such issues. Whether ethical acceptability becomes a significant factor in judging the permissibility of initiating certain lines of basic research remains to be seen. Judging the ethical value of basic research prospectively and preemptively would be a considerable departure from current practices.

Cook-Deegan's record of the project's prenatal history identifies the contending forces that shaped the debate. These include the competing research interests and priorities among the "power" and "fringe" scientists, the similar tensions in the executive agencies governing biomedical research, and the jurisdictional sensibilities of congressional committees. Even though the project gained official sanction, debate over it lingers and threatens to flare up and polarize the constituencies needed for the project's support.

One of the most disturbing threats stems from the biomedical science community's still divided views concerning the project's merit, particularly in view of its perceived impact on traditional ways of supporting science; the simplistic view of this challenge is "Big Science versus Little Science." This debate is exacerbated by the current dismal research funding situation and the bleak prospects for any remedies. The present and next year's genome budgets can hardly be responsible for the current crisis. We can anticipate that unless the virtues and benefits of the early-phase mapping studies, the availability of clone banks, and the development of improved sequence technology are seen to benefit all scientists, the sniping will continue. Moreover, if the genome budget rises to its projected steady state—$200 million per year—while the research grant crisis worsens, the project's continuation will be jeopardized. Alternatively, funding for the genome project could be stretched out, as was done in the space program.

The case study does not indicate the extent to which the scientist activists, various advisory panels, or government agencies seriously considered the consequences of a fiscal crisis on Congress's ability or willingness to support the genome initiative. Perhaps this is because throughout the debate it was assumed that the project would be funded by supplemental (incremental) appropriations to NIH and DOE. Even though explicit assurances of the validity of those assumptions were never made, discussions and negotiations seemed to proceed as if the project's funding would not detract from support of investigator-initiated research in areas unrelated to the genome project.

The current funding crisis for projects unrelated to the genome project and the subsequent reactions of scientists and Congress indicate that neglecting the possibility and consequences of a funding shortfall was a serious deficiency in the planning. Perhaps that oversight stems from the pace with which the project was launched. Hindsight suggests that a more deliberate review, particularly by "disinterested" participants, could have led to contingency planning to contend with present or future difficulties in biomedical science funding.

Commentary

Ernest R. May

This story begins in the mid-1980s. More or less at once, a number of geneticists and molecular biologists saw the possibility of mapping and sequencing the entire human genome. A few developed visions of an immense and expensive project, making an analogy with the space program. The analogy the case brought to my mind was the opening of Africa in the nineteenth century and the response of Victorian imperialists such a Cromer, Curzon, and Rhodes.

For these visions to become reality, several things were needed. One was wide approval among knowledgeable scientists. Another was evidence that something appropriate could be done both bureaucratically and politically. Could any agency do it? Would the taxpayers countenance it?

The first requirement was satisfied. Despite reserved commentary in *Science* and *Nature*, the visionaries succeeded in winning wide backing from their peers. An NAS panel, together with advisory committees in both DOE and NIH, helped measurably.

Meanwhile, DOE-NIH competition helped both agencies come to readiness to do something on a large scale. OTA, abetted by or abetting key congressional staffers, worked out means such that the competition could end in cooperation rather than paralysis.

In the larger world, local interests of New Mexico, Florida, and California enabled congressional leaders to push the project. Appeals to the sense of

---

Ernest R. May is Charles Warren Professor of History at Harvard University.

what might make a legislator's name live in history also helped. Watson's inspired decision to commit a percentage of project budgets to the study of ethical issues defused possible opposition.

If this is the story—more or less—what are its lessons? Henry Kissinger used to say that no proposition was interesting unless one could imagine an intelligent person arguing the exact opposite. One way of asking about the lessons of the genome case is to ask what interesting propositions it speaks to. I see three.

The first is the proposition that there should be consensus among scientists *before* efforts are made to construct science policy. The affirmative brief would say that otherwise, policy could be constructed on erroneous premises and/or be vulnerable in the public arena because of evidence of expert differences. The negative brief would argue, among other things, that policy may never get made if it waits for scientific consensus and perhaps science policy is too important to be left to scientists.

The genome case seems to support this latter brief. The development of policy proceeded while scientists were still actively disagreeing. DOE/Office of Energy Research and OMB defined objectives, mechanisms, and tentative funding levels at a time when, according to the case, a poll of attendees at the Cold Spring Harbor conference would have voted against any early undertaking. Of course, the policy choices defined in mid-1986 were later to change, but the later effort would have been slower and different without this spadework.

The second proposition is that scientists, in the process of developing a large, pathbreaking project, should think about the bureaucratics of the project as well as about the science. Affirmative: the key question is not just what to do but how, in what sequence, and by whom. Negative: what to do is a large enough question, and it is the only one that most scientists are competent to consider.

Here, too, the genome case seems evidence for the negative. The efforts of the NAS panel to deal with bureaucratic implementation were, says the case, appallingly naive. It didn't matter. The bureaucracy, OTA, and congressional committees understood implementation issues. They dealt with them.

The third proposition is that, in developing such a project, scientists should think about politics—that is, about the types of citizen concerns that might surface once commitment of public money enters open debate. The affirmative case is summarized in the charter for this Institute of Medicine committee. The negative case is rather like that for the second proposition—too complicated, not scientists' strong suit, someone else (more expert) should carry the can.

On this third proposition, the genome case testifies for the affirmative as well as the negative. DeLisi got as far as he did in part because he recognized, and could take advantage of, New Mexicans' concern about the future of Los Alamos. Watson clearly pushed a hurdle out of his way by manifesting awareness of fears that the genome project might awaken. But the case, as written, does not show that thought about politics needed to be a major component of debate among scientists. So long as a few key figures kept the public in mind, that sufficed.

Origins of the Medicare Kidney Disease Entitlement: The Social Security Amendments of 1972

Richard A. Rettig

In the final days of the 1972 presidential campaign, Congress passed and sent to President Richard M. Nixon the Social Security Amendments of 1972. Nixon signed the bill on Monday, October 30, just one week before he was overwhelmingly reelected in his race against Senator George McGovern.

The 1972 social security legislation had begun its journey the previous year in the U.S. House of Representatives as H.R. 1. One of its chief elements had been welfare reform, a response to the administration's proposed family assistance plan. The other principal element, however, was a review and extension of Medicare and Medicaid, the first time since the 1965 enactment of Medicare that Congress had returned to that historic legislation to improve on its earlier works. (In fact, as we shall see, the Medicare and Medicaid provisions that were part of the social security amendments had almost become law in 1970.)

An eleventh-hour Senate floor amendment to the bill became Section 2991 of the final legislation. For more than 90 percent of the nation's population, this provision extended Medicare coverage to those with chronic kidney failure. The language of this brief amendment is found in an appendix.

Richard A. Rettig is a member of the professional staff of the Institute of Medicine, National Academy of Sciences. He has written extensively about the Medicare End-Stage Renal Disease program.

The purpose of this paper is to review how and why Congress enacted this historic entitlement, the first (and perhaps the last) designed to cover a particular diagnosis.

A HISTORICAL FOOTNOTE

I was asked to write this paper in the fall of 1989. Because I had previously written about the antecedents to and legislative history of the 1972 Medicare kidney amendments (Rettig, 1976), I was able to suggest the approach that has resulted in this paper. A workshop was held on December 18-19, 1989, at the National Academy of Sciences, with the principals involved in the 1972 legislation.[1] The workshop was chaired by Carl W. Gottschalk and supported by Institute of Medicine (IOM) staff. Participants were provided with historical materials before the meeting; several brought additional documents from personal files. The discussion focused on how Congress came to adopt the Medicare kidney disease entitlement. The meeting transcript was used to prepare a draft of this paper. The draft paper was reviewed by all participants and was also discussed at a meeting of the project committee at the National Academy of Sciences Beckman Center in March 1990.

Memories are often unreliable sources of details about events that occurred many years ago. As a result, specific factual claims have been corroborated from documented sources. The workshop basically served as a lengthy interview with a number of key individuals that clarified the major assumptions, underlying processes, and contextual factors that influenced the legislative outcome.

ANTECEDENTS TO THE 1972 LEGISLATION

A brief review of the evolution of federal government policy regarding hemodialysis and kidney transplantation is useful at this point. An extended treatment can be found in the literature (Rettig, 1981,1982). In 1944, in Nazi-occupied Holland, Willem Kolff first succeeded in prolonging the life of a patient using his primitive artificial kidney machine. (The surviving individual was his seventeenth attempt, all the others having died.) After the war, Kolff sent four of his machines to Europe and the United States, where they provided a basis for successful treatment of acute renal failure in the Korean War.

In 1960, Belding Scribner of the University of Washington in Seattle, working with Wayne Quinton, an engineer, invented a permanent vascular access device and placed his first patient on long-term, continuous, intermittent hemodialysis. That patient, Clyde Shields, lived 11 years. In 1963, when the hemodialysis procedure for treating chronic kidney failure was barely three years old, the Veterans Administration (VA) announced its intention to establish approximately 30 dialysis treatment units in VA hospitals across the country. These efforts, among others, would later prompt the Bureau of the Budget to question the fiscal implications of dialysis. In fact, when the Gottschalk Committee was formed in the mid-1960s, for example, Pierre Palmer, the Budget Bureau staff officer assigned to it, was the examiner for the VA hospital program.

The National Institutes of Health (NIH), through the National Institute of Allergy and Infectious Diseases, established a program in transplant immunology in 1964 in response to the discovery that immunosuppressive drugs prevented rejection of transplanted kidneys. In 1965 the National Institute of Arthritis and Metabolic Diseases initiated the artificial kidney/chronic uremia program, one year after the establishment of an artificial heart program in the National Heart Institute.

Also in 1965 the Public Health Service (PHS) started the Kidney Disease Control Program (KDCP). The program awarded 12 grants to establish dialysis centers across the country on a declining, step-funded basis. Alarmed by the cost implications of center dialysis, it then awarded 14 home dialysis contracts in 1966. Still seeking to dodge the fiscal implications of even this least costly treatment, in 1969 it let seven organ procurement contracts for organ procurement and combined kidney transplantation/home dialysis programs. In 1969 the PHS KDCP was administratively transferred to the Regional Medical Program, a transfer ratified by legislation in 1970.

Several years after the VA dialysis program had begun, and as various plans for a PHS dialysis program were being debated within the executive branch, the Bureau of the Budget, prompted by the White House Office of Science and Technology Policy, established an expert committee to review growing federal government obligations in the treatment of end-stage renal disease (ESRD). The group, later known as the Gottschalk Committee, after its chairman, issued the *Report of the Committee on Chronic Kidney Disease* in 1967 (Bureau of the Budget, 1967). The effect of that report is examined below.

The culmination of these events, for the purposes of this paper, was the enactment by Congress, in the Social Security Amendments of 1972 (P.L. 92-603), of Section 2991. This legislation authorized Medicare entitlement for individuals with a diagnosis of chronic renal failure who were fully or currently insured under social security: it also authorized coverage for the spouse and dependent children of fully or currently insured individuals. Persons with a diagnosis of chronic renal failure were "deemed to be disabled" for purposes of coverage under Parts A and B of Medicare.

The Influence of the Gottschalk Report

One question of great historical interest that has been asked repeatedly was whether the Gottschalk report influenced the events of 1972. Gottschalk, chairman of the expert committee, and George Schreiner, a member, elaborated on the 1967 report during the December 1989 workshop; the other participants dealt with the legislative events of 1972. The question posed at the workshop was this: Is there any evidence that the Gottschalk report influenced the thinking of any major actors in 1972 or that it influenced the 1972 congressional deliberations in any way?

The answer has three basic parts. First, the key congressional staff had not read the Gottschalk report; indeed, they were unaware of its existence. This lack of awareness extended to the members of Congress. Second, the report greatly influenced the medical community. Prepared by a distinguished committee, it essentially declared that hemodialysis and kidney transplantation were established therapies for the treatment of ESRD, thus resolving the debate about the "experimental versus established" status of these treatments. It also sanctioned the work of many clinicians who were then treating patients. Third, the 1967 report recommended a Medicare entitlement for chronic kidney failure patients that was quite similar to the entitlement that was adopted in 1972. The particulars of the report anticipated many features both of the legislation and of the program that was later established.

What explains the report's lack of influence on the key congressional actors of the drama? For one thing, the Bureau of the Budget established this expert committee as a secret group. Although its existence and the identity of its members became known in a short time, it was not a public body (Medical World News, 1967). Therefore, when the committee submitted its confidential report to the Budget Bureau in September 1967, the members were graciously thanked by letter by the director, Charles L. Shultze, but they were not publicly acknowledged.

The report was "released" in November by the National Institute of Arthritis and Metabolic Diseases, which had reproduced copies of the report for limited public distribution. The audience, however, was a medical research and public health one and not strongly connected to the new Medicare program. In addition, the National Kidney Foundation at that time had no Washington representative to publicize the report's conclusions. The report, therefore, did not reach enough of the right people.

Furthermore, the Medicare establishment had other concerns. The Bureau of Health Insurance of the Social Security Administration was preoccupied with the initial tasks of administering the fledgling Medicare program. The House Ways and Means Committee and the Senate Finance Committee were also concerned mainly with Medicare and Medicaid start-up problems. Receptivity to expanding Medicare to individuals under age 65 for treatments that very recently had been regarded as experimental was low.

Setting the Legislative Stage

The "Big Four" in dialysis in the 1960s included George Schreiner, Willem Kolff, John Merrill, and Belding Scribner. Kolff had invented the artificial kidney machine, and Scribner had invented the vascular access device that made continuous dialysis possible. Merrill led the nation's premier kidney transplant group at the Peter Bent Brigham Hospital in Boston. Schreiner conducted research and ran a major nephrology training program at Georgetown University in Washington, D.C. In addition, he was a founder of the American Society for Artificial Internal Organs in 1954, served as its president in 1959-1960, and for 29 years edited the *Transactions* of its annual meeting. He was also a founder of the American Society of Nephrology in 1967. In 1966 and 1967, he served as a member of the Gottschalk Committee.

Of these four, Scribner and Schreiner played important political roles in the development of federal government policy, the former as the outside advocate, the latter as the Washington strategist and tactician. Scribner, within a few months after his first three patients were rehabilitated by chronic hemodialysis, became the country's leading spokesman for treating patients by dialysis. His efforts resulted in Seattle's receiving the first dialysis center grant from the PHS in 1964, thus paving the way for the creation of the KDCP the following year. Seattle also pioneered home dialysis treatment, setting the stage for a PHS home dialysis contract program in 1966 and 1967.

Schreiner, in addition to bearing the above responsibilities, was also active in the National Kidney Foundation, serving as its president from 1968 to 1970. After that, he served several years as chairman of its legislative committee. In 1969, he hired Charles Plante, his next-door neighbor, as Washington representative of the foundation. Plante had worked on Capitol Hill for the senators from his home state of North Dakota from 1954 to 1966 and had spent two years in the Peace Corps before returning to Washington in 1969.

An initial step taken by the Schreiner-Plante team was to hold a meeting in 1969 and develop a five-year plan of legislative activity. The plan emphasized several courses of action: increasing NIH funding for kidney research and obtaining a new kidney institute; establishing ESRD-related activities, and securing funding for them in the Regional

Medical Program of the PHS, the Vocational Rehabilitation Program, and the crippled children's program; and obtaining coverage for the treatment of ESRD.

Bills to increase the federal government's role in financing the treatment of kidney disease were introduced in every session of Congress from 1965 onward. Most bills proposed to amend the Public Health Service Act; several pertained to vocational rehabilitation and other federal programs. Scribner's advocacy, for example, found strong support from the two powerful Washington State senators, Warren G. Magnuson and Henry M. Jackson. From 1965 onward, Jackson routinely submitted legislation to finance treatment of ESRD.[2] In addition, others, like Senator John Tower (R-Tex.) and Congressman Edward Roybal (D-Calif.) consistently sponsored kidney legislation during these years. Clearly, kidney disease became an item on the legislative agenda of the U.S. Congress during this time.

It was not until 1970, however, when the Heart Disease, Cancer, and Stroke Amendments of 1965 were modified by the inclusion of "and Kidney Disease" in the law's title and throughout its text that this activity resulted in legislation. Another important feature of the process was that no congressional hearings on kidney disease were held during this period (1965-1970), revealing the deliberateness with which Congress approached this issue.

In the 1960s several things were occurring simultaneously in the field of kidney disease treatment. The formation of the American Society of Nephrology in 1966 reinforced the development of the nephrology specialty within medicine. The Gottschalk Committee report, in 1967, sanctioned dialysis and transplantation as established therapies, thus resolving the conflict between clinicians who wished to treat patients and researchers who thought dialysis experimental. These several stimuli resulted in an increase in the number of physicians entering nephrology as opportunities for treating uremic patients grew.

The number of treatment centers was also steadily increasing. The Seattle Artificial Kidney Center, founded in 1962, pioneered the development of dialysis treatment centers. In 1963 the VA committed itself to developing 30 treatment centers. A number of centers were directly supported by the PHS from 1965 through 1968, and still more were later assisted by planning efforts of the PHS Regional Medical Program. Most centers were financed through a patchwork of funding sources— PHS programs, NIH grants, state kidney programs (being enacted in Illinois, for example, and elsewhere), and community fund-raising drives.

Relations between treatment units and academic medical centers, which provided most of the physicians for such facilities, proved complicated. In Seattle, the University of Washington sought to limit its involvement in dialysis, a policy that gave rise to the Seattle Artificial Kidney Center. In Minneapolis, the Regional Kidney Disease Program at Hennepin County Hospital, predominantly a dialysis effort, reflected the resistance of the University of Minnesota School of Medicine to housing the effort on their premises. John S. Najarian, chairman of surgery, believed that kidney transplantation was a cure but dialysis only a holding procedure.[3] In Boston, a controversial breakaway from Harvard University's Peter Bent Brigham Hospital resulted in the establishment of National Medical Care, Inc. But whatever the local reasons, the nation's dialysis treatment capacity continued to grow during this time.

Most important, the number of patients was also increasing. Nephrologists trooped to Seattle in the early 1960s to learn how to perform dialysis, and programs sprang up across the country, each growing over time as means were found to finance treatment. During the time the Gottschalk Committee was at work,[4] there were fewer than 1,000 patients being dialyzed in the entire country, but that number had increased to approximately 10,000 by the time the 1972 legislation was adopted.

As the number of physicians, treatment facilities, and patients increased, so too did local newspaper and television coverage of dialysis and kidney transplantation. In turn, members of Congress heard from and about constituents who needed dialysis, much of the information coming through local newspapers. Individual physicians, of course, made their views known to their own representatives and senators. The foundation for political action was being laid.

The National Kidney Foundation, through the efforts of Schreiner and Plante, focused these developments in the legislative arena much like a parabolic reflector gathers signals from many sources and focuses them on a single point. The foundation provided full-time professional representation of its cause to members of Congress and their staff, supplied them with continuous information, and pursued all available legislative and executive opportunities to advance the cause of kidney disease.

THE SOCIAL SECURITY AMENDMENTS OF 1972, SECTION 2991

The section above notes the stimuli to the 1972 legislation. What can be said about other "receptor sites" in Congress? Were representatives and senators prepared to hear from the advocates of kidney disease?

The Legislative Process

The legislative process in 1972 differed greatly from that of today. Power was concentrated in committee chairmen to a much greater extent than is now true, both for legislation and for appropriations. Congressional staff agencies, which are now prominent features of the scene, were much less important. The General Accounting Office (GAO) was beginning to shift from a traditional audit and accounting emphasis to one of program and management analysis. In the Library of Congress, the Legislative Reference Service provided strong constituent support to individual congressmen; the current Congressional Research Service, by contrast, provides professional staff support to committees. The Office of Technology Assessment was created in 1972.

Most important, the 1974 Budget Reform Act had not yet been passed. Consequently, the Senate and House budget committees were not yet in existence and thus had not yet disrupted relations between legislative and appropriations committees. The annual budget reconciliation process of today had not been established, and the Congressional Budget Office, which was authorized by this law, did not exist. The end result was that a more deliberate, patterned approach to legislation and fiscal matters occurred in 1972.

In this context, the Committee on Ways and Means was clearly the most powerful committee of the House of Representatives. In addition to its legislative authority, until the early 1970s the chairman and his Democratic colleagues on the committee had the authority to make all committee assignments for House Democrats. Wilbur Mills (D-Ark.), its chairman, was arguably the most powerful member of the House Democratic leadership. Understandably, assignment to the Ways and Means Committee was highly prized and went only to individuals who had shown themselves to be responsible legislators over several terms in the House.

The legislative jurisdiction of Ways and Means included the Internal Revenue Act (the tax code), international trade and tariffs, general revenue sharing, and the Social Security Act (including old age, survivors, and disability insurance, cash assistance programs, and Medicare and Medicaid). As one workshop participant said, the Ways and Means Committee, together with the Senate Finance Committee, "raised all of the federal government's revenue and spent half of it."

The House Ways and Means Committee had, and still has, an important advantage over the Senate Finance Committee. The Constitution stipulates that all revenue legislation must originate in the House of Representatives. That requirement was extended over time to include all those matters under its jurisdiction. Administration proposals affecting taxes, social security, and Medicare, for example, are submitted first to the Ways and Means Committee. It serves as the architect, one might say, for legislation that reaches the Senate.

In 1970, the House of Representatives, following the lead of its Ways and Means Committee, sent to the Senate the proposed Social Security

Amendments of 1970. The Senate Finance Committee deliberated at length, adopted a bill that the Senate passed, and returned a substantially amended bill to the House in the week between Christmas 1970 and the new year. The Senate announced, however, that it had no time to go to conference to resolve differences. It was "take it or leave it" politics. Although the legislation contained many provisions desired by members of the House, they rejected the Senate proposal rather than yield on such a fundamental procedural matter. No bill was passed as the ninety-first Congress adjourned.

Under Wilbur Mills, the Ways and Means Committee's style was well known. There were no subcommittees; all committee work was done by the full committee. Deliberately, every three or four years, the committee took up one of the major statutes under its jurisdiction—tax, international trade, social security, or Medicare. It then devoted great attention to the issues before it (many of which had accumulated since the last time they had been addressed), holding extensive hearings on any given subject. Members debated general legislative issues in executive session until consensus on the main provisions was established, and then, within an agreed-upon framework, the legislative and executive branch staff wrote language that could be implemented.

Mills seldom sponsored legislation himself. Rather, he allowed a bill to emerge from the deliberative processes of the committee. The legislation that went to the floor of the House had a bipartisan seal of approval; Mills took great care to ensure that John Byrnes (R-Wis.), the ranking minority member, and all of the committee Republicans agreed to it.[5] Mills's objective was to achieve unanimity of the committee as a preliminary step to carrying the full House.

One tradition of the Ways and Means Committee was to hear any citizen who wished to address the committee. Mills did not engage in selective hearings that were restricted to those advocating a point of view or to organizations representing major constituent interests. Consequently, hearings of the Ways and Means Committee always included statements by a number of interested individuals.

The Senate Finance Committee had comparable legislative jurisdiction, which was exercised under the chairmanship of Russell B. Long (D-La.). (Long, however, did not play the same political role in the Senate Democratic leadership as Mills played in the House.) The Committee was organized into subcommittees in the early 1970s, and the Subcommittee on Health was chaired by Herman Talmadge (D-Ga.), who worked closely with the chairman.

The Senate Finance Committee lacked the internal cohesion of the House Ways and Means Committee. On welfare reform, for example, a major element of the social security legislation in 1972, Long favored a fiscally conservative bill that emphasized work by welfare recipients. Abraham Ribicoff (D-Conn.), although supporting the work provision, favored a financially more generous bill. The administration's original proposal, the family assistance plan authored by Secretary of Labor Daniel P. Moynihan, represented an intermediate position. Each of the three parties had roughly one-third of the Senate votes. No one was prepared to compromise to assemble a majority, and the resulting three-way deadlock defeated welfare reform.

Finally, it is important to note that congressional staff, although fewer in number than today, exercised great influence and were a tightly knit group with close ties to the executive branch. William Fullerton joined the Ways and Means Committee in 1970 as its first professional staff person; in 1972, he was the only such staff attached to the committee. His counterpart in the Senate, Jay Constantine, had joined the Senate Finance Committee in 1966 as its first professional staff person on Medicare, Medicaid, and welfare. In 1972, he was aided, especially in the ESRD amendment, by James Mongan, a physician, and Paul Rettig from the Social Security Administration (SSA), who worked at the Senate Finance Committee on a daily basis during this time.

Congressional staff ties to the SSA's Bureau of Health Insurance were strong. Irwin Wolkstein, the bureau's deputy director for policy, had worked on health insurance issues since before the 1965 enactment of Medicare and Medicaid. Fullerton had worked for him at SSA, as had Rettig. In 1969, Constantine recruited Fullerton from the Legislative Reference Service of the Library of Congress to coauthor *Medicare and Medicaid: Problems, Prospects, and Alternatives*. This report greatly influenced the proposed legislation of 1970, which, although not enacted at that time, was basically adopted in 1972. In short, both committees' staff constituted a group of individuals with strong personal and professional ties to each other and with effective working relationships to the executive branch.

The Policy Context

Several features characterized the setting in which the 1972 legislation was enacted. First, there was a strong commitment among the members of Congress to pass a bill. They had no desire to repeat the experience of 1970 when legislation was not passed because the Senate refused to go to conference. Second, the policy debate focused much attention on national health insurance. Senator Edward M. Kennedy (D-Mass.) had become chairman of the Subcommittee on Health of the Senate Committee on Labor and Public Welfare in January 1971 and immediately began to discuss national health insurance. The Nixon

White House responded with legislation of its own. In a message to Congress on February 18, 1971, President Nixon proposed the National Health Insurance Partnership Act of 1971, one of the most important of the many proposals put forward at that time (U.S. Congress, House, Committee on Ways and Means, 1971b). There is some feeling that Nixon's action came out of his fear of the possibility of a Kennedy candidacy for the presidency the following year (Rettig, 1977).

Reflecting this interest in national health insurance, the House Ways and Means Committee, after passing H.R. 1 in the summer of 1971, held 21 days of hearings in October and November on national health insurance proposals, including that of the administration (U.S. Congress, House, Committee on Ways and Means, 1971a). In February 1972, the administration submitted extensive amendments to its original proposal (U.S. Congress, House, Committee on Ways and Means, 1972). In the Senate, although Finance Committee Chairman Long did not favor comprehensive health insurance measures, he did advocate insurance against the catastrophic costs of health care, indicating the broad interest in expansion of the existing Medicare and Medicaid programs.

The legislative agenda in 1971 and 1972, however, was dominated by H.R. 1, not by national health insurance. This legislation, as noted earlier, dealt with social security, Medicare, and welfare reform. Perhaps the bill's most important amendment to Medicare, marking its most significant expansion since 1965, was the extension of Medicare coverage to the disabled. President Lyndon Johnson had proposed such an extension in 1967, two years after Medicare had been enacted, but then it was regarded as too soon to be seriously considered. In 1970, however, it had been part of the bill that failed enactment for procedural reasons. Its passage in 1972 was a foregone conclusion.

The Senate Finance Committee first considered H.R. 1 in July and August 1971, as soon as the bill was sent over by the House (U.S. Congress, Senate, Committee on Finance, 1971). These hearings were limited to administration witnesses and focused mainly on the family assistance plan. Senator Long noted with asperity that two-thirds of the bill consisted of Senate amendments adopted in 1970. He noted that the most controversial feature of the legislation was the welfare reform proposal of the administration, as modified by the House.

The Senate committee resumed hearings again in January and February 1972, and the opening statements of Long and Ribicoff foreshadowed the welfare reform deadlock mentioned above (U.S. Congress, Senate, Committee on Finance, 1972a). That deadlock, and the ensuing controversy and behind-the-scenes negotiations, delayed Senate action on the bill until members had returned to Washington from the summer recess.

Despite these maneuverings, the facts were that major legislation amending the Social Security Act was proceeding through both the House and the Senate in 1971 and 1972, and the Nixon administration was participating in all aspects of the process. There was no uncertainty about whether there would be legislation. The only question was the kind of bill a Democratic Congress would send to the White House and its acceptability to a Republican president.

The Adoption of Section 299I

The formal legislative history of Section 299I is quite brief. The provision was not considered by the House Ways and Means Committee in hearings or in any executive session on H.R. 1. The Senate kidney amendment was added to H.R. 1 on the Senate floor, with no prior hearings, on a Saturday morning, September 30, 1972. The joint House-Senate conference committee agreed to the Senate amendment barely two weeks later. On October 30, the brief kidney provision was included in the 300-page bill signed by the President. The informal legislative history, however, is far more complicated.

Ways and Means: November and December 1971

The House Ways and Means Committee, as part of its hearings on national health insurance, devoted the end of the morning of November 4, 1971, to testimony about ESRD (U.S. Congress, House, Committee on Ways and Means, 1971c). It particular, it heard from representatives of the National Association of Patients on Hemodialysis (NAPH). These included Shep Glazer, vice president of the group and a dialysis patient from New York; William Litchfield, a dialysis patient from Houston; Roland Fortier, an NAPH member from Connecticut; Peter Lundin, a medical school student who was also a dialysis patient and NAPH member from California; June Crowley, a dialysis patient from New York; and Abraham Holtz, a dialysis patient from New York.

Glazer made an official statement for NAPH, and then spoke about his personal situation:

> I am 43 years old, married for 20 years, with two children ages 14 and 10. I was a salesman until a couple of months ago until it became necessary for me to supplement my income to pay for the dialysis supplies. I tried to sell a non-competitive line, was found out, and was fired. Gentlemen, what should I do? End it all and die? Sell my house for which I worked so hard, and go on welfare? Should I go into the hospital under my hospitalization policy, then I cannot work? Please tell me. If your kidneys failed tomorrow, wouldn't you want the opportunity to live? Wouldn't you want to see your children grow up? (U.S. Congress, House, Committee on Ways and Means, 1971b)

The most dramatic moment of the hearing, however, came when Glazer was briefly dialyzed before the committee. This event was widely publicized afterwards and was believed by many to have been decisive in the decision of Congress to enact the kidney disease entitlement.

In fact, great ambivalence surrounded this dialysis "session." The hearing record, for example, mentions only that a dialysis machine was brought to the hearing room but not that Glazer was dialyzed (U.S. Congress, House, Committee on Ways and Means, 1971b). The session had been arranged by Glazer and Ways and Means Chief Counsel John M. Martin, who consulted William Fullerton, the committee staff person for health. Neither was enthusiastic; indeed, Martin was afraid of what might happen if Glazer died in front of the committee. Nor did the other members or their staff think it was especially appropriate. Plante remembers that the senior staff aide to Barber Conable (R-N.Y.), when he saw Glazer being dialyzed, exclaimed "What the f— is going on here?" But the committee had a tradition of hearing anyone who wished to testify, and it chose not to change its rules in this instance.

Glazer, at a New York NAPH press conference on November 3, the day before the hearing, had announced his intention to undergo dialysis before Chairman Mills and the Ways and Means Committee. The National Kidney Foundation opposed the effort—directly in discussions with Glazer and indirectly through Eli Friedman, advisor to NAPH. Schreiner and Plante had been lobbying Congress assiduously, seeking support for kidney treatment programs from all sources—the tax committees, the health legislative committees, and the appropriations committees. They feared that an accident would cancel all the progress they had made, and Schreiner stressed this possibility when he tried to dissuade Glazer from dialyzing before the committee. Given these activities, Schreiner's incredulity was all the greater when he received a telephone call at home on the evening before the hearing. Glazer had arrived in Washington, D.C., from New York, and was calling to ask Schreiner if a Georgetown University dialysis machine could be brought to the hearing room the next morning for use at that time (Institute of Medicine, 1989). Schreiner, suppressing his anger, trucked a machine over to the Longworth House Office Building on Capitol Hill. Barred from attending the hearing by the National Kidney Foundation, which did not wish him to lend its prestige to the event, he sent a Georgetown nephrology fellow, James Carey, to act as attending physician. If any untoward event occurred, Carey was instructed by Schreiner to clamp the blood lines, turn off the machine, and declare that the dialysis session was over.

Several years later, Carey disclosed to Schreiner that Glazer had gone into ventricular tachycardia during the dialysis session before the committee. Carey had immediately clamped the lines. The "treatment" was very short, perhaps five minutes in all, long enough to open the blood lines but hardly a dialysis session. Nevertheless, the few members of the committee who were present characterized the episode as "excellent testimony." They were thinking broadly about national health insurance at the time, however, not about doing something special for dialysis patients. Indeed, Fullerton recalls that a parent of a child with hemophilia made a far greater impression on the committee. The national press, on the other hand, had been handed a dramatic story and publicized it widely. The myth that Glazer's treatment had been decisive in the decision by Congress to enact Section 2991 had been established.

On November 11, one week later, Schreiner and William J. Flanigan, a nephrologist from the University of Arkansas in Little Rock, hometown to Wilbur Mills, testified before the committee on behalf of the National Kidney Foundation (U.S. Congress, House, Committee on Ways and Means, 1971d). Flanigan cited the disparity between the few patients with end-stage renal failure who were actually being treated and the many who could benefit, adding the following:

Just over two decades ago we did not have the artificial kidney machine, and kidney transplant became a technique just one decade ago. Today we have both therapies because of research, both with and without Government support. These life saving procedures cost money and they save lives. It seems to those of us who each day work in the field of kidney disease that too many years have already gone by without a national program of catastrophic insurance or a National Health Insurance Act with provisions for catastrophic coverage.

The events of the previous week were neither mentioned by the National Kidney Foundation representatives nor raised in the perfunctory questioning after the testimony. The testimony simply added one more statement to the hearing record in behalf of national health insurance.

It was noteworthy, then, when Mills introduced a personal bill, H.R. 12043, on December 6, 1971, to amend the Social Security Act and provide financing for individuals with chronic kidney disease. The bill proposed to amend Title XVII rather than Title XVIII (Medicare) or Title XIX (Medicaid), as would have been more appropriate. (Fullerton remembers modeling the bill after Title V, which applies to maternal and child health.)

This proposed bill, far more than the amendment enacted in late 1972, reveals Mills's thinking about this issue. The purpose of the bill was "to assure that any individual who suffers from chronic renal disease will have available to him the necessary life-saving care and treatment for such disease and will not be denied such treatment because of his inability to pay for it." The bill provided for a budgeted program, not an entitlement; it authorized appropriations of "such sums as may be necessary" to financially assist U.S. citizens or "aliens lawfully admitted . . . for permanent residence." Financial assistance was to be "for any part of such costs which [such individuals] are unable to pay from funds otherwise available to them," but only to the extent that such payments "do not exceed the cost of the least expensive form of dialysis which is or would be medically sufficient." In addition, a project grant program was proposed to assist in the development "of new and improved methods of treatment, with emphasis on less costly methods," "the establishment of hemodialysis centers, but including only those centers which make home dialysis equipment available to those who require" it, training of personnel, and educational programs regarding the prevention of chronic renal disease.

What was going on? There were probably at least two things operating. First, Mills, who practically never submitted a personal bill, was signaling his sympathy for action on kidney disease. The degree of his commitment to the precise language of H.R. 12043 was unclear at that time. Mills had heard from Arkansas constituents and individuals across the country, however, and recognized a genuine problem that needed attention. Fullerton recalls that the chairman began to get calls during this time from people about to die who needed help. Mills's administrative assistant, Gene Goff, handled the Arkansas constituents and took a personal interest in the issue; Fullerton dealt with the others. It bothered Mills, as it did Fullerton, that the congressman had to get involved with life-and-death matters (Institute of Medicine, 1989).

Second, it was about this time that Mills decided to seek the Democratic presidential nomination, a decision he announced a few months later. Coincidentally, perhaps, substantial legislation emerged from the Committee on Ways and Means during 1971 and 1972—expansion of Medicare to include the disabled and general revenue sharing—flowing from a congressional consensus that Mills was powerful in shaping.

Senate Finance Committee: 1972

The Senate Finance Committee held hearings on H.R. 1 in July and August 1971 and again in January and February 1972. During this time, the supplemental security income benefit was developed on the Senate side. The Senate Finance Committee did not report out a bill, however, until September (U.S. Congress, Senate, Committee on Finance, 1972b). In the intervening period, discussions went forward on all aspects of the proposed legislation.

Although neither the House nor the Senate version of H.R. 1 contained a kidney disease provision, the summer of 1972 was an active one for the National Kidney Foundation. For example, the 1972 Republican Party platform included a plank on the coverage of kidney failure treatment. Unbeknownst to the foundation, Bryce Harlow at the Nixon White House apparently had been responsible for this plank provision on behalf of Mamie Eisenhower, then a member of the Kidney Foundation board.

More important, Schreiner, Plante, and other foundation officials had had contact with Senate Finance Committee Chairman Long and with Herman Talmadge (D-Ga.), chairman of the Senate Subcommittee on Health. Following a February 1972 visit, E. Lovell Becker, then president of the National Kidney Foundation, wrote to thank Long for meeting with him, Plante, and another Kidney Foundation physician. In a letter dated February 28, 1972, Becker included "some basic information on the incidence of kidney disease and the costs of hospital dialysis, home dialysis and transplantation."

In the early months of 1972, Charles Plante had his first encounter with Vance Hartke (D-Ind.), during which the senator indicated his support for the Kidney Foundation's legislative agenda. On February 22, Hartke introduced S. 3210 on behalf of himself and Alan Cranston (D-Calif.), a bill to amend the Public Health Service Act "to provide assistance to certain non-Federal institutions, agencies, and organization for the establishment and operation of cooperative community programs for patients with kidney disease for the conduct of training related to such programs, and to provide financial assistance to individuals suffering from chronic kidney disease who are unable to pay the costs of necessary treatment" (U.S. Congressional Record, 1972a). Hartke's action foreshadowed the events of September, although S. 3210 would amend the Public Health Service Act, not the Social Security Act.

Plante maintained regular contact with Constantine and Mongan on the Senate subcommittee staff and with Fullerton on Ways and Means during the spring and summer of 1972. The staff of both committees, in turn, were in touch with Irwin Wolkstein in the SSA Bureau of Health Insurance. Although no kidney provision was formally under consideration, it was being discussed as part of a much larger, more comprehensive package of Medicare amendments.

The key discussions at the Senate Finance Committee staff level occurred during this period. Constantine was inclined against a kidney disease amendment. Why favor this treatment, he asked, over the long-term treatment of cancer? Mongan, the physician, counseled against opposing a kidney provision. It was the one situation, he argued, where the only thing separating individuals from life and death was money. He suggested that it be looked at as a pilot for catastrophic health insurance. Constantine yielded; he would not recommend against such a provision if it were offered.

Notwithstanding Hartke's earlier expression of interest, there was little indication by late summer that he might offer a kidney disease amendment to H.R. 1 on the Senate floor. When that possibility arose in early September, Schreiner went to Long, concerned that Long—not Hartke—should receive credit. Long replied, according to Schreiner, "Do you want to credit me or to have a bill? Let Hartke do it; we may need him for something else."

The Senate Finance Committee report of September 26 revealed the complexity of legislation that dealt, among other things, with old age, survivors, and disability insurance, Medicare, Medicaid, maternal and child health, social security benefits, supplemental security income, jobs for families, child care, aid to families with dependent children, and general revenue sharing; the document was nearly 1,300 pages long. Listed first among the health-related provisions of the House bill that were basically adopted without change by the Senate was the extension of Medicare coverage to disability beneficiaries (U.S. Congress, Senate, Committee on Finance, 1972b).

In this provision, the committee was responding to the obvious needs of the disabled, who used medical services at greater rates than those who were not disabled but who were also much less well off financially. On the other hand, by requiring that an individual be disabled for 24 months before Medicare eligibility began, the provision regulated the share of the costs to be borne by Medicare.

The Finance Committee added 49 provisions to the House bill. The two most prominent were professional standards review organizations and coverage of maintenance drugs by Medicare. The former would be enacted; the latter would be rejected. There was no provision for kidney disease included in the bill reported out by the committee. However, in a section at the very end of the report entitled "Additional Views of Senator Vance Hartke," Hartke discussed kidney disease (U.S. Congress, Senate, Committee on Finance, 1972b).

In what must be the most tragic irony of the twentieth century, people are dying because they cannot get access to proper medical care. . . . More than 8,000 Americans will die this year from kidney disease who could have been saved if they had been able to afford an artificial kidney machine or transplantation. These will be needless deaths—deaths which should shock our conscience and shame our sensibilities. . . . We have the opportunity now to begin a national program of kidney disease treatment assistance administered through the Social Security Administration, and I propose that we take that opportunity so that more lives are not lost needlessly.

The last sentence clearly anticipated the events that would follow in swift succession.

The National Kidney Foundation representatives—Schreiner, Plante, and Lovell Becker, the current president—had no reason to expect that a kidney provision would be included in the Senate bill as the Finance Committee took it to the Senate floor in the final week of September. They flew off to San Francisco on Friday, September 29, to attend a major conference on kidney transplantation organized by Samuel Kountz, the transplant surgeon at the University of California, San Francisco. Before leaving, they made a precautionary check and were assured that nothing was likely to happen.

On their arrival in San Francisco, however, the foundation representatives received a telephone call from Washington indicating that Long had agreed to let Hartke offer a kidney entitlement amendment the following morning, Saturday, September 30, and their presence was requested. Schreiner, who was already committed to a dinner at Norman Shumway's, the Stanford heart transplant surgeon, and scheduled to deliver a paper at the transplant meeting, remained in San Francisco. Plante took the "red-eye" flight back to Washington.

Plante arrived at the Senate early Saturday morning and remembers the day as "dark and stormy." He first helped Howard Marlow, Hartke's staff aide, prepare the senator's remarks for introducing the amendment on the floor. He also discussed with Mongan the precise wording of the amendment, which had not been entirely worked out.

The Senate, after perhaps 30 minutes of floor debate, voted 52 to 3 in favor of the Hartke amendment, with 45 senators absent and not voting (Rettig, 1976). Dissenting votes were cast by Wallace Bennett (R-Utah), the ranking minority member of the Finance Committee, James Buckley (R-N.Y.), and Sam Ervin (D-N.C.).

Was the Senate action capricious or a considered step of the world's greatest deliberative body? From the discussion at the Institute of Medicine's December 1989 workshop, several factors stand out. First, the extension of Medicare coverage to the disabled was an essential prerequisite for a kidney disease amendment. Without it, a special provision for kidney disease would have violated basic equity. Given the disability framework, however, chronic kidney failure could be viewed as a disabling, life-threatening condition.[6]

Second, Russell Long's long-standing interest in insuring people against the costs of catastrophic health problems made him responsive to the financial implications of kidney disease, especially for working individuals. Of the staff, Mongan was pivotal. He persuaded Constantine to treat the issue as a "pilot" for catastrophic health insurance. Together, with substantial help from the Kidney Foundation, they persuaded Long.

Third, the kidney entitlement was adopted at a time when national health insurance, or at least catastrophic insurance, was anticipated shortly. The kidney amendment, although consistent with this broader agenda, was an issue that deserved immediate attention. As Long put it on the Senate floor:

> *The next Congress will tackle health insurance issues, and I am sure during that debate we will deal with health insurance problems in general, and I hope that specifically we will deal with the problem of insuring against catastrophic illness. I am cosponsoring this proposal at this time because these very unfortunate citizens with chronic renal failure cannot wait for Congress to debate these broader issues. They need help—it is critical—and that help must come now as many of them, without assistance, simply will not be alive for another two years. (U.S. Congressional Record, 1972c)*

Finally, the human face of the issue that presented itself to Long and his colleagues, and to Wilbur Mills and other members of Congress, was that of a working member of the community, married, a father, and a responsible citizen—the Shep Glazers of the world. The only thing between them and death was money. That, at least, could be supplied by the Congress of the United States. For Long, providing life-saving benefits to these individuals was consistent with his commitment to catastrophic health insurance, his emphasis on work, and his general populist outlook.

The Joint House-Senate Conference Committee: 1972

Both the Senate and House were determined to send a bill to the White House before election day, but time was short. The staff prepared a report for the Joint House-Senate Conference Committee that analyzed both the House and Senate bills, focusing on the differences between them (U.S. Congress, Conference Committee, 1972). In addition, House Ways and Means Committee staff prepared a provision-by-provision document solely for the benefit of the House members.

The conference began on Thursday, October 12, and continued through Saturday evening, October 14. Amendment number 328, providing coverage of "certain specified drugs, purchased on an outpatient basis, which are necessary in the treatment of the most common, crippling or life-threatening disease conditions of the aged," had been added by the Senate (U.S. Congress, Conference Committee, 1972). The administration, however, opposed the coverage of drugs. Indeed, some observers thought that this amendment alone, if accepted, risked a presidential veto. The administration and the pharmaceutical industry, which also opposed the provision, lobbied strongly against it with Mills and his House colleagues. As the provision was not in the Ways and Means bill, and would have cost a great deal, the House resolved before the conference to reject this proposed amendment.

The Senate bill also included the kidney disease amendment, but the House bill did not. Mills was sympathetic to the kidney provision, as he had indicated at the end of 1971; he was quite unsympathetic to the drug provision. As Long presented the case for the drug provision, Fullerton recalls whispering to Mills, "Tell him that if they are prepared to recede on this one, we're ready to talk turkey on the kidney provision." Mills conveyed that message, and Long yielded. Although he believed strongly in the drug benefit, he knew he did not have the votes. He also knew that the Ways and Means Committee was prepared to accept the kidney provision.

Soon the conference turned to the kidney provision. Discussion was brief. The Hartke amendment had included a six-month waiting period between the application for entitlement (following the first treatment for chronic kidney failure) and the period of eligibility for benefits. The House proposed to shorten that to three months, which the conference accepted.

Thus, the conference included Section 299I in the Social Security Amendments of 1972, at that time the longest single piece of legislation Congress had ever adopted. After adoption by both the House and Senate, the bill was sent to the White House and signed by President Richard M. Nixon on October 30, 1972.

ESTIMATES OF COST

One persistent criticism of the ESRD program has been that its total costs were grossly underestimated. What lies behind this criticism? In retrospect, the basic misestimation involved the incidence and prevalence of individuals with permanent kidney failure. Although "unit costs," as measured in Medicare expenditures per patient treatment year, have always been high, usually in the range of $25,000 to $30,000 nominal dollars (unadjusted for inflation), the steady growth in the patient population has driven program costs higher and higher. Even though these unit costs have been controlled in an impressive way over time, total Medicare expenditures are substantial. In addition, initial estimates in 1972 dollars have usually been compared with nominal dollars in later years.

The basic reason for the criticism, however, is that initial Medicare ESRD costs were wrong, or not reported, or not inclusive of induced costs, and exceeded initial expectations. The kidney disease amendment of October 1972 was an obscure event to most Washington observers. After all, a presidential election dominates news and public awareness both inside and outside the Washington beltway. Not until January 1973, when the *New York Times* carried a story about the low estimates and ran an editorial, "Medicarelessness," was this issue forcefully injected into public consciousness. Let us attempt to disentangle this complex aspect of the story.

First, Senator Hartke was the only source of public information about estimates. On the Senate floor on September 30, drawing heavily on information from the National Kidney Foundation, he discussed costs at length:

In terms of indirect costs of mortality—lost future income—kidney disease is the highest ranking killer, costing the country $1.5 billion annually. Additionally, more that $1 billion has to be spent each year for hospital and nursing home care, professional services, and drugs. Surprisingly, this amount exceeds the annual medical services costs for maternity care, or for all forms of cancer. (U.S. Congressional Record, 1972b)

Hartke added information about the epidemiology of the disease and the insurance coverage of its victims:

Approximately 55,000 Americans are now suffering from chronic renal disease. Twenty to 25,000 of these people are prime candidates for dialysis or other life-saving kidney treatment. Of these people, less than one-third have any insurance coverage of their own, and most of these people have coverage for no more than 2 years.

Although the unit costs of dialysis were high, the senator was optimistic that technological advance could be expected to bring them down:

The cost of dialysis is $22,000 to $25,000 per year per patient in a hospital; $17,000 to $20,000 in a hospital-related dialysis center; and $19,000 in the first year of home dialysis with a subsequent cost of about $5,000 per year. There is substantial evidence available, however, indicating that these costs will continue to go down each year with new advances in the technology of artificial kidney care.

Remarkable success in transplantation, coupled with declining costs, would also affect total program costs:

Perhaps more exciting is the remarkable success that transplant surgeons are having with kidney transplants. It is estimated that over 2,000 procedures will be performed this year in the United States. Of these, 85 percent will be successful. It is also important to point out that the 15 percent rejection rate means kidney mortality and not human mortality. These people are placed back on the artificial kidney machine to await another tissue-typing for another transplant. At the present time, the average costs of a transplant are $15,000. Again, we can look at the substantial reductions in the cost of transplantation. For example, Dr. Sam Kountz,[7] a transplant surgeon at the University of California, has reduced his costs to $8,000 per transplant or no more than any major surgical procedure.

Treatment, Hartke argued, would rehabilitate a major proportion of the patients:

Sixty percent of those on dialysis can return to work but require retraining and most of the remaining 40 percent require no retraining whatsoever. These are people who can be active and productive, but only if they have the lifesaving treatment they need so badly.

Then, regarding program costs, the senator stated the following:

Final cost estimates for this vital amendment are now being worked out. Preliminary estimates indicate an annual cost of approximately $250 million at the end of 4 years with the first full year cost at about $75 million.

It is possible that these costs could be covered by the slight actuarial surplus in the hospital insurance trust fund and the slight reduction in costs now estimated for the regular Medicare program for the disabled. However, if it is finally determined—and I think it can be, before these considerations of H.R. 1 are concluded—that a Medicare tax increase of a small amount is necessary, it would be quite normal.

When the actuaries complete their work, and if they indicate the need for an increase in the Medicare tax, I would be more than glad to propose a further amendment to that effect in the interest of responsible legislating.

The need for this amendment is urgent. We will do what is required to pay these costs.

That is what the pending amendment provides—a chance for thousands of Americans to remain alive and be productive. The $90 to $110 million that this amendment will cost each year is a minor cost to maintain life. And it is a minor cost when compared to the rewards which society will reap from people who can return to the workforce rather than wither and die.

I think this is one instance in which medical technology has given its blessing to a wonderful Nation, and what we need now is to implement this blessing, to make sure that the amendment is adopted.

Where did Hartke get his numbers? The National Kidney Foundation supplied him with figures from the spring of the year onward. The low estimates on dialysis came mostly from Scribner in Seattle, who was advocating home dialysis as the right course. In addition, Samuel Kountz, a kidney transplant surgeon at the University of California, San Francisco, an enthusiastic advocate for transplantation, was predicting falling transplant costs over time. Furthermore, the discussions of cost invariably reflected the expectation that technological change would lead to falling costs. In short, much of Hartke's information came from the advocates for treatment, fiscally responsible individuals themselves, who argued that treatment could be done economically. The situation was one in which few epidemiological data existed; the Gottschalk report analyses, which might have been updated, were basically unknown by key policymakers; and political action clearly overtook expenditure estimation.

The statements by Hartke on the Senate floor, then, stand as the most "official" estimates of the expenditure impact of the kidney provision. In fact, a more formal estimation process did exist. When major legislation was being considered by Congress, it was customary for the appropriate officials in the executive branch to consult closely on the probable costs of such legislation. Today, the Congressional Budget Office, established by the Congressional Budget Reform Act of 1974, provides estimates to congressional committees on pending legislation. In the case of the Social Security Amendments of 1972, this responsibility fell to the Office of the Actuary of the SSA. The health actuaries of the SSA worked with the House Ways and Means Committee, the Senate Finance Committee, the Joint Committee on Taxation, and the conference committee to cost out the various provisions under consideration.

In 1972, as today, the focus of cost calculations for amendments to the Social Security Act was the amount of increase in the Federal Insurance Contributions Act (FICA) payroll tax that was required to finance new provisions. The FICA (or social security) tax consists of two parts: the social security contribution and the health insurance contribution. The estimated increase in the FICA tax required to finance new or expanded benefits is called the "percent of payroll"; payroll refers to the national wage base against which the tax is applied. Thus, for members of the House Ways and Means and Senate Finance committees, the estimates question is embedded in the larger issue of how much the FICA tax must be increased to finance program expansion. This question differs from that of how much has to be appropriated in the budget for programs financed out of general revenues.

The numerous provisions of H.R. 1 required a good deal of actuarial work to estimate. Substantial calendar time was available, however, to cost out the House provisions, as H.R. 1 was completed in mid-1971 and the joint conference committee did not meet until October 1972. Moreover, many of the House provisions remained unchanged from the aborted 1970 legislation, and the Senate had already agreed to many of these. The health actuaries also worked closely with the Senate Finance Committee in the summer of 1972. As the provisions of the Senate bill became clearer, they received appropriate attention.

The full Senate bill was not reported out of the Finance Committee until September 26, early in the week that it went to the Senate floor. Neither the Senate nor the House bill contained the kidney provision, so estimates had not been prepared for this last-minute amendment. Gordon Trapnell, director of health insurance studies in the Office of the Actuary, SSA, recalls that he had never heard of ESRD before that week.

Consequently, not until Thursday evening, September 28, did Trapnell hear from Mongan, asking for an estimate.[8] Hartke, Mongan informed

Trapnell, had introduced a provision that would cover patients for dialysis or kidney transplantation after a six-month waiting period. The National Kidney Foundation had estimated the cost of the proposal at $35 million to $75 million in the first year. Could Trapnell get back to the committee staff within 24 hours with some idea of what the cost of such a provision might be?

Trapnell called Mongan the following afternoon. The estimate was difficult to make, he said, "both because of the poor data that was available and because of the unusually large number of highly volatile variables involved, such as technological advance, [and the] very expensive nature of transplant operations and dialysis." The SSA Office of the Actuary estimated the first-year cost, on an incurred basis, in the range of $100 million to $500 million, increasing substantially in later years to a level several times the initial amount (Trapnell, 1973).

The working assumption, shared by legislative and executive branch officials (including the actuaries), was that Senate floor amendments to social security legislation were usually symbolic gestures of support for particular constituencies. Such amendments were regarded as prime candidates for removal from a bill in conference with the House. In this case, however, it became clear after the Senate action on September 30 that the kidney amendment had a good chance of being adopted (Trapnell, 1973).

Consequently, in the first week of October, the health actuaries were asked by both committees for estimates for the conference committee. Trapnell recalls preparing these for zero, three-, and six-month waiting periods and projecting these estimates 25 years into the future. His staff then computed the average tax rate required to finance the hospital insurance cost of the provision, the resulting average annual cost, and the cash cost in each of the first five years (using the zero, three-, and six-month waiting periods).[9]

How did Congress respond to the uncertain cost estimates? Trapnell's memorandum provides a useful glimpse of the scene:

The conferees met to resolve the differences between the Senate and House versions of H.R. 1 toward the end of the next week and discussed the kidney disease provision on Saturday night, October 14, 1972, around 9 o'clock in the evening. When the staff brought out the provision, Chairman Mills looked up and said, "I have the greatest sympathy for those people; what does it cost?" He and Senator Long had in front of them a piece of note paper on which appeared the first year incurred cost (for HI [Hospital Insurance] and SMI [Supplementary Medical Insurance] together) and the average tax rate for HI for a zero, three months, and six months waiting periods. I was summoned to the end of the table opposite Mr. Mills and Senator Long by Mr. Ball [Commissioner of Social Security Robert Ball] to answer their questions. I pointed out that the cost was expected to increase many times over the 25 year period for which hospital cost tax rates are set and that this was why the average cost provided was so much higher than the first year costs. I also pointed out that the Senate provision effectively had no waiting period due to the impossibility of determining when the onset of chronic kidney [disease] occurred; but dialysis would substantially reduce the costs, as indicated in the estimates provided (average cost of .09% with no waiting period, .06% with a three month waiting period, and .05% with a six month waiting period). I further explained that the relatively larger drop from a zero to 3 month waiting period than from a 3 month to 6 month waiting period was due to the concentration of inpatient dialysis in the first month or so and that nearly all transplants occurred six months or more after the beginning of dialysis. I also explained that there was a very large difference between inpatient, outpatient, and home dialysis care. Mr. Mills selected the 3 month waiting period as being the most cost effective and turned to Long (who nodded) and then to the other conferees saying "that's all right with you, isn't it?"—and they nodded. Thus the care of persons suffering from chronic kidney disease became law.

Several further comments are warranted about the estimation process. One concerns what was being estimated. Technically, the actuaries' estimates pertained to the narrow language of the kidney amendment, which established a Medicare benefit for individuals *under 65 years of age*, not for those who were 65 or older. It was presumed that the benefit existed for the elderly, however, because a Medicare benefit could not be established for those under 65 and not be available for the elderly. In fact, very few elderly persons were being dialyzed at that time and none were receiving transplants. Although the Bureau of Health Insurance had answered several inquiries in the previous year, the nature and extent of coverage for the elderly had not been clarified. Estimates by the actuaries of the cost of the entitlement were for those under 65 and failed to account for the "induced cost" that would result from increased treatment by the elderly as services expanded. Similarly, estimates of the impact on Medicare focused on the costs of treating kidney disease, not on the use of additional Medicare resources for other than renal conditions. Yet the entitlement was to individuals with ESRD for Medicare benefits—not just for kidney disease treatment.

Finally, the working problem for the actuaries and Congress was whether the increase in payroll tax was sufficient to cover the expenditure impact of the new provision. Trapnell remembers that the revenue side of the bill actually included more funds than were necessary. This was not widely publicized, however, because the actuaries discovered afterward that another, more costly provision in the legislation had been underestimated.

The demands of complex legislation like H.R. 1 for estimates of expenditure impact and the corresponding increases required in the

FICA tax are substantial. Estimates must often be developed in a short time. All decision makers, whether they be actuaries, committee staff, or members of Congress, consequently reduce decisions to their simplest form and limit analysis to the bare minimum. For the kidney entitlement, the actuaries prepared their estimates in the final stages of the legislative process. They did so quickly and did not publish them widely. This was costly to the ESRD program for two reasons. The "estimates" used by Senator Hartke, which were provided by Scribner and Kountz and transmitted by the National Kidney Foundation, seriously underestimated the costs of the program. Neither the actuaries nor the congressional staff took them seriously; yet no one challenged them, and they became the only available public numbers.

Second, a controversy broke out in January 1973 between the Office of the Assistant Secretary of Health (OASH), an agency that felt considerably stronger after Nixon's landslide victory over George McGovern in early November, and the Democratic Congress. The leadership and staff of OASH harbored partisan distrust of the SSA Bureau of Health Insurance and of the close ties between the bureau's Medicare professionals and the key congressional committee staff. The front page of the *New York Times* was the arena for the clash (Altman, 1973; Lyons, 1973; *New York Times*, 1973). The controversy resulted in a new set of "estimates" by OASH that called into question the Hartke numbers. The political damage created by this challenge affected supporters of the legislation and stalked the program for years to come.

SUMMARY AND CONCLUSIONS

How did it happen that Congress enacted the kidney entitlement as one of the Social Security Amendments of 1972? In a previous paper I suggested a "tipping" process was at work, borrowing the concept from Schelling's discussion of changes in neighborhood composition (Schelling, 1972). "It was necessary," I wrote, "for the cumulative effect of an increasing number of government programs to be felt. Moreover, it appears that widespread publicity of lives lost for lack of scarce medical resources was necessary, including specific dramatization of identified lives at stake. Finally, the number of patients being kept alive had to increase to the point where they simply could not be ignored" (Rettig, 1976). The growth in patients, physicians, and treatment centers created strong momentum for government action.

Broad-scale, across-the-board advocacy for kidney disease characterized the efforts of the National Kidney Foundation. It assembled the demands of patients and physicians and focused them on the PHS, including the research programs of NIH, vocational education, and the crippled children's program. The effort was neither one of scattershot nor one of reliance on hitting a single target but rather one designed to advance the cause.

And Congress was receptive. It had already authorized limited programs in the PHS. Furthermore, members had been hearing from constituents without the means to pay for life-saving treatment, and they had introduced numerous legislative proposals over a relatively long period of time. Authority over the Medicare statute involved a few representatives and senators, and a small set of staff aides, who effectively managed a broad legislative consensus that could not be resisted. The deliberate cycle of the policy process, in which issues accumulated and were addressed every three or four years, facilitated consideration of specific matters as part of major legislation like H.R. 1.

If the Medicare kidney entitlement had not been adopted in the Social Security Amendments of 1972, what would have happened? One can only speculate about the answer to this question. History is the record of the contingent possibilities that were selected and the vapor trail of those that were not. I believe that some public policy responsive to the needs of kidney disease patients would have been adopted. It might not have taken the form of a Medicare entitlement. In any event, it would have represented a peculiarly American adaptation to this country's particular dual "system" of publicly financed care for the elderly, the poor, and the disabled, and privately financed health insurance for the working population. One can imagine many scenarios.

Was equity violated by favoring kidney disease patients over others with arguably comparable claims? In retrospect, it appears so. At the time, however, as noted in this paper, it was widely expected that national health insurance or at least some form of catastrophic health insurance would be enacted within a few years of the 1972 legislation. Moreover, the extension of Medicare coverage to the disabled was seen by all key participants as a sine qua non justification of Section 2991.

What importance should attach to the estimates of program costs? Practically speaking, better estimates might have barred or slowed congressional action. But how are good estimates made about an unknown future under circumstances in which data are few, time is short, the agenda is long, and the fundamental political, not technical, issue is "What is to be done?"

And what kind of question is the estimation question in the first place? It would be strange indeed if the world were suddenly purged of the public and private programs that had involved serious early cost misestimates. Even though we aspire to rationality in the conduct of human affairs, it is hard to imagine a more draconian social decision-making criterion than adherence to predictions about unknown futures.

The estimation question, in fact, is more an issue about outcomes. The Medicare ESRD program reflects the benefits and burdens of modern medical technology. It is characterized by moderately high program expenditures, and thus genuine opportunity costs, with very high "unit costs" for a relatively few but nontrivial number of beneficiaries. It represents effective, life-saving treatment for many patients, but such treatment is transmuted into merely life-prolonging therapy for others with serious complications and comorbidities and low quality of life (as "objectively" measured by external observers) (Evans et al., 1985). These "outcomes" are sufficiently complicated to induce thoughtful reflection by all observers.

Finally, we must ask whether the medical, moral, and political bases for policy were sound. Medically, two effective treatments existed that saved lives and palliated symptoms but did not cure the underlying disease. Morally, this technology was financed to save lives. It is hard to conceive of a public justification for failing to intervene. Politically, Congress was responding to genuine constituent needs by providing funds from the public fisc, insuring individual citizens against one form of catastrophic illness, hardly an unreasonable thing to do. The bases were sound but vulnerable to repeated challenge. The kidney disease entitlement remains a focus for debate about the relative benefits and burdens of medical technology.

AFTERWORD

In June 1990, I interviewed former Senator Russell B. Long in his Washington, D.C., law office. The following summarizes my notes of Long's responses in that interview.

"It was clear from the beginning that government health insurance would involve costs beyond what anyone was telling you at the time. I thought, how do we move into this thing? It was clear that we would do something like England and other nations. To what extent can we keep it in the private sector? To what extent do we need to do it by the government?

"For starters, I thought we should do catastrophic cases. I sponsored legislation. It was not original with me; Paul Douglas [former Democratic senator from Illinois] had the idea long ago. But I could not have given a reliable estimate of the cost of cancer, heart disease, stroke. A majority of the committee were not willing to vote to report a catastrophic bill or bring it to the floor.

"Jay Constantine or Jim Mongan, or both, came to me to say that Senator Hartke was going to sponsor a kidney amendment. They thought it was meritorious and that I was well advised to accept it and perhaps join as a cosponsor. If the time is right, why not join? is my view. If you are for something, why not cosponsor it? Otherwise, I would have had to oppose it, defeat it, and explain why. It is one thing to say that something is premature. It is another thing if you are going to have to vote on the record. Often you would rather vote for something than explain why you voted against it.

"I can recall testimony by a doctor that impressed me. He testified that he had patients with kidney failure—hardworking people, good, responsible citizens, honest, salt-of-the-earth people. 'What are my possibilities?' they would ask. 'Kidney transplant, dialysis, or death,' he would reply. 'What does it cost?' was their next question. When told, they responded, 'There is no way to raise that kind of money. What am I to do?' "As chairman [of the Senate Finance Committee], I sat there and thought to myself: We are the greatest nation on earth, the wealthiest per capita. Are we so hard pressed that we cannot pay for this? A life could be extended 10 to 15 years. You're not going to make any money that way. But it struck me as a case of compelling need.

"My attitude on Medicare and catastrophic was that the government shouldn't start out paying bills that people were able to pay themselves. The overwhelming majority of middle-income people needed some help to pay the bills, but it was better to help them than to pay the bill. On catastrophic, though, it was an area where it was appropriate for the government to say 'We'll take care of you.'

"My attitude at the time, probably not expressed on the floor but in committee or conference, was that the kidney amendments would give us some sense for the cost and impact of coverage for catastrophic illness. If it turned out a lot worse than the estimates, that ought to give us some basis for thinking about catastrophic illness. The cost of catastrophic will jolt you. Kidney may be a jolt, but it will be nothing compared to all catastrophic. For advocates of action, cost is not important. It is the right thing to do. If you have responsibility for paying the bill, though, it is a different matter."

[Question: What estimate were you given?]

"They gave me an estimate of approximately $1 billion a year. On estimates, look at the original Medicaid estimate of $200 million. A few years down the line it was at $20 billion. They initially looked at what the states were doing at the time. A minor change in the regulations can change things in a major way."

[Question: In retrospect, do you have any second thoughts, any reservations, about the kidney amendment?]

"On this one, no. It was an idea whose time had come. It has done a lot of good. It has brought some of the same problems as Medicare and catastrophic, cost control problems. But it was something that the government should have been involved in."

APPENDIX

Public Law 92-603, 92nd Congress, H.R. 1
October 30, 1972

Chronic Renal Disease Considered to Constitute Disability

Sec. 299I. Effective with respect to services provided on and after July 1, 1973, section 226 of the Social Security Act (as amended by section 201(b)(5) of the Act) is amended by redesignating subsection (e) as subsection (f), and by inserting after subsection (d) the following new subsection:

"(e) Notwithstanding the foregoing provisions of this section, every individual who—

"(1) has not attained the age of 65;

"(2) (A) is fully or currently insured (as such terms are defined in section 214 of this Act), or (B) is entitled to monthly insurance benefits under title II of this Act, or (C) is the spouse or dependent child (as defined in regulations) of an individual who is fully or currently insured, or (D) is the spouse or dependent child (as defined in regulations) of an individual entitled to monthly insurance benefits under title II of this Act; and

"(3) is medically determined to have chronic renal disease and who requires hemodialysis or renal transplantation for such disease;

shall be deemed to be disabled for purposes of coverage under parts A and B of Medicare subject to the deductible, premium, and copayment provisions of title XVIII.

"(f) Medicare eligibility on the basis of chronic kidney failure shall begin with the third month after the month in which a course of renal dialysis is initiated and would end with the twelfth month after the month in which the person has a renal transplant or such course of dialysis is terminated.

"(g) The Secretary is authorized to limit reimbursement under Medicare for kidney transplant and dialysis to kidney disease treatment centers which meet such requirements as he may by regulation prescribe: *Provided*, That such requirements must include at least requirements for a minimal utilization rate for covered procedures and for a medical review board to screen the appropriateness of patients for the proposed treatment procedures."

NOTES

1. Workshop participants, with historical identities noted, included Carl W. Gottschalk, M.D., who had chaired the Bureau of the Budget Committee in

1966-1967 that prepared the *Report of the Committee on Chronic Kidney Disease*, Washington, D.C., 1967; Jay Constantine, staff director of the Subcommittee on Health, Senate Finance Committee; William D. Fullerton, professional staff, House of Representatives, Committee on Ways and Means; David McCusick, assistant actuary (for Medicare), Social Security Administration (SSA); Charles L. Plante, Washington representative of the National Kidney Foundation (NKF); George E. Schreiner, M.D., past president and chairman of the committee on legislation, NKF; Gordon R. Trapnell, chief actuary (for Medicare), SSA; Irwin Wolkstein, deputy director (for policy), Bureau of Health Insurance, SSA; and James J. Mongan, M.D. (who participated by telephone), professional staff to the Subcommittee on Health, Senate Finance Committee.

2. Senator Jackson had a personal interest in Scribner's work. In 1964, a close grammar school friend of Jackson's, Ms. Kay Sloane, had become one of Scribner's patients. She began dialysis in 1967 and lived until 1977.

3. Noteworthy of Najarian's efforts in this regard was the sponsorship in 1972 by Senator Walter F. Mondale (D-Minn.) of legislation that emphasized kidney transplantation.

4. Even with the small number of patients in 1967, the Gottschalk Committee deemed both dialysis and transplantation to be established treatments that were no longer experimental.

5. Byrnes, an avid fan of the Green Bay Packers, was informed of the status of a key Packer with kidney disease by the treating nephrologist in Neenah, Wisconsin.

6. Constantine credits Paul Rettig with inventing the formula that permanent kidney failure patients were "deemed to be disabled for purposes of coverage under Parts A and B of Medicare," thus making the kidney amendment part of the larger disability provisions.

7. Kountz was also prominent as the only black transplant surgeon in the country. Moreover, he had come to San Francisco from Little Rock, Arkansas, his home state, and was known to Mills and his staff.

8. David McCusick, Trapnell's assistant, recalls receiving a call from Mongan at 9 a.m. on Saturday, September 30, before the amendment was taken to the floor, asking for an estimate. He recalls saying that within 10 years the provision would cost $2 billion a year, an estimate that Mongan, according to McCusick, did not believe. Mongan does not recall this conversation. No documentation exists to check these differing recollections about an obviously hectic time.

9. Gordon Trapnell's January 18, 1973, memorandum included attachments indicating estimates for the kidney disease provision of 25-year costs to the hospital insurance portion of the program and the cash cost for the first five program years. These attachments were missing from the copy of the memorandum that was available to me.

REFERENCES

Altman, L. 1973. Kidney foundation criticizes articles on care costs. New York Times, January 19, p. 30.

Bureau of the Budget. 1967. Report of the Committee on Chronic Kidney Disease. Washington, D.C.

Evans, R., D. L. Manninen, L. P. Garrison, Jr., L. G. Hart, C. R. Blagg, R. A. Gutman, A. R. Hall, and E. G. Lowrie. 1985. The quality of life of patients with end-stage renal disease. New England Journal of Medicine 312:553-559.

Institute of Medicine. 1989. Workshop on the Kidney Disease Entitlement. Washington, D.C., December 18-19.

Lyons, R. 1973. Program to aid kidney victims faces millions in excess costs. New York Times, January 11, p. 1.

Medical World News. 1967. Secret panel weights U.S. kidney policy. August 15, pp. 36-38.

New York Times. 1973. Medicarelessness. January 14, p. 16.

Rettig, R. A. 1976. The policy debate on patient care financing for victims of end-stage renal disease. Law and Contemporary Problems 40:196-230.

Rettig, R. A. 1977. Cancer Crusade: The Story of the National Cancer Act of 1971. Princeton, N.J.: Princeton University Press.

Rettig, R. A. 1981. Formal analysis, policy formulation, and end-stage renal disease. Case Study #1 in Background Paper #2: Case Studies of Medical Technologies; The Implications of Cost-Effectiveness Analysis of Medical Technology. Contractor report for the Office of Technology Assessment, U.S. Congress. Washington, D.C.

Rettig, R. A. 1982. The federal government and social planning for end-stage renal disease: Past, present, and future. Seminars in Nephrology 2:111-133.

Schelling, T. 1972. A process of residential segregation: Neighborhood tipping. In Racial Discrimination in Economic Life, Anthony Pascal, ed. Lexington, Mass.: Lexington Books.

Trapnell, G. R. 1973. Memorandum concerning cost estimates furnished to the Congress during consideration of H.R. 1 for the cost of chronic kidney disease amendment. January 18.

U.S. Congress, Conference Committee. 1972. H.R. 1, Social Security Amendments of 1972: Brief Description of Senate Amendments (prepared for the use of the conferees). Conference committee print, 92nd Congress, 2nd Session, October 11, pp. 13-14.

U.S. Congress, House, Committee on Ways and Means. 1971a. National Health Insurance Proposals. Hearings, 92nd Congress, 1st Session, October 19, 20, 26-29, November 1-5, 8-12, 15-19, Parts 1-13.

U.S. Congress, House, Committee on Ways and Means. 1971b. National Health Insurance Proposals. Hearings, 92nd Congress, 1st Session, October 19 and 20, Part 1 of 13 parts, pp. 218-236.

U.S. Congress, House, Committee on Ways and Means. 1971c. Statement of Shep Glazer, Vice President, National Association of Patients on Hemodialysis, et seq., National Health Insurance Proposals. Hearings, 92nd Congress, 1st Session, November 4, part 7 of 13 parts, pp. 1524-1546.

U.S. Congress, House, Committee on Ways and Means. 1971d. National Health Insurance Proposals. Hearings, 92nd Congress, 1st Session, November 11, Part 10 of 13 parts, pp. 2226-2228.

U.S. Congress, House, Committee on Ways and Means. 1972. Material Relating to Amendments to the Administration's National Health Insurance Partnership Act. Committee Print, 92nd Congress, 2nd Session, February 10.

U.S. Congress, Senate, Committee on Finance. 1971. Social Security Amendments of 1971. Hearings, 92nd Congress, 1st Session, July 27, 29, August 2 and 3.

U.S. Congress, Senate, Committee on Finance. 1972a. Social Security Amendments of 1971. Hearings, 92nd Congress, 2nd Session, January 20, 21, 24, 25, 27, 28, and 31, February 1-3, 7-9, Parts 2-6.

U.S. Congress, Senate, Committee on Finance. 1972b. Social Security Amendments of 1972. 92nd Congress, 2nd Session, Report No. 92-1230, September 26 (legislative day, September 25).

118 U.S. Congressional Record 4840-4842, 1972a.

118 U.S. Congressional Record 33003, 1972b.

118 U.S. Congressional Record 33009, 1972c.

Commentary

Carl W. Gottschalk

The circumstances of this case are unique in at least two regards. Patients with chronic renal failure are a cohort of identified individuals with an inexorable progress of their disease to a fatal outcome. There is absolute certainty that the disease process will be fatal unless patients are treated by one of the two available treatment modalities, which are potentially either curative (kidney transplantation) or palliative (chronic dialysis). Either can prolong survival for many years. The other unique feature of this case is that Section 2991 of the Social Security Amendments of 1972 is the only entitlement for a specific disease process, namely, chronic kidney failure.

Richard A. Rettig presents a fascinating account of the enactment of Medicare coverage for patients with chronic kidney failure. At his initiative, for the first time, many of the principals, legislative assistants, officials of the Social Security Administration, and leading advocates for the program who were involved in passage of the legislation were assembled for a candid discussion of the events immediately preceding the adoption of the program in October 1972. The context of those events was multifaceted. Two very expensive treatment modalities had been painstakingly developed, largely at taxpayer expense, but they were essentially inaccessible except to the

Carl W. Gottschalk is a Career Investigator of the American Heart Association and Kenan Professor of Medicine and Physiology at the University of North Carolina at Chapel Hill. He chaired the Gottschalk Committee.

very wealthy because of the great discrepancy between supply and demand. The equity issue was agonizing. The proceedings of "life or death committees," as they struggled with rationing these services in the few centers in which they were available, received widespread media attention.

Advocacy groups consisting of patients, their families, and physicians, as well as the National Kidney Foundation, worked vigorously to stimulate federal and state governments to provide financial coverage for treatment. The issue of equity became even more sharply focused when in 1963 the Veterans Administration announced its intention to establish treatment units in VA hospitals across the country. The Public Health Service also established a number of treatment centers as demonstration units with decreasing funding. The widespread public visibility of these issues and the major fiscal considerations led the President's Office of Science and Technology Policy to prompt the Bureau of the Budget to establish an expert committee to consider all aspects of the problems posed by chronic kidney disease and to make recommendations that addressed these problems. The committee's recommendations were not pursued.

The 1967 report of this committee in effect resolved the debate about the experimental versus established nature of the two treatment modalities and recommended a federal program involving Medicare entitlement for chronic kidney failure patients similar to the provision that was eventually adopted. Although the report was well known to nephrologists, members of Congress and key congressional staff were totally unaware of it.

Why was a national program adopted in 1972? Simply, the time was right. As the media extensively and effectively told the public, a serious health care problem existed, with many thousands dying each year because there was no access to scarce and costly treatment modalities. The unrelenting lobbying effort of several individuals was instrumental in creating a growing awareness of this need among members of Congress and their staff. Support for the proposed program abetted the political aspirations of certain powerful legislators, and at the time there was much congressional support for national catastrophic health insurance. The kidney legislation was viewed as a pilot program.

All of these factors came together in the push toward completing action on the amendments to the social security legislation. There was little time for staff assistants and Social Security Administration actuaries to develop estimates of cost and the number of patients involved, and they were unaware of the detailed projections in the Bureau of the Budget report. Nevertheless, by a kind of political alchemy, the program was adopted with minimal public debate and signed into law by President Nixon one week before the 1972 presidential election.

The hastily assembled cost estimates quickly proved to be seriously underestimated, and today costs continue to escalate. In 1987 they were $2.8

billion, and equaled 3 percent of total Medicare costs. Ironically, the original legislation called for quality control surveillance that could have helped in cost control, but this feature has never been implemented.

The great quandary when the legislation was enacted was whether to proceed with a less than perfect treatment program for the fatally ill or wait for a research breakthrough that would cure or preferably prevent the occurrence of chronic renal failure. Twenty-eight years later, this quandary persists. Thousands of lives have been extended for very significant periods of time. The extent of rehabilitation and the quality of life have been variable, but few have opted to drop out of the program. Techniques have improved and unit costs of transplantation and dialysis have decreased, but no research breakthrough is in sight. This commentator believes that such policy decisions should be based on the public's opinion as implemented by their informed elected officials.

Commentary

Stanley Joel Reiser

The funding of kidney dialysis and transplantation through the federal budget of the United States in 1972 was a landmark decision in modern health care policy. As such, it has suffered a fate characteristic of landmark events—to be often cited but rarely understood. We are then indebted to Richard Rettig for the clarification his essay offers.

Why it should count as a landmark is perhaps the most interesting facet of this tale of policy and a question to be engaged shortly. But first let us proceed to other features of this story, beginning with the influence of a frequently used instrument of policy—the advisory committee report. Here, it is represented by the 1967 *Report of the Committee on Chronic Kidney Disease*, which is known commonly, taking the name of its chair, as the Gottschalk report.

The advisory committee is now a commonly used instrument of policy in the United States. Its stated purpose generally is to sort out in a controversial subject the true state of events, which it accomplishes through a panel of learned and often uninvolved parties. Such reports, however, are often commissioned or used after they are written for extrascientific purposes such as gaining support for a particular political position, pacifying critics, or postponing action. Rettig indicates that the report scientifically resolved the ques-

Stanley Joel Reiser is the Griff T. Ross Professor and Director of the Program on Humanities and Technology in Health Care at the University of Texas Health Science Center, Houston.

tion of whether dialysis and transplantation were effective in favor of the therapy and recommended the payment mechanism that was eventually decided upon for it—Medicare entitlement. Yet his research indicates that the report was virtually unknown to key policymakers who ultimately fashioned the 1972 kidney legislation.

This situation is a typical fate of policy papers. Those for whom the paper is significant or even intended often do not see it. How to get such relevant data to decision makers is a problem that requires attention. Just as pressing an issue, however, is the fact that such documents are rarely designed for the multiple purposes to which they will ultimately be put. Here we can learn much from the British, who have a long history of policymaking through their version of advisory committees, the royal commission.

The congressional hearing is a second feature of this story. Like the advisory committee, it is a vehicle for knowledge seeking, but as a forum for Congress, political purpose openly pervades its use. Rettig sheds a revealing light on the true events occurring on November 4, 1971, when the House Ways and Means Committee provided a forum for testimony on kidney disease therapy and allowed the dialysis of a patient before members of Congress and the press. By this time, the dialysis machine had become a potent symbol of the power of the emerging technology of medical rescue; technology that could make both biologically secure and socially productive life possible. Just as penicillin stood for the progress medical science was making through drugs when it was introduced in the 1940s, so the kidney dialysis machinery had become for the 1970s the epitome of medicine's ability to turn away death with advanced machines that could substitute for critical biological functions. Politicians found support of such innovation attractive and, in the end, easy to give—as long as their cost was not prohibitive.

It is here that miscalculation crept in, for the ground under the long-term estimates of a new technology's cost cannot be trusted to sustain the weight of future uses. No one foresaw in 1972 the magnitude of the growth in dialysis and transplantation because no one could anticipate how future clinicians would expand the clinical indications for the technology. Time and again, projections of a technology's use are based on indications from the present continuing into the future. New developments that improve the effectiveness and safeness of a technology, clinical experience with its use, and changes in reimbursement policy are some of the many facts that inevitably influence the way a technology is applied. Such uncertainties should be recognized and cited in the development and announcement of projected costs.

As the costs of treating kidney disease have passed the $2 billion mark and are creeping toward $3 billion per year, many wonder at the wisdom of the initial policy and recommend caution in introducing federal financing of disease-specific therapy. It is in this negative sense that the kidney treatment program is cited as a landmark—of a policy not wisely calculated from a fiscal perspective and of a disease-specific approach that is inappropriate for the public financing of medical care because it is unfair to those who suffer from other ailments.

It must be understood, however, that the approach of the United States to coverage of population groups for medical care has followed an incremental and sometimes disease-based pattern. For example, in the nineteenth and twentieth centuries, public facilities for treatment of mental illness and mental retardation were made available. Thus, the kidney treatment legislation was within the realm of American policy tradition for health care. Furthermore, this is not the first time that long-term program costs have been underestimated by government. We do it continually, with the overruns on Medicare and Medicaid as even more dramatic examples of our failings.

Thus, a misreading of the traditions of American health policy accounts for one source of criticism of federal funding of kidney disease treatment. But there is another facet that helps explain the place of the kidney legislation as a cautionary tale in the lore of health policy—the ambivalent feelings generated in us by its technological mainstay, the dialysis machine. It is a power that saves and a power that costs; it makes life possible, but that life can be a source of misery. The evocation of such multiple and conflicting images creates ambiguity and perplexity regarding appropriate clinical use and public policy. The dialysis machine has become a metaphor for modern technological medicine, and deciding the right response to this whole new area of treatment continues to elude the makers of policy and holders of political power in the United States.

Deliberations of the Human Fetal Tissue Transplantation Research Panel

James F. Childress

This case study focuses on the deliberations of the Human Fetal Tissue Transplantation Research Panel during the period September-December 1988. It analyzes the major debates that occurred about conflicting principles and values as a majority of the panel reached the conclusion that the use of human fetal tissue in transplantation research, following deliberate abortions, is "acceptable public policy" if certain "guidelines" are in place. The panel's deliberations occurred in an evolving context that comprised medical-scientific, social-political, legal, and cultural factors. To interpret the panel's deliberations and recommendations, it is necessary to discuss aspects of this context and the background to the panel's efforts.

In addition to drawing on the references and other bibliographic materials listed below, the author held telephone conversations in June 1990 with several people who had been involved at the National Institutes of Health (NIH) and the Department of Health and Human Services (DHHS) in decision making, question formation, panelist selection, and other activities involved with human fetal tissue trans-

James F. Childress is the Edwin B. Kyle Professor of Religious Studies and Professor of Medical Education at the University of Virginia. He served on the Human Fetal Tissue Transplantation Research Panel.

plantation research. The author is most appreciative for helpful comments from the following: Jay Moskovitz, Charles McCarthy, Miriam Davis, Barbara Harrison, Judy Lewis, and LeRoy Walters. Of course, they are not responsible for errors of fact or interpretation in the case study.

BACKGROUND AND CONTEXT

By the mid-1980s, promising animal research on fetal tissue transplantation that had been under way for some time both in the United States and abroad had led several researchers in other countries to experimentally transplant human fetal tissue, following elective or spontaneous abortions, into human patients with Parkinson's disease. In addition, in the United States, NIH had awarded an extramural grant to Hans Sollinger of the University of Wisconsin to study transplantation of human fetal pancreatic cells into patients with diabetes. In late 1987 NIH received a request from intramural investigators at the National Institute of Neurological and Communicative Disorders and Stroke for permission to undertake research transplanting human fetal neural tissue, following elective abortions, into patients with Parkinson's disease. Even though he had the legal authority to approve this research—and some members of his staff urged him to do so—James B. Wyngaarden, the director of NIH, sought approval from the Office of the secretary of DHHS to "permit maximum review of this sensitive area of research" (Office of Science Policy and Legislation, 1988). Wyngaarden's memorandum of October 23, 1987, to Robert Windom, then assistant secretary for health, noted that the proposed research had "the potential for publicity and controversy" and "may be characterized in the press as an indication that the Department is encouraging abortions," even though the "research will in no way be a factor in a woman's decision to have an abortion and no Federal funds will directly or indirectly support abortion." The memorandum also stressed NIH's conviction that "on balance . . . the importance of this research outweighs any potential for adverse publicity."

In a March 22, 1988, memorandum to the director of NIH, the assistant secretary for health declared a moratorium on the use of federal funds to support human fetal tissue transplantation research (hereafter, HFTTR) that used tissue from induced abortions until NIH could convene "special outside advisory committees" to hear testimony, deliberate, and offer their recommendations. His memorandum identified 10 questions that such committees should address (see Appendix A), which focused mainly on the connection or linkage between abortion and the use of human fetal tissue in research. The assistant secretary's staff developed the questions on the basis of an analysis of the existing literature and after consultation with three academic bioethicists. Whereas the NIH director's memorandum focused on the public controversy that might result from the federal government's sponsorship of such research, the assistant secretary's staff perceived the problem as largely ethical.

There are several relevant features of the context of the deliberations of NIH, DHHS, and the HFTTR panel. First, there had been earlier research that used human fetal tissue, and many of these projects had support from NIH. In fiscal year 1987, NIH awarded 116 grants and contracts (estimated at $11.2 million) for research that involved the use of human fetal tissue (Office of Science Policy and Legislation, 1988). Most of this research, however, had no direct therapeutic intent and did not involve transplantation. One widely reported earlier example of the use of human fetal tissue in research was in the development of the polio vaccine. Some commentators (e.g., Nolan, 1988) distinguish using cadaveric fetal tissue to *develop* a treatment from using it *as* a treatment.

Second, animal research had shown that transplantation of human fetal neural tissue might provide therapeutic benefits for patients with Parkinson's disease. Fetal tissue has special features that make it potentially useful in this case—for example, it is immunologically more naive than developed tissue, and it grows and differentiates rapidly. Furthermore, fetal tissue is widely available from the 1.5 million abortions performed in the United States each year.

Third, the U.S. Supreme Court decision in *Roe* v. *Wade* in 1973 overturned restrictive abortion laws but failed to resolve the serious moral and political debate and conflict about abortion in the United States. Opponents of abortion have been quite active since then and have regularly challenged practices, policies, or laws that appear to encourage abortions.

Fourth, beyond the legal framework for abortion, the transfer of human cadaveric tissue is governed by the Uniform Anatomical Gift Act (UAGA), which was adopted by all 50 states and the District of Columbia in the late 1960s and early 1970s. In general, the UAGA permits either parent, subject to the known objection of the other, to donate fetal tissue, following spontaneous or deliberate abortions, for research, education, or transplantation. However, some states restrict the use of fetal materials following induced abortions in some research (DHHS/NIH, 1988; see vol. 1, p. 11, and vol. 2, app. F). Federal regulations permit research "involving the dead fetus, macerated fetal material, or cells, tissue, or organs excised from a dead fetus . . . in accordance with any applicable State or local laws regarding such activities" (45 CFR 46.210). Many of the existing federal regulations focus on research involving the living fetus rather than on the use of tissue derived from fetal remains. Also of relevance is the National Organ Transplant Act of 1984 with subsequent amendments, which will be discussed later.

PROCESS

During early summer 1988, NIH appointed the HFTTR panel to meet in the fall to respond to Assistant Secretary Windom's questions and then to submit its finished report to the NIH Director's Advisory Committee, a diverse outside group that advises NIH on policy matters. NIH had reason to expect that a favorable recommendation from the panel and the advisory committee would lead to DHHS authorization to NIH to approve the research. On the recommendation of an internal, informal ad hoc committee, NIH appointed Arlin Adams, a retired federal judge from Philadelphia, to chair the fetal tissue panel; as a Republican opposed to abortion, he was considered an ideal choice. In addition, NIH appointed special panel chairpersons for scientific issues (Kenneth J. Ryan, a physician and scientist) and ethical and legal issues (LeRoy Walters, an ethicist).

Members of Congress, members of the executive branch, and organizations with an interest in the research, among others, submitted nominations for the 21-person panel; the various categories of nominations were ethicists, lawyers, biomedical researchers, clinical physicians, public policy experts, and religious leaders. The ad hoc committee (which included the panel's chair and co-chairs and a member of the NIH Director's Advisory Committee) considered the nominations in early July, emphasizing in their selections the qualifications of proposed panelists and the need for more women and minority panel members. There was vigorous outside support for particular nominees, much of which centered on opponents of abortion; three—James Bopp, James Burtchaell, and Daniel Robinson—were selected. In a departure from the nominations model being used, one senator asked to review the proposed list and personally discussed the proposed panelists with NIH officials prior to their invitation to serve. One of the conditions for serving on the panel was that the prospective panelist had to agree to be available for the first meeting, which was already planned for September 16-18, 1988. After the members of the panel were announced, defenders of HFTTR worried about the presence of strong opponents of abortion on the panel; critics of HFTTR, on the other hand, thought they discerned an overall bias among the panel in favor of such research. (For a list of panelists, see Appendix B.)

Just prior to the panel's first meeting, the White House leaked a draft executive order that proposed a ban on transplantation research using human fetal tissue following elective abortions. Otis Bowen, then secretary of health and human services, responded that he would not impose new curbs on HFTTR until the advisory committees could make their final recommendations or until he received a direct order from the President. Over the next several weeks, 50 members of Congress wrote to the President urging him to promulgate the executive order that would signify his commitment to protecting unborn lives; several hundred physicians and others also wrote, offering their strong support for the proposed order. However, no action was taken.

In September 1988, the HFTTR panel convened to hear scientific, legal, and ethical views from more than 50 invited speakers as well as testimony from representatives of public interest groups. All meetings of the panel were opened to the public after an initial announcement of several closed, executive sessions drew a vigorous negative reaction. When it became clear that the three-day meeting would not be sufficient for the panel to complete its deliberations and offer its response, a second meeting was set for October 20-21. In a draft report considered at the second meeting, the panel offered relatively brief responses to the assistant secretary's questions but little justification for them. During the meeting there was discussion about whether such justifications could be developed without a third meeting; the panel decided to submit only what had been developed and accepted by the time of adjournment. But at the end of the second meeting, James Bopp and James Burtchaell brought in a long dissent to the report. Several other panelists were concerned that this long dissent would overwhelm the brief responses in the report, especially considering that the recommendations were left without sufficient justification. A third meeting was scheduled for December 5, with members of the panel preparing and circulating in advance drafts of "considerations" for each response to the assistant secretary's 10 questions. At that meeting the report was put into final form: it contains the responses and considerations, along with the panel vote, for each question; a brief summary of the current scientific literature relevant to HFTTR; three concurring statements (Judge Arlin Adams; Aron Moscona, joined by two other panelists; and John Robertson, joined in whole or in part by ten other panelists); two dissenting statements (by David Bleich and by James Bopp and James Burtchaell); and a final dissenting letter (Daniel Robinson). Volume 2 of the report contains the written testimony submitted to the panel.

After observing the meetings, science writer Jeffrey Fox described the panel's process: "Despite the diversity of views held by members of the *ad hoc* panel, the group steadfastly tried to follow a consensual approach during its deliberations. Although consensus was difficult to achieve, the panel members consistently tried to accommodate one another's respective positions. Thus, in most cases, very disparate philosophical positions were melded into a coherent stance that was deemed acceptable by a substantial majority of the panel. However, neither of these observations should be taken to suggest that the debate within the panel was somehow constrained by the majority viewpoint, as indeed it was not" (Fox, 1988). The panelists spent a great deal of time debating and modifying the wording of particular responses to gain as much consensus as possible. The majority frequently compromised on the exact wording, but the minority often voted against the response that had been carefully worked out through compromise.

The panel experienced other constraints, including the pressure to complete a report as quickly as possible and the lack of staff and resources; originally the panel had been expected to offer a report on the basis of one meeting. The tight schedule, the pressure for a prompt report, and the limited resources all contrasted sharply with the arrangements for other bodies dealing with ethical issues in science and health care, such as the National Commission for the Study of Ethical Problems in Biomedical and Behavioral Research, the President's Commission for the Study of Ethical Problems in Medicine, and the Task Force on Organ Transplantation. Another major constraint was the 10 questions raised by the assistant secretary. As noted earlier, these questions focused on issues related to abortion rather than on issues parallel to transplantation of other cadaveric tissue. Thus, it is not surprising that the panel's deliberations concentrated to a great extent on ethical and societal concerns about abortion without directly addressing the morality of abortion.

THE MORAL STATUS OF THE FETUS AND THE MORALITY OF ABORTION

With this sketch of the background, context, and process of the panel's deliberations and recommendations, we can now turn to an examination of the major explicit and implicit issues it faced. One of the major issues involved the status of fetal life—for example, whether the fetus should be viewed as tissue, as a potential human life, or as a living human being. Certainly the members of the panel differed greatly in their individual views on this question, which required some of them to oppose the use of fetal tissue following abortions. Others contended that it was possible to separate, morally and practically, abortions and the use of fetal tissue, despite the fact that elective abortions provide the bulk of tissue for HFTTR.

Some panel members contended that their acceptance of various guidelines or safeguards to separate abortion decisions from decisions about the use of fetal tissue did not imply that they viewed abortion as immoral. The recommended guidelines were intended to reduce the likelihood that the possibility of donation would influence the pregnant woman's decision to abort. Even if abortion were not viewed as immoral, these guidelines could be accepted for various reasons, including (1) the desire to allay the moral controversy in our society about abortion, or (2) the desire to reduce the vulnerability of some pregnant women to exploitation and coercion because of the need for fetal tissue. These reasons are sufficient to justify the guidelines, without the presupposition that abortion is immoral.

Thus, while accepting the proposition that "it is of moral relevance that human fetal tissue for research has been obtained from induced abortions," the majority of the panel nevertheless held that, in view of the significant medical goals of HFTTR and the legality of abortion, "the use of such tissue is acceptable public policy." In the consideration it noted for this response, the panel observed that "a decisive majority of the panel found that it was acceptable public policy to support transplant research with fetal tissue either because the source of the tissue posed no moral problem or because the immorality of its source could be ethically isolated from the morality of its use in research" (DHHS/ NIH, 1988:2). Thus, the panelists who voted for using fetal tissue for research subscribed to one of two views: (1) that abortion is morally acceptable and the use of aborted fetal tissue for HFTTR is morally acceptable; or (2) that abortion is "immoral or undesirable," although legal, and HFTTR can be morally separated from abortion and can proceed with appropriate safeguards. The majority rejected the position that HFTTR should be prohibited from receiving federal funds because it is, morally speaking, inextricably linked to or would lead to immoral abortions.

COMPLICITY, COLLABORATION, AND COOPERATION IN MORAL EVIL

During the panel's deliberations, James Burtchaell, a theologian at Notre Dame University, invoked the language of complicity, collaboration, and cooperation in the moral wrongdoing of others to stress what he considered the impossibility of separating, at least in practice, the use of fetal tissue from the (immoral) abortions that produced it (Bopp and Burtchaell, 1988:63-70). Particularly important for Burtchaell was a form of indirect association that implied moral approval. Cooperation that involves casual actions—for example, driving the getaway car after a robbery—must be distinguished from actions that only symbolize, convey, or express approval but do not materially contribute to the actions themselves. Burtchaell invoked various analogies. One involved the banker in a town in Florida who decided to accept deposits from participants in the drug trade on the grounds that this action would benefit the community and that the drug trade would continue regardless of what the banker did. Another was of the researcher who visits an abortionist each week to obtain fetal tissue but who each time expresses his disapproval while planning to return the next week. Burtchaell contends that these actions involve complicity in the moral wrongdoing of others, whether drug trafficking or abortion.

According to written testimony from the Bishops' Committee for Pro-Life Activities of the National Conference of Catholic Bishops, "it may not be wrong in principle for someone unconnected with an abortion to make use of a fetal organ from an unborn child who died as the result of an abortion; but it is difficult to see how this practice can be institutionalized [including arrangements to ensure informed consent] without threatening a morally unacceptable collaboration with the abortion industry" (DHHS/NIH, 1988:E42; for a slightly different version, see G1). What may be possible in the abstract, in principle, or in theory is not possible in practice because of the institutionalization of abortion and the way fetal tissue is currently procured. James Bopp and James Burtchaell write in their dissent: "Our argument, then, is that whatever the researcher's intentions may be, by entering into an institutionalized partnership with the abortion industry as a supplier of preference, he or she becomes complicit, though after the fact, with the abortions that have expropriated the tissue for his or her purposes. It is obvious that if research is sponsored by the National Institutes of Health, the Federal Government also enters into this same complicity" (Bopp and Burtchaell, 1988:70).

There are at least two responses to the charge of moral cooperation in the wrongdoing of others. One is to deny that the primary action, in this case, abortion, is morally wrong; another is to deny that the use of aborted fetal tissue implies approval of abortion. The panel did not try to resolve the debate about the morality of abortion, but the majority insisted that it is at least possible to draw a moral line between the use of fetal tissue and the abortions that make the tissue available in such a way as to ensure that unacceptable moral cooperation does not occur (DHHS/NIH, 1988:2). The majority of the panel noted that it is possible to use organs and tissues from homicide and accident victims without implying approval of homicides and accidents and without diminishing efforts to reduce their occurrence (Robertson, 1988:31-32). Even if one were to accept that abortion is immoral, "it does not follow that use of fetal remains makes one morally responsible for or an accomplice in abortions that occur prior to or independent of later uses of fetal remains" (Robertson, 1988:31). In addition, the majority statement underlined the fact that abortions are already being performed with the result that fetal tissue that could benefit others is being discarded rather than used.

Several members of the panel strongly objected to the analogies to Nazi research on living subjects invoked by James Bopp and James Burtchaell to illustrate moral complicity in the wrongdoing of others (Bopp and Burtchaell, 1988:63-70). Critics contended that there are several morally relevant differences between the use of tissue from dead fetuses following debatably immoral abortions and the clearly immoral actions of Nazi investigators who experimented on living subjects against their will (Robertson, 1988:32-33; Moscona, 1988:27-28). In a concurring statement, a majority of the panelists noted that the complicity claim "is considerably weakened when the act making the benefit possible is legal and its immorality is vigorously debated, as is the case with abortion. Given the range of views on this subject, perceptions of complicity with abortions that will occur regardless of tissue research should not determine public policy on fetal tissue transplants" (Robertson, 1988:33).

Panelists also noted that the loose concept of complicity in the moral wrongdoing of others could be turned in other directions, perhaps even against the positions held by those who invoked it in the context of HFTTR. For example, critics of the application of the concept of complicity in HFTTR argued that a failure to provide sex education, contraceptives, and social support for pregnant women could be construed as modes of complicity and cooperation in the actions of abortion. In this instance, the alleged complicity or cooperation is the material contribution of causal factors through omission.

Recognizing that some potential participants in research, whether as patients or as professionals, might want to avoid any connection and thus any felt complicity with abortion, the panel recommended that "potential recipients of such tissues, as well as research and health care participants, should be properly informed as to the source of the tissues in question" (DHHS/NIH, 1988:1-2).

INCREASE IN THE NUMBER OF ABORTIONS

One fundamental question in the fetal tissue controversy is whether its use in transplantation research would result in an increase in the number of abortions and if so, whether it would still be justified. Answers to this question hinge in part on matters that should be resolvable by empirical data—the reasons why women have abortions. The panel's report noted that "the reasons for terminating a pregnancy are complex, varied, and deeply personal" and "regarded it highly unlikely that a woman would be encouraged to make this decision [to abort] because of the knowledge that the fetal remains might be used in research" (DHHS/ NIH, 1988:3). In addition, the panel noted the lack of any evidence that, over the past 30 years, the possibility of donating fetal tissue for research purposes had resulted in an increase in the number of abortions (DHHS/NIH, 1988:3). Furthermore, according to the panel majority, it is possible to set up guidelines or safeguards to reduce the likelihood of an impact on the incidence of abortion. Defenders of the minority position argue, however, that knowledge of this possibility of benefit from the provision of fetal tissue would make a difference in some, perhaps even many, cases. There are several possible scenarios addressed by the critics and defenders of HFTTR; they are organized below more systematically than in the HFTTR panel's report.

General Altruism

First, would the possibility of donating fetal tissue to benefit unrelated and unknown patients through transplantation play a role in a woman's decision to abort? Neither the defenders nor the critics of HFTTR can find strong evidence for their claims about the potential impact of this possibility on individual abortion decisions (DHHS/NIH, 1988:3). The debate thus hinges on speculations about women's abortion decisions and on answers to the moral question about which way society should err in such a situation of doubt.

Critics charge that HFTTR would reduce some pregnant women's ambivalence about abortion so that the possibility of an altruistic act— what could be called "general altruism"—would probably lead to some abortions that would not otherwise have occurred. Defenders of HFTTR respond that such a claim is speculative: there is only sketchy evidence about women's decision making about abortion and no evidence that the long-time possibility of donating fetal tissue to benefit others through research (although only rarely through transplantation research) has led to any abortions that would not otherwise have occurred (DHHS/NIH, 1988:3). Even if it was known that the possibility of donating fetal tissue provided a "motivation, reason, or incentive for a pregnant woman to have an abortion," this would not constitute a prohibited "inducement" (under federal law) because it is not a promise of financial reward or personal gain and is not coercive (DHHS/NIH, 1988:4).

In such complex personal decisions as abortion, it is difficult to determine the role of various motives, such as general altruism, and particularly whether these motives are necessary or sufficient for an action. In the case of panel members, however—whether their motives were to protect the fetus, to prevent exploitation and coercion of pregnant women, or to allay moral controversy—the majority of them proposed guidelines to reduce the likelihood that HFTTR would lead some women to abort when they would not otherwise have done so. These guidelines include efforts to prevent the stimulation or encouragement of general altruistic motives on the part of pregnant women.

According to the panel, "the decision and consent to abort must precede discussion of the possible use of the fetal tissue and any request for such consent as might be required for that use," and "informed consent for an abortion should precede informed consent or even the preliminary information for tissue donation," except when the pregnant woman requests such information (DHHS/NIH, 1988:3-4). Ideally, the request and the decision to donate should follow the abortion decision itself, but because postmortem tissue deteriorates quickly and cryogenic storage is not possible for many transplants, "the pregnant woman must be consulted before the abortion is actually performed" (DHHS/NIH, 1988:10).

In a concurring statement prepared largely by John Robertson and joined, at least in part, by 10 other panel members, a majority of the panelists allow that even an increase in the number of abortions would not be a decisive reason for rejecting federal support of HFTTR: "Yet even if *some* increase in the number of family planning abortions due to tissue donation occurred, it would not follow that fetal tissue transplants should not be supported. Surely it does not follow that *any* increase in the number of abortions makes fetal tissue transplants unacceptable" (Robertson, 1988:34). Drawing a distinction between means, ends, and consequences, this argument denies that an increase in the number of elective abortions is a means to the end of HFTTR. Instead, an increase in the number of elective abortions is a possible consequence, a risk, of the use of HFTTR. Risk is a probabilistic notion and includes the probability of a negative outcome. It is thus necessary to judge the likelihood of a negative outcome along with its magnitude. The risk of an increase in fetal deaths is comparable to other losses of life in the pursuit of important societal goals, such as automobile design, highway engineering, and bridge building. According to Robertson's concurring statement, "[t]he risk that *some* lives will be lost, however, is not sufficient to stop those projects when the number of deaths is not substantial, when the activity serves worthy goals and when reasonable steps to minimize the loss have been taken" (Robertson, 1988:34). Furthermore, a "more stringent policy is not justified for fetal tissue transplants just because the risk is to prenatal life from *some* increase in the number of legal abortions" (Robertson, 1988:34-35).

Noting that the risk of an increase in the number of abortions is speculative at best, the report's concurring statement stresses that similar speculative and tenuous risks that the society might encourage, as well as legitimate deaths resulting from homicide, suicide, and accidents, to gain organs for transplantation are not viewed as a sufficient reason to stop using organs from these sources (Robertson, 1988:35 [fn. 23]). In a later response (Mason, 1990), Assistant Secretary for Health James Mason contended that in the argument above, the concurring statement simply disregarded moral and ethical considerations. Nevertheless, its signers view it as offering a different balance of moral and ethical considerations instead of a denial of those considerations. In addition, the panel maintained that its recommended guidelines would reduce the probability of an increase in the number of abortions.

A different risk-benefit calculation appears in the dissent by J. David Bleich, who holds that "these mitigating safeguards [the ones proposed by the panel] notwithstanding, intellectual integrity compels recognition that the goal of preventing an increment in the total number of abortions performed is not totally attainable" (Bleich, 1988:39). He interprets the majority's proposals as an effort to balance interests "through a policy of damage containment" (Bleich, 1988:40). By contrast, he notes that the duty to rescue human life through fetal tissue transplants is diminished because the studies at issue are *research* protocols with uncertain, distant benefits rather than certain immediate good for identified lives, and because the "moral harm" of the increase in the number of abortions is certain and immediate. Hence, "on balance, the duty to refrain from a course of action that will have the effect of increasing instances of feticide must be regarded as the more compelling moral imperative" (Bleich, 1988:43). This formulation appears to leave open the possibility of a different balance if the procedure reached the point, without federally funded research, of providing an immediate, certain benefit. By contrast, the majority of the panel held that the increase in the number of abortions was not certain and immediate and could be avoided at least in part through the proposed guidelines.

Specific Altruism

The second scenario raises the possibility that a pregnant woman (or a woman contemplating pregnancy) might donate fetal tissue to help a family member or acquaintance, which could result in abortions that would not otherwise have occurred. In contrast to the motivation of general altruism considered above, this motivation might be called specific altruism, that is, beneficence toward specific known individuals. Because of dramatic proposals by a few women to become pregnant in order to abort and donate fetal tissue to help a beloved family member, and its recognition of the strength of specific altruistic motives, the panel recommended this guideline: "There should be no Federal funding of experimental transplants performed with fetal tissue from induced abortions provided by a family member, friend, or acquaintance. Absent such prohibition, the potential benefits to friends and family members might encourage abortion or encourage pregnancy for the purpose of abortion—encouragements that the panel strongly opposed" (DHHS/NIH, 1988:8). Another formulation reads: "The pregnant woman should be prohibited from designating the transplant-recipient of the fetal tissue" (DHHS/NIH, 1988:3). In yet another recommendation with the same import, the panel held that "anonymity between donor and recipient shall be maintained, so that the donor does not know who will receive the tissue, and the identity of the donor is concealed from the recipient and transplant team" (DHHS/NIH, 1988:4).

These recommendations clearly reflect the panel's concerns about maternal welfare as well as concerns about the morality of abortion. Moreover, they are based on the lack of evidence that "a prohibition against the intrafamilial use of fetal tissue would affect the attainment of valid clinical objectives" (DHHS/NIH, 1988:8). For example, in fetal tissue transplants for diabetes, it would be medically contraindicated to use intrafamilial transplants, but no definitive conclusions can be drawn at this time about other conditions for which fetal tissue transplantation may be a possibility. Nevertheless, in the considerations it noted for its response, the panel referred to expert testimony that "if circumstances change . . . there may be reasons to modify the prohibition . . . it was strongly urged that the Secretary for Health and Human Services review these recommendations at regular intervals" (DHHS/NIH, 1988:8). In the last section of the concurring statement, which was prepared by John Robertson and signed by ten other panelists (with the exception of this section, in which one of the ten did not concur), this position is elaborated: "If the situation changes so that the supply of fetal tissue from family planning abortions proves inadequate, the ban on donor designation of recipients and aborting for transplant purposes should be re-examined. The ethical and legal arguments in favor of and against such a policy would then need careful scrutiny to determine whether such a policy remains justified" (Robertson, 1988:38).

Incentives of Financial Gain

In a third way—beyond general and specific altruism—the possibility of HFTTR could provide another motive for abortion in the shape of financial incentives for the provision of fetal tissue. Congress had already addressed this issue by passing an amendment (which Ronald Reagan signed into law) to the National Organ Transplant Act that prohibited the transfer of human organs (including fetal organs and their subparts) for "valuable consideration, or payment." The panel's report supported this position, stressing that "it is essential . . . that no fees be paid to the woman to donate, or to the clinic for its efforts in procuring fetal tissue (other than expenses incurred in retrieving fetal tissue)" (DHHS/ NIH, 1988:9). As is true of several of the panel's other recommendations, this one could be justified as a way to protect fetuses from abortion, to protect women from exploitation and coercion, to reduce moral controversy, and even to help avoid societal commodification of "human" body parts.

SOCIETAL LEGITIMATION OF ABORTION DECISIONS AND PRACTICES

Although the topic of societal legitimation tends to collapse into issues of complicity in and encouragement of abortions, it may be useful to consider it separately. According to Dorothy Vawter (1990), "to legitimate an act or practice is to justify or promote it in such a manner that others will become more inclined to regard it as acceptable and to engage in it." On the one hand, critics contend that federally funded HFTTR following elective abortions would tend to legitimate abortion because of the difficulty—or even the impossibility—of distinguishing within the expenditure of federal funds (1) approval of the use of fetal tissue from elective abortions and (2) approval of the elective abortions that produced the fetal tissue. Rabbi David Bleich argued in the panel's report that "[f]ederal funding conveys an unintended message of moral approval for every aspect of the research program" (Bleich, 1988:40[fn. 2]). By contrast, defenders of the research could argue that the approval of the use of federal funds in treatment of end-stage renal disease through organ transplantation does not constitute approval of the homicides, suicides, and accidents that provide the occasions for organ donation (Robertson, 1988:35[fn. 23]). Furthermore, they might note that there is no evidence that efforts to reduce such events have abated in order to maintain the supply of needed organs.

A second version of the societal legitimation argument focuses on society's acceptance of the benefits of human fetal tissue donations following elective abortions rather than on government funding. It would be difficult, perhaps even impossible, critics argue, for society to accept the benefits of HFTTR without becoming increasingly inclined to accept as legitimate the abortions that make the benefits possible. (Such a legitimation would be likely to occur even if no federal funds were used to support HFTTR protocols.) Thus, if HFTTR were to confer substantial benefits in the form of new life-saving or life-enhancing procedures, society would become less likely to delegitimate abortion by declaring many acts of abortion illegal (provided future Supreme Court decisions make such declarations more possible). It is not likely that society will renounce either the benefits of HFTTR or the decisions and practices that make the benefits possible.

Because of the panel's focus on federal funding, it only addressed the first version of the societal legitimation argument. The panel maintained that this symbolic societal legitimation could be avoided by the separation measures it proposed (see the earlier discussion of complicity). The second version of the societal legitimation argument focuses more on society's acceptance of abortion decisions and practices rather than on individual decisions, and it may not be directly countered by the panel's arguments that its proposed separation measures would reduce the likelihood that HFTTR would encourage abortion decisions by particular women.

A final criticism of societal legitimation appears in the panel's report in the dissenting letter by Daniel Robinson, who argued "that induced abortion is a moral wrong and that it cannot be redeemed by any actual or potential 'good' secured by it. Thus, the possible medical benefits held out by research tissues obtained by such measures cannot be exculpatory" (Robinson, 1988:73). This argument was offered after the report was completed, but the panel could have responded that it attempted to *separate* abortion decisions and practices from decisions and practices regarding the use of fetal tissue. HFTTR using fetal tissue from elective abortions in no way redeems or exculpates the abortions themselves. It only involves the use of tissue that would otherwise be discarded or incinerated, without implying approval (or, for that matter, disapproval) of the abortions themselves, just as the use of tissue from adult cadavers does not imply approval of—or redeem or exculpate— the homicides or negligent accidents that resulted in death.

DISPOSITIONAL AUTHORITY OVER FETAL REMAINS

The fourth question posed by Assistant Secretary Windom was as follows: "Is maternal consent a sufficient condition for the use of the tissue, or should additional consent be obtained? If so, what should be the substance and who should be the source(s) of the consent, and what procedures should be implemented to obtain it?" This question engendered one of the most divisive debates of the HFTTR panel as members wrestled with the problem of dispositional authority over fetal tissue following abortions, including the authority to transfer fetal tissue for use in transplantation research. The vote in favor of the sufficiency of maternal consent (within limits) was 17 yes, 3 no, and 1 abstention, the smallest majority of any answer to any question.

The argument surrounding this question also focused on ways to separate the abortion decision of the pregnant woman from the decision about the use of fetal tissue. The majority held that "fetal tissue from induced abortions should not be used in medical research without the prior consent of the pregnant woman. Her decision to donate fetal remains is sufficient for the use of tissue, unless the father objects (except in cases of incest or rape)" (DHHS/NIH, 1988:60). Critics of this view contended that when the pregnant woman "resolves to destroy her offspring, she has abdicated her office and duty as the guardian of her offspring, and thereby forfeits her tutelary powers" (Bopp and Burtchaell, 1988:47). From this perspective the abortion decision deprives the pregnant woman of any subsequent authority over the disposition of the fetus. Thus, this viewpoint requires a total separation between the decision to abort and the decision to use or transfer tissue for use; this separation is put into practice by disqualifying the woman who decides to abort from making a decision about fetal tissue use.

Of the several possible modes of transfer of fetal tissue—donation, abandonment, expropriation, or sales—the panel recommended donation, which is the dominant method of transfer of cadaveric organs and tissues in the United States. Donation is carried out mainly in the form of *express donation* by the decedent or by the decedent's next of kin but also by *presumed donation* for corneas in several states. "Express donation by the pregnant woman after the abortion decision is the most appropriate mode of transfer of fetal tissue because it is the most congruent with our society's traditions, laws, policies, and practices, including the Uniform Anatomical Gift Act and current Federal research regulations" (DHHS/NIH, 1988:6). (The panel heard some evidence that fetal tissue probably has been viewed at times as abandoned and has been used without maternal consent [DHHS/NIH, 1988:11].) The panel further argued that a woman's choice of a legal abortion does not disqualify her legally and should not disqualify her morally from serving as "the primary decisionmaker about the disposition of fetal remains, including the donation of fetal tissue for research." Against arguments that the decision to abort leaves only biological kinship, without any moral authority, the panel concluded

that disputes about the morality of her decision to have an abortion should not deprive the woman of the legal authority to dispose of fetal remains. She still has a special connection with the fetus and she has a legitimate interest in its disposition and use. Furthermore, the dead fetus has no interests that the pregnant woman's donation would violate. In the final analysis, any mode of transfer other than maternal donation appears to raise more serious ethical problems. (DHHS/NIH, 1988:6)

A concurring statement (written by John Robertson and signed by a majority of the panelists) disputed the guardianship model affirmed by the Bopp-Burtchaell dissent, contending that it "mistakenly assumes that a person who disposes of cadaveric remains acts as a guardian or proxy for the deceased, who has no interests, rather than as a protector of their own interests in what happens to those remains" (Robertson, 1988:36). (Of course, where the deceased has expressed his or her wishes, then the situation is different.)

Although the panel accepted the structure of the UAGA (revised, 1987) as generally adequate, it recommended a modification in policy for the donation of fetal tissue in federally funded research. The UAGA allows either parent to donate fetal tissue unless the other parent objects. The panel concluded, however, that "the pregnant woman's consent should be *necessary* for donation—that is, the father should not be able to authorize the donation by himself, and the mother should always be asked before fetal tissue is used. In addition, her consent or donation should be *sufficient*, except where the procurement team knows of the father's objection to such donation" (DHHS/NIH, 1988:7). Affirming that there is no legal or ethical obligation to seek the father's permission, the panel nevertheless held that there is "a legal and ethical obligation not to use the tissue if it is known that he objects (unless the pregnancy resulted from rape or incest)" (DHHS/NIH, 1988:7). In its recommendations on federal funding of HFTTR, the panel also stressed the importance of compliance with state laws and noted that at least eight states have statutes that prohibit the experimental use of cadaveric fetal tissue from induced abortions (DHHS/NIH, 1988:13; Smith, 1988).

LIMITS ON DISCLOSURE OF INFORMATION AND DECISION MAKING

Several times during its deliberations the panel addressed questions of the disclosure of information, as well as the specificity of the woman's decision to donate. On the one hand, the panel concluded that no information about the donation and use of fetal tissue in research should be provided prior to the pregnant woman's decision to abort, *unless* she specifically requested that information (DHHS/NIH, 1988:3, 4). Donation, in contrast to informed consent in medicine and research, generally does not presuppose the disclosure of detailed information. Yet, in addition to the requirement of informed consent for the research subject, that is, the recipient of the transplant, the woman having the abortion and donating fetal tissue is herself a research subject insofar as she provides a medical history and undergoes tests relevant to the research transplant. Any research protocol reviewed by the institutional review board (IRB) in a given situation will therefore involve procedures and consent documents that pertain to the woman as a research subject, and the IRB must determine the adequacy of the information disclosed to her when she is considering "whether to consent to tests (e.g., for antibody to the human immunodeficiency virus) to determine the acceptability of the fetal tissue for transplantation research" (DHHS/NIH, 1988:7). Within the model of stages of disclosure of information and decision making about the separate acts of abortion and donation, it is thus necessary to disclose information about tests to determine the acceptability of fetal tissue as part of the research protocol. Other issues include what to disclose to the pregnant woman about the test results.

For various reasons that have already been identified—the desire to separate the abortion decision from the donation decision, the desire to protect pregnant women from exploitation and coercion, and the desire to avoid fanning the flames of the abortion controversy—the panel recognized several limits on the pregnant woman's autonomy without restricting the abortion decision itself. In the UAGA there is no obligation to accept donated tissue and organs; hence, the woman's right to give fetal tissue does not engender an obligation on the part of anyone else to accept the gift. The pregnant woman has a right, the panel argued, to request and receive information about donation of fetal tissue prior to her abortion decision, but that information should not be disclosed to her as a matter of course if she does not request it. Here again, the rationale is to separate the two decisions to reduce the likelihood that knowledge of the possibility of donating will influence the decision to abort. In addition, the panel recommended that "the timing and method of abortion should not be influenced by the potential uses of fetal tissue for transplantation or medical research" (DHHS/NIH, 1988:4). In response to the assistant secretary's questions about potential pressure to modify the timing and method of abortion to secure older fetuses, the panel stressed that, according to the evidence it had received, there were no pressures for later abortions. It further insisted that, "to the extent that Federal sponsorship or funding is involved, no abortion should be put off to a later date nor should any abortion be performed by an alternate method entailing greater risk to the pregnant woman in order to supply more useful fetal materials for research" (DHHS/NIH, 1988:14).

Stressing the express donation model embodied in the UAGA, the panel's recommendations would allow the pregnant woman to choose whether to donate fetal tissue for research or some other purpose and to receive as much information as she needed regarding donation after she had decided to abort, without allowing her to know or to designate the recipient. By contrast, the 1989 report of Britain's Committee to Review the Guidance on the Research Use of Fetuses and Fetal Material (the so-called Polkinghorne report) recommended indeterminate donation to the extent of providing "no knowledge of what will actually happen to the fetus or fetal tissue"—to make it even less likely that the possibility of beneficial use of tissue will influence the woman's decision to have an abortion—and not allowing her "to make any direction regarding the use of her fetus or fetal tissue" (p. 10). Reflecting differences in sociocultural context, the British report does not emphasize the disclosure of information to the pregnant woman to the same extent as the U.S. panel report does. Similarly, the U.S. panel recommended the disclosure of the source of the tissue—that is, that it came from a fetus or fetuses provided by induced abortion—so that the potential recipient of the transplant could choose not to participate; the British report recommended against such disclosure. However, both reports recommended disclosure of information about the tissue source to health care professionals.

OTHER ISSUES AND RECOMMENDATIONS

A few other issues and panel recommendations merit attention before we turn to other developments, including recent public policy responses. The panel insisted on procedures that would accord dead human fetuses "the same respect accorded other cadaveric human tissues entitled to respect" (DHHS/NIH, 1988:1).

Although the panel did not discuss the implications of this recommendation, the principle entails that the dead human fetus not be subjected to procedures that are undignified or that show disrespect toward "cadaveric human tissue." This position does not presuppose that the fetus is a full human being; instead it may rest on other convictions—for example, that the fetus is a potential human being and has symbolic significance even when dead, or that respect for human fetal tissue is appropriate to avoid offending those who view the fetus as a full or potential human being. At any rate, the principle of equal respect implies that if it is justifiable to use any "cadaveric human tissue" in transplantation research—for example, after accidents or homicides—then it is justifiable to use cadaveric fetal tissue after abortions.

Throughout its deliberations the panel recommended institutional procedures and arrangements to avoid conflicts of interest, that is, situations in which parties might have some incentive to encourage pregnant women to abort to provide fetal tissue. The panel concluded that concerns about the impact of the use of fetal tissue on the practices of abortion clinics could be "best addressed by strict adoption of a number of safeguards; safeguards that would eliminate or at least radically reduce profit motives and tendencies toward commercialization, and safeguards that would ensure the greatest possible separation between abortion procedures, facilities, and personnel on the one hand, and fetal-tissue research procedures, facilities and personnel on the other" (DHHS/NIH, 1988:10). These safeguards included the insistence, in accord with current federal law and many state laws, that no fees be paid to the abortion clinic "for its efforts in procuring fetal tissue (other than expenses incurred in retrieving fetal tissue)" (DHHS/NIH, 1988:9; see also p. 10); in addition, however, the panel recognized that, in order "to prevent abortion clinics from making profits from fetal tissue donation, specific rules for what counts as a reasonable payment for retrieval expenses may be required" (DHHS/NIH, 1988:12). In accord with the spirit of the panel, other commentators have recommended additional precautions to separate the practices; for example, Annas and Elias (1989) argue that "to avoid any conflict of interest there should be no academic incentive (such as co-authorship of publications or grant support) or other incentive for the physician performing the abortion or anyone else involved in the woman's care, to obtain her agreement for the use of fetal tissue."

Another major set of issues centers on the justification of human fetal tissue transplantation *research*, particularly from the standpoint of potential recipients. According to federal regulations and common practice, ethically justified research must satisfy several criteria, including favorable benefit-risk ratios (Levine, 1986). Such benefit-risk analyses presuppose careful laboratory and animal studies before research involving human subjects can be justified. In response to Assistant Secretary Windom's question about whether animal studies justify HFTTR for certain diseases, the panel concluded that "there is sufficient evidence from animal experimentation to justify proceeding with human clinical trials in Parkinson's disease and juvenile diabetes," but not enough evidence from animal studies to justify proceeding with HFTTR for other diseases (DHHS/NIH, 1988:14; see also pp. 19-20). The panel did not have the research protocol that had been submitted to NIH and thus did not approve or disapprove a specific research protocol as a peer review process or institutional review board would have done.

OTHER DEVELOPMENTS AND PUBLIC POLICY RESPONSES

This case study has focused on the deliberations and recommendations of the HFTTR panel. The panel's report was submitted to the Director's Advisory Committee of NIH on December 14, 1988, with oral presentations by nine of the ten panel members who attended (another absent panel member's statement was entered into the record). The report of the Director's Advisory Committee, *Human Fetal Tissue Transplantation Research* (December 14, 1988), notes that the advisory committee members and NIH council representatives quickly concluded that the panel's report was "an impressive and skillfully crafted document" that reflected "extensive and thoughtful work." "[G]iven the divisiveness underlying our society on the issues related to the topic under consideration, the report represented a remarkable consensus" (Advisory Committee to the Director, NIH, 1988:4). After reviewing and discussing the panel's report, the advisory committee unanimously approved three recommendations:

- to accept the report and the recommendations of the panel as written;
- to recommend that the assistant secretary for health lift the moratorium on federal funding of human fetal tissue transplantation research utilizing tissue from induced abortions; and
- to accept current laws and regulations governing human fetal tissue research with the development of additional policy guidance as appropriate, to be prepared by NIH staff to implement the recommendations of the panel (Advisory Committee to the Director, NIH, 1988).

The panel's report and the advisory committee's report were not forwarded to DHHS until January 1989, just before the end of the Reagan administration, which took no action on the reports. After President Bush's inauguration, controversy developed over his nominee for secretary of health and human services, in part because of concerns about his stand on abortion and related issues, including HFTTR. Hearings on Louis Sullivan's nomination included attention to these matters, and during the hearings Sullivan commented that he had not read the two reports an HFTTR and could not respond until he had done so (Rich, 1989; Tolchin, 1989). The reports were not released to the public until April 1989.

Then, on November 2, 1989, in a letter to acting NIH director William F. Raub, Secretary Sullivan informed NIH of his decision to continue indefinitely "the moratorium on Federal funding of research in which human fetal tissue from induced abortions is transplanted into human recipients." Stressing his office's discretion in the matter, as well as the extensive review and public discussion, he identified several substantive considerations. First, the administration and Congress had made it clear that DHHS should not fund activities that encouraged or promoted abortion, and Sullivan was persuaded that "permitting the human fetal research at issue will increase the incidence of abortion across the country." He continued: "I am particularly convinced by those who point out that most women arrive at the abortion decision after much soul searching and uncertainty. Providing the additional rationalization of directly advancing the cause of human therapeutics cannot help but tilt some already vulnerable women toward a decision to have an abortion." In support of his position he notes that 18 of the

21 members of the panel agreed to begin their report with the statement that "[i]t is of moral relevance that human fetal tissue has been obtained from induced abortions." However, he did not examine the different meanings this statement about "moral relevance" had to the different panelists or consider the significance of the fact that the three dissenters from this part of the report were also opposed to HFTTR and dissented from the report as a whole.

Second, Secretary Sullivan doubted that the desired "strict wall" between the abortion decision and the donation decision could be erected, however clear it might be in theory, because it "may be necessary to consult pregnant women before the abortion is actually performed" to be able to utilize postmortem tissue promptly. This consultation could influence the woman's decision making process.

Third, Sullivan noted that if the research proved successful, there would be a demand for more fetal tissue. He seemed to suggest that there would be a subsequent demand for more abortions, but did not address the question of whether the current rate of abortions would be sufficient to provide the needed tissue.

Finally, he noted that HFTTR can be continued in the private sector to generate "whatever biomedical knowledge" might emerge. There has been some privately funded HFTTR—for example, during fall 1988, at the University of Colorado and Yale University, and it continues there and perhaps elsewhere in the United States as well as abroad; yet some people express the fear that without federal funding the field will not grow rapidly or attract the best researchers. In addition, Sullivan's acceptance of private HFTTR did not address the concern expressed by Judge Arlin Adams, chairman of the HFTTR panel, who opposes abortion except in very limited situations:

> Without government funding there undoubtedly would be many efforts to use fetal tissue for medical research that would be completely unsupervised and not governed by any guidelines. Thus if the National Institutes of Health proceeds cautiously, and with carefully articulated safeguards and a program of periodic reviews, there would be much greater assurance that carefully crafted guidelines will be in place as an absolute condition to any research procedures. Such an arrangement would protect pregnant women and fetuses in a far more circumspect and intelligent manner than if the NIH did not participate in any way. (Adams, 1988:26-27)

James Mason, assistant secretary for health, reiterated and further amplified the views of DHHS, as expressed by Secretary Sullivan. In particular, he averred that "if just one additional fetus were lost because of the allure of directly benefiting another life by the donation of fetal tissue, our department would still be against federal funding. . . .

However few or many more abortions result from this type of research cannot be erased or outweighed by the potential benefit of this research" (Mason, 1990:17). He stressed moral and ethical factors (mainly having to do with abortion) that had to be weighed with the potential benefits of the research and called for a common effort to "find alternatives to fetal tissue transplantation" and "explore other research paths that lead us to the same ends." After the announcement of the indefinite extension of the moratorium, some abortion opponents indicated that they would apply pressure to eliminate not only transplantation research but all federally funded research involving human fetal tissue (Kolata, 1989).

In view of the subsequent disregard by Secretary Sullivan of the panel's conclusions, some panelists have indicated that they should have pressed for stronger language—for example, in contending that HFTTR is not only "acceptable public policy" but also "ethically acceptable"—because the numerous efforts to find compromise language to gain the support of more panelists left the report vulnerable at points and subject to neglect, misuse, and misquotation. To take one instance, Assistant Secretary Mason claimed that the majority of the panelists indicated that "moral and ethical considerations were not central to their view of the issue" (Mason, 1990:17). Yet rather than denying the centrality of "moral and ethical considerations," the panelists in the majority arguably had a different view of the dictates of morality and ethics and offered a different balance of such considerations.

Critics have sharply challenged DHHS's indefinite extension of the moratorium. Thirty-two medical research and education organizations, including the American Medical Association, the Association of American Medical Colleges, and the American Academy of Pediatrics, wrote Secretary Sullivan on January 4, 1990: "It is clear to us that the potential for good to result from this research outweighs the concerns about the impact on the abortion rate in this country, concerns that are at best speculative. Continuing the moratorium ignores the suffering of millions of Americans" (Hilts, 1990). After reviewing some documents and requesting others, Congressman Ted Weiss (D-N.Y.) contends that DHHS has offered no documentation that HFTTR would increase the number of abortions. In addition, he notes, even a member of DHHS's Office of General Counsel conceded that an extension of the ban would have a "shaky legal base" unless it was made permanent in the proper way through public notice with public comment and then by establishing a rule (Hilts, 1990). "The so-called indefinite moratorium," Congressman Weiss continues, "is a thinly veiled scheme to ban Federal funds for fetal tissue transplant research while avoiding the public outrage and scientific and legal scrutiny that would result from establishing a permanent ban. . . . I am hopeful Secretary Sullivan will be able to get beyond these abortion litmus tests to promote the crucial research that could be saving the lives of thousands of seriously ill Americans" (Hilts, 1990).

Similar themes emerged in the April 2, 1990, hearings on human fetal tissue research before the House Subcommittee on Health and the Environment of the Committee on Energy and Commerce, chaired by Congressman Henry Waxman. Following testimony from several members of the HFTTR panel, as well as by the assistant secretary for health, bioethicist John Fletcher accused the federal government of "moral recklessness" in the suppression and repression of several forms of research relating to the fetus and the embryo. He also noted the oddity of DHHS officials maintaining that it would be wrong for the federal government to fund HFTTR without condemning (and even apparently accepting) HFTTR funded through private sources.

CONCLUSION

In light of recent reports of the success of HFTTR for a Swedish (Lindvall, 1990) and a U.S. (Freed, 1990) patient with Parkinson's disease, the debate about the moral justifiability of the moratorium can be expected to continue. One former panelist, LeRoy Walters, has noted that the position taken by the panel, in contrast to the moratorium by DHHS, is in accord with the international ethical consensus on HFTTR using tissue from electively aborted fetuses. He observes that the recommendations of various committees or deliberative bodies around the world, which numbered at least nine by December 1988 and have been increased by several others since then, display "remarkable similarities." In fact, Walters says, there is "an impressive international consensus on the ethical standards that should govern the use of fetal tissue for research. The positions adopted in the panel's report are located squarely in the middle of this international consensus" (Walters, 1988; see also his testimony on April 2, 1990, before the Subcommittee on Health and the Environment). While conceding that there is no guarantee that such an international consensus is itself "ethically correct," Walters stresses that "we are less likely to make a serious moral mistake when numerous groups of conscientious men and women from around the world have sought to study the issue with great care and have reached virtually identical conclusions about appropriate public policy" (Walters, 1988). Within the United States, similar proposals, with minor variations, have emerged in the last two years from such groups as the Stanford University Medical Center Committee on Ethics (Greely et al., 1989) and the Councils on Scientific Affairs and on Ethical and Judicial Affairs of the American Medical Association (1990).

This case study has offered in passing several comparisons with other reports and actual or proposed policies in other countries, particularly the proposals of the Polkinghorne Committee in the United Kingdom in 1989. Several distinctive features of the social-political-cultural context in each nation account for differences in specific guidelines even within a strong international consensus on ethical standards. Obviously one major difference is the political strength of various groups that press certain moral visions or interests, such as the right-to-life movement in the United States. In addition, some concerns about HFTTR may be particularly appropriate in the United States because of special factors. First, many European countries have abortion laws that are more restrictive than those of the United States and thus may have less reason to fear the impact of HFTTR on abortion decision making and on the societal acceptance of abortion (Clendon, 1989). Second, there may be important differences in the commercialization and regulation of abortion clinics and of tissue procurement. For example, it could be argued that the HFTTR panel in the United States did not pay sufficient attention to actual institutional pressures (Annas and Elias, 1989), whereas the Polkinghorne report, which also recommended the separation of *decisions* regarding abortion and the use of fetal tissue, called for an intermediary as a mechanism of separation of the practice of abortion and the use of fetal tissue. (If there were more than one tissue bank, they would all function under a single intermediary organization.)

Sociocultural differences may lead to such variations in guidelines and approaches, even within a strong international consensus about the relevant ethical standards. One important question in the United States is whether, as some critics claim, public policy regarding HFTTR is being held hostage to the society's uneasiness about abortion, or whether the recommendations of the HFTTR panel or similar recommendations will be found to reflect an acceptable balance of ethical concern for fetuses, prior to and after their deaths; for pregnant women; for professionals and researchers; for patients who lack effective therapies and are potential beneficiaries of HFTTR; and for social integrity, including the democratic process. The debate is in part about how to proceed in a situation of doubt; thus, it also becomes a question of which side has the burden of proof when there is a lack of irrefutable evidence that it is possible to separate abortion decisions and practices sufficiently from decisions and practices regarding the use of fetal tissue following abortions. Because of the lack of irrefutable evidence, the panel recommended that the secretary of health and human services review the proposed guidelines at appropriate intervals. As of this writing, the moratorium continues to be defended by the secretary, and

Congress is considering legislation that would require a lifting of the ban. There is no doubt that this issue will continue to be argued on moral, ethical, legal, political, and medical grounds for some time.

EDITOR'S NOTE: A bill (H.R. 5661) that would lift the ban on federally approved fetal tissue transplantation research failed passage near the end of the 101st Congress. In January 1991, the American College of Obstetrics and Gynecology and the American Fertility Society announced they will form a national advisory board to monitor embryo and fetal tissue research in the absence of federal guidelines.

APPENDIX A

Appendix A is a March 1988 memorandum from the assistant secretary for health to the director of the National Institutes of Health. The memo lists 10 questions that should be addressed by a Human Fetal Tissue Transplantation Research Panel, once it is appointed and convened.

DEPARTMENT OF HEALTH & HUMAN SERVICES

Public Health Service
National Institutes of Health

Memorandum

Date   MAR 2 2 1988

From   Assistant Secretary for Health

Subject   Fetal Tissues in Research

To   Director, National Institutes of Health

I have given careful thought to your request to perform an experiment calling for the implantation of human neural tissue from induced abortions into Parkinson's patients to ameliorate the symptoms of this disorder.

This proposal raises a number of questions--primarily ethical and legal--that have not been satisfactorily addressed, either within the Public Health Service or within society at large. Consequently, before making a decision on your proposal, I would like you to convene one or more special outside advisory committees that would examine comprehensively the use of human fetal tissue from induced abortions for transplantation and advise us on whether this kind of research should be performed, and, if so, under what circumstances.

Among other questions, I would like the advisory committee(s) to address the following:

1. Is an induced abortion of moral relevance to the decision to use human fetal tissue for research? Would the answer to this question provide any insight on whether and how this research should proceed?

2. Does the use of the fetal tissue in research encourage women to have an abortion that they might otherwise not undertake? If so, are there ways to minimize such encouragement?

3. As a legal matter, does the very process of obtaining informed consent from the pregnant woman constitute a prohibited "inducement" to terminate the pregnancy for the purposes of the research--thus precluding research of this sort, under HHS regulations?

4. Is maternal consent a sufficient condition for the use of the tissue, or should additional consent be obtained? If so, what should be the substance and who should be the source(s) of the consent, and what procedures should be implemented to obtain it?

B1

Page 2 - Dr. Wyngaarden

5. Should there be and could there be a prohibition on the donation of fetal tissue between family members, or friends and acquaintances? Would a prohibition on donation between family members jeopardize the likelihood of clinical success?

6. If transplantation using fetal tissue from induced abortions becomes more common, what impact is likely to occur on activities and procedures employed by abortion clinics? In particular, is the optimal or safest way to perform an abortion likely to be in conflict with preservation of the fetal tissue? Is there any way to ensure that induced abortions are not intentionally delayed in order to have a second trimester fetus for research and transplantation?

7. What actual steps are involved in procuring the tissue from the source to the researcher? Are there any payments involved? What types of payments in this situation, if any, would fall inside or outside the scope of the Hyde Amendment?

8. According to HHS regulations, research on dead fetuses must be conducted in compliance with State and local laws. A few States' enacted version of the Uniform Anatomical Gift Act contains restrictions on the research applications of dead fetal tissue after an induced abortion. In those States, do these restrictions apply to therapeutic transplantation of dead fetal tissue after an induced abortion? If so, what are the consequences for NIH-funded researchers in those States?

9. For those diseases for which transplantation using fetal tissue has been proposed, have enough animal studies been performed to justify proceeding to human transplants? Because induced abortions during the first trimester are less risky to the woman, have there been enough animal studies for each of those diseases to justify the reliance on the equivalent of the second trimester human fetus?

10. What is the likelihood that transplantation using fetal cell cultures will be successful? Will this obviate the need for fresh fetal tissue? In what time-frame might this occur?

Page 3 - Dr. Wyngaarden

Based on the findings and recommendations of the advisory
committee(s), I would like you to reconsider whether you would
like to proceed with this kind of research, and, if so,
whether you wish to make any changes, regulatory or otherwise,
in your research review and implementation procedures for both
extramural and intramural programs.

Pending the outcome of the advisory committee(s)' assessment
and your subsequent review, I am withholding my approval of
the proposed experiment, and future experiments, in which
there is performed transplantation of human tissue from
induced abortions. You will note that this does not include
research using fetal tissues from spontaneous abortions or
stillbirths. However, I would like the special advisory
committee(s) to consider whether current research procedures
are adequate for the appropriate ethical, legal and scientific
use of tissue from these other sources.

I believe that greater input from outside professionals and
also from the public will enhance protections for research
participants and will help assure greater public confidence in
our work.

Robert E. Windom, M.D.

B3

APPENDIX B

Human Fetal Tissue Transplantation Research Panel

Arlin M. Adams *(Chair)*, Schnader, Harrison, Segal & Lewis, Philadelphia, Pennsylvania

Kenneth J. Ryan *(Chair, Scientific Issues)*, Chairman, Department of Obstetrics & Gynecology, Brigham and Women's Hospital, Boston, Massachusetts

LeRoy Walters *(Chair, Ethical and Legal Issues)*, Director, Center for Bioethics, Kennedy Institute of Ethics, Georgetown University, Washington, D.C.

J. David Bleich, Professor of Law, Cardozo Law School, New York, New York

James Bopp, Jr., Brames, McCormick, Bopp, and Abel, Terre Haute, Indiana

James T. Burtchaell, Professor of Theology, Department of Theology, University of Notre Dame, Notre Dame, Indiana

Robert C. Cefalo, University of North Carolina School of Medicine, Chapel Hill, North Carolina

James F. Childress, Chairman, Department of Religious Studies, University of Virginia, Charlottesville, Virginia

K. Danner Clouser, Professor, Hershey Medical Center, Pennsylvania State University, Hershey, Pennsylvania

Dale Cowan, Hematologist/Oncologist, Marymount Hospital, Garfield Heights, Ohio

Jane L. Delgado, President and Chief Executive Officer, National Coalition of Hispanic and Human Services Organizations, Washington, D.C.

Bernadine Healy, Chairman, Research Institute, Cleveland Clinic Foundation, Cleveland, Ohio

Dorothy I. Height, President, National Council of Negro Women, Alexandria, Virginia

Barry J. Hoffer, Professor of Pharmacology, Department of Pharmacology, University of Colorado, Denver, Colorado

Patricia A. King, Professor of Law, Georgetown University Law Center, Washington, D.C.

Paul Lacy, Professor of Pathology, Washington University School of Medicine, St. Louis, Missouri

Joseph B. Martin, Chief, Neurology Service, Massachusetts General Hospital, Boston, Massachusetts

Aron A. Moscona, Professor, Department of Molecular Genetics and Cell Biology, University of Chicago, Chicago, Illinois

John A. Robertson, Baker & Botts Professor of Law, University of Texas School of Law, Austin, Texas

Daniel N. Robinson, Chair, Department of Psychology, Georgetown University, Washington, D.C.

Charles Swezey, Annie Scales Professor of Christian Ethics, Union Theological Seminary, Richmond, Virginia

REFERENCES

Adams, A. B. 1988. Concurring statement. Pp. 25-28 in Report of the Human Fetal Tissue Transplantation Research Panel, vol. 1 (December). Bethesda, Md.: Department of Health and Human Services/National Institutes of Health.

Advisory Committee to the Director, National Institutes of Health. 1988. Human Fetal Tissue Transplantation Research. Bethesda, Md., December 14, 1988.

Annas, G. J., and S. Elias. 1989. The politics of transplantation of human fetal tissue. New England Journal of Medicine 320 (April 20):1079-1082.

Bleich, J. D. 1988. Fetal tissue research and public policy (dissenting statement). Pp. 39-43 in Report of the Human Fetal Tissue Transplantation Research Panel, vol. 1 (December). Bethesda, Md.: Department of Health and Human Services, National Institutes of Health.

Bopp, J., and J. T. Burtchaell. 1988. Human fetal tissue transplantation research panel: Statement of dissent. Pp. 45-71 in Report of the Human Fetal Tissue Transplantation Research Panel, vol. 1 (December). Bethesda, Md.: Department of Health and Human Services, National Institutes of Health.

Clendon, M. A. 1989. A world without Roe: How different would it be? Hastings Center Report 19 (July-August):22-37.

Committee to Review the Guidance on the Research Use of Fetuses and Fetal Material. 1989. Review of the Guidance on the Research Use of Fetuses and Fetal Material. London: Her Majesty's Stationery Office.

Councils on Scientific Affairs and on Ethical and Judicial Affairs. 1990. Medical applications of fetal tissue transplantation. Journal of the American Medical Association 263 (January 26):565-570.

Department of Health and Human Services/National Institutes of Health. 1988. Report of the Human Fetal Tissue Transplantation Research Panel. Bethesda, Md.: National Institutes of Health, vol. 2, December 1988.

Fox, J. 1988. Overview of panel meetings. Appendix A in Report of the Human Fetal Tissue Transplantation Research Panel, vol. 2 (December). Bethesda, Md.: Department of Health and Human Services, National Institutes of Health.

Freed, C. 1990. Transplantation of human fetal dopamine cells for Parkinson's disease. Archives of Neurology 47 (May):505-512.

Greely, H. T., T. Hamm, R. Johnson, C. R. Price, R. Weingarten, and T. Raffin. 1989. The ethical use of human fetal tissue in medicine. New England Journal of Medicine 320 (April 20):1093-1096.

Hilts, P. J. 1990. U.S. aides see shaky legal basis for ban on fetal tissue research. New York Times, January 30, 1990.

Kolata, G. 1989. More U.S. curbs urged in the use of fetal tissue. New York Times, November 19, 1989, pp. 1, 38.

Levine, R. J. 1986. Ethics and Regulation of Clinical Research, 2nd ed. Baltimore, Md.: Urban and Schwarzenberg.

Lindvall, O. 1990. Grafts of fetal dopamine neurons survive and improve motor function in Parkinson's disease. Science 247 (February 2):574-577.

Mason, J. O. 1990. Should the fetal tissue research ban be lifted? Journal of NIH Research 2 (January-February):17-18.

Moscona, A. A. 1988. Concurring statement. Pp. 27-28 in Report of the Human Fetal Tissue Transplantation Research Panel, vol. 1 (December). Bethesda, Md.: Department of Health and Human Services, National Institutes of Health.

Nolan, K. 1988. Genug ist genug: A fetus is not a kidney. Hastings Center Report 18 (December):13-19.

Office of Science Policy and Legislation, Office of the Director, National Institutes of Health. 1988. Fact sheet: NIH fetal tissue research. Bethesda, Md.: Department of Health and Human Services, National Institutes of Health, July 22, 1988.

Rich, S. 1989. Senate panel recommends Sullivan for HHS. Washington Post, February 24, 1989, A4.

Robertson, J. A. 1988. Concurring statement. Pp. 29-43 in Report of the Human Fetal Tissue Transplantation Research Panel, vol. 1 (December). Bethesda, Md.: National Institutes of Health.

Robinson, D. N. 1988. Letter to Dr. Jay Moskowitz. P. 73 in Report of the Human Fetal Tissue Transplantation Research Panel, vol. 1 (December). Bethesda, Md.: National Institutes of Health.

Smith, D. H. [Poynter Center]. 1988. Using human fetal tissue for transplantation and research selected issues. Appendix F in Report of the Human Fetal Tissue Transplantation Research Panel, vol. 2 (December). Bethesda, Md.: National Institutes of Health.

Tolchin, M. 1989. Bush choice backed for health chief after an apology. New York Times, February 24, 1989, A1 and A13.

Vawter, D. E. 1990. The use of human fetal tissue: Scientific, ethical, and policy concerns. A report of phase 1 of an interdisciplinary research project conducted by the Center for Biomedical Ethics, University of Minnesota, January 1990.

Walters, L. 1988. Statement. In Human Fetal Tissue Transplantation Research, Advisory Committee to the Director. Bethesda, Md.: National Institutes of Health, December 14, 1988.

ADDITIONAL BIBLIOGRAPHY

Burtchaell, J. T. 1988. University policy on experimental use of aborted fetal tissue. IRB: A Review of Human Subjects Research 10 (July-August):7-11.

Burtchaell, J. T. 1989. The use of aborted fetal tissue in research: A rebuttal. IRB: A Review of Human Subjects Research 11 (March-April):9-12.

Cefalo, R. C., and H. T. Engelhardt, Jr. 1989. The use of fetal and anencephalic tissue for transplantation. Journal of Medicine and Philosophy 14 (February):25-43.

Fine, A. 1988. The ethics of fetal tissue transplants. Hastings Center Report 18 (June-July):5-8.

Forum: Neural fetal tissue transplantation scientific, legal, and ethical aspects. 1988. Clinical Research 36:187-222.

Freedman, B. 1988. The ethics of using human fetal tissue. IRB: A Review of Human Subjects Research 10 (November-December):1-4.

Hansen, J. T., and J. R. Sladek, Jr. 1989. Fetal research. Science 246 (November 10):775-779.

Lafferty, K. J. 1990. Should the fetal tissue research ban be lifted? Journal of NIH Research 2 (January-February):16, 18.

Landau, W. M. 1990. Artificial intelligence: The brain transplant cure for Parkinsonism. Neurology 40:733-740.

Levine, R. J. 1989. An IRB-approved protocol on the use of human fetal tissue. IRB: A Review of Human Subjects Research 11 (March-April):7-12.

Mahowald, M. B., J. Silver, and R. A. Ratcheson. 1987. The ethical options in transplanting fetal tissue. Hastings Center Report 17 (February):9-15.

McCullagh, P. 1987. The Foetus as Transplant Donor. New York: John Wiley & Sons.

Miller, R. B. 1989. On transplanting human fetal tissue: Presumptive duties and the task of casuistry. Journal of Medicine and Philosophy 14:617-640.

Robertson, J. 1988. Fetal tissue transplant research is ethical. IRB: A Review of Human Subjects Research 10 (November-December):5-8.

Robertson, J. 1988. Rights, symbolism, and public policy in fetal tissue transplants. Hastings Center Report 18 (December):5-12.

Sparks, R. C. 1990. Ethical issues of fetal tissue transplantation: Research, procurement, and complicity with abortion. Paper presented at the annual meeting of the Society for Christian Ethics, Arlington, Va., January 20.

Commentary

Patricia A. King

Since the early 1970s, complex ethical, social, legal, and scientific controversies generated by scientific and medical advances have been referred increasingly to national commissions, committees, boards, or panels. The case study of the HFTTR panel[1] underscores the need to assess in a systematic way the goals, structure, and processes of such bodies if they are to continue to successfully resolve significant questions posed by the biomedical sciences. This need is particularly acute with respect to the consensus style that has been the hallmark of these groups.

Although the efforts of these groups have sometimes been described as "doing ethics,"[2] it would be more accurate to characterize their activities as developing public policies in the tradition of courts, legislatures, and regulatory agencies. These bodies have been so successful that thoughtful observers such as LeRoy Walters, director of bioethics at Georgetown University's Kennedy Institute of Ethics, have concluded that, although these groups "are not likely to replace the work of legislators, government agencies, and the courts, . . . periodic committee statements and reports may become the preferred mode of public oversight and social control for at least certain areas of biology and medicine."[3] The perceived success of these bodies can be attributed to many factors. I believe that three considerations deserve special note.

Patricia A. King is professor of law at Georgetown University Law Center and was a member of the HFTTR panel.

First, the issues posed for these policymaking bodies involve complex social dilemmas that appear to require more flexible and more extensive analysis than that permitted by the institutional restraints placed on courts, legislatures, and regulatory agencies. Typically, these issues are highly controverted and often seem incapable of resolution. While creation of these bodies may allow legislatures and agencies to avoid or defer acting on a difficult matter,[4] many issues are amenable to thoughtful resolution by these interdisciplinary groups. For many controversies, extensive, detailed consideration may be necessary before effective guides for action can be established, especially when existing principles and methods of analysis are inadequate to the task. Indeed, fundamental concepts and ways of thinking may first need to be reexamined.

Second, despite the seemingly intractable nature of the issues, the members of these bodies in many instances have been able to reach consensus on their advice or recommendations. This ability to bring order out of chaos gives their reports a compelling quality that facilitates their incorporation into relevant areas of law and public policy.

Third, these bodies have explicitly and self-consciously incorporated ethical premises into their deliberations. Their membership or staff (or both) often includes ethicists, philosophers, and theologians. These individuals articulate perspectives that are not ordinarily associated with policy development but that are essential to resolution of these complex issues.[5] The inclusion of ethical premises makes clear that the issues under scrutiny are not solely medical or technical in nature and require more than technical expertise to resolve. Success in including ethical premises, however, has obscured the fact that a range of perspectives—social, political, and economic, to name a few—is required for full resolution of these issues.

Successful inclusion of ethical premises has also tended to foster the illusion that these bodies have achieved consensus at the level of ethical principle or even ethical analysis. In fact, the consensus usually comes at the level of practice and policy. Moreover, it is not clear whether an effort to reach consensus at the level of principle is either possible or desirable. As Alexander Morgan Capron pointed out in connection with the work of the President's Commission for the Study of Ethical Problems in Medicine and Biomedical and Behavioral Research, "[t]he issues presented by modern medicine and research involve too many of the central facets of human existence . . . to be summed up by a few simple principles."[6]

Clearly, however, ethical principles and concepts are incorporated in the work of these groups, both as a part of a detailed analysis of the dilemmas under scrutiny and as a mechanism to facilitate the acceptance of the bodies' conclusions by persons with diverse religious, cultural, and ethical views. Stephen Toulmin summarizes the utility of appeal to principle in this way: "Principles serve less as foundations, adding intellectual strength or force to particular moral opinions, than they do as corridors or curtain walls linking the moral perceptions of all reflective human beings, with other, more general positions—theological, philosophical, ideological, or *Weltanschaulich*."[7]

The HFTTR panel was created and operated in the tradition of these preexisting national bodies with certain critical differences noted in the case study (staffing, timing, etc.). Significantly, the panel reached consensus on its responses to the questions presented to it. Nevertheless, the careful procedural and substantive examination of the HFTTR panel's operation presented in the case study makes clear that the panel's creation and work, as well as the operation of other such national bodies, need thoughtful scholarly analysis before they can become "the preferred mode of public oversight." At least two questions posed by the panel's work require critical examination.

The first involves the nature and importance of achieving consensus, especially in a context that touches on abortion. Weisbard and Arras put the problem succinctly when they ask: "[W]hat does `consensus' or `unanimity' signify, when it is achieved on deeply controversial questions in a society as pluralistic as our own?"[8] Unlike courts, legislators, and regulatory agencies, national bodies like the HFTTR panel have no means to enforce their conclusions or recommendations but instead depend on persuasion for impact. The force of their conclusions seems to depend on whether the body was able to reach consensus. Morris Abram, chairman of the President's Commission, makes this point powerfully, stating that "a commission requires agreement that is as close to unanimity as possible, to have any effect at all. Without such virtual unanimity, the commission members simply voice powerful arguments; with it, the commission can persuade."[9]

As the case study notes, the drive to achieve consensus was central to the HFTTR panel's work, and, indeed, consensus was achieved. Yet I believe that ultimately the product is not particularly persuasive. The fact that the panel's recommendations were not adopted by the Department of Health and Human Services is not the test of their persuasiveness. Rather, a clue lies in the fact that James Childress's discussion of the panel's deliberations in the case study is more coherent and consistent than that of the panel. I believe the HFTTR panel report lacks persuasive import because it failed to make clear how persons holding radically different views about abortion could nonetheless agree that the use of fetal tissue from induced abortion is "acceptable public policy" under specified conditions. It was probably necessary to describe the process that resulted in acceptance of this point rather than merely stating it.

In part, the HFTTR panel's failure to explain its conclusions adequately can be attributed to some of the events described in the case study, especially to the fact that the majority initially developed responses and not justifications for its conclusions. Yet I believe there is a deeper problem lurking here. Perhaps in the drive to achieve consensus, the panel gave insufficient attention to diverse views, to raising new questions, to stimulating debate, and to furthering societal discussion of controversial matters. Perhaps consensus was achieved at the expense of other functions that these national bodies ought to perform.[10] I suggest that one such function would be to reexamine traditional societal values in relation to a given modern dilemma to determine their present-day usefulness. A national group should draw on a variety of sources about norms, methodologies, and culturally informed perspectives in these deliberations. In so doing, it could develop new or revised analytical frameworks within which to examine contemporary issues. If the HFTTR panel had been permitted to engage in this type of effort, its conclusions might ultimately have been more persuasive.[11] They surely would have been more coherent.

In part, the panel's failure to develop new or revised analytical frameworks is related to its mandate. That point brings me to the second issue that needs critical examination, namely, the nature and structure of the mandate and the mandate's impact on the character of group deliberations. Every good lawyer (and teacher) knows the importance of formulating the right questions because in part the form of the question has implications for the nature of the answer. The HFTTR panel's mandate was in the form of 10 questions it had to answer. As discussed in the case study, these questions focused the group's attention on the connection between fetal tissue transplantation research and abortion.

Let us consider, for a moment, what product might have resulted if the question had been something like the following: Under what circumstances, if any, should the federal government support human fetal tissue transplantation research? Several possibilities come to mind. First, the HFTTR panel might have articulated new or revised analytical frameworks that would have helped clarify how persons holding different perspectives could reach consensus at the level of policy recommendations. For example, a person who held that the fetus was mere tissue and a person who held that the fetus was a person might be able to agree that the woman should give consent to the tissue donation. The first person might reach this conclusion because the woman was giving consent to use of her bodily tissue. The other might conclude that the next-of-kin should always give consent to the use of tissue from cadavers where wishes were unknown and where the purpose of the consent was not to further the best interests of the fetus.

Second, a more neutrally constructed question that resulted in the articulation of a new or revised analytical framework might have helped clarify the relationship between ethical analysis and policy development. It is not sufficient to ask whether a proposed practice is ethical. There is no necessary symmetry between ethics and public policy. As was evident in the HFTTR panel's work, it is possible to contend that abortion is morally wrong without also contending that the law should prohibit abortion or the use of fetal tissue from abortion in research. Moreover, it is possible to consider an act morally acceptable without concluding that it ought to be legal. Ultimately, ethical principles and ethical analysis may be too abstract to provide sufficiently specific guidance for conduct. There are many other considerations that must be taken into account, such as efficiency, cultural pluralism, public sensibilities, and uncertainty about risk, before policies can be developed.

If the relationship between ethical analysis and public policy formulation had been better understood, reviewers of the report might have appreciated some of the points about cost-benefit analysis that were made in John Robertson's concurring statement. Moreover, if members of the panel had focused their attention on policy judgments as well as ethical analysis, we might have paid closer attention to such factors as the scientific basis for fetal tissue transplantation research.

Finally, a new or revised analytical framework might have helped the panel avoid undue reliance on precedents with their accompanying arguments, stereotypes, and biases. I was often frustrated in the course of the HFTTR deliberations by what I perceived to be an antifemale bias, particularly during the discussions about whether fetal tissue transplantation research would encourage abortion and maternal consent. In my view, stereotypes originating in the abortion discussion obscured the need to better understand the implications of the linkage between the pregnant woman and the fetus in contexts that did not involve abortion directly.

There are many other issues associated with the efforts of national bodies that need critical attention.[12] In view of the untimely demise of the congressionally created Bioethics Board and the Biomedical Ethics Advisory Committee, which the Bioethics Board established,[13] in part over the abortion controversy, undertaking a critical assessment of the structure and processes of these national bodies assumes new urgency. The case study on the deliberations of the HFTTR panel is an important step in this assessment.

NOTES

1. I served as a member of the HFTTR panel. My observations are a product of that experience as well as service on the National Commission for the Protection of Human Subjects of Biomedical and Behavioral Research, the President's Commission for the Study of Ethical Problems in Medicine and Biomedical and Behavioral Research, and the Recombinant DNA Advisory Committee.

2. For an example, see the reference to remarks of Albert R. Jonsen in Alexander Morgan Capron, "Looking Back at the President's Commission," *Hastings Center Report* 13, no. 5 (October 1983):8.

3. Suzanne Wymelenberg for the Institute of Medicine, *Science and Babies: Private Decisions, Public Dilemmas* (Washington, D.C.: National Academy Press, 1990), p. 154.

4. Michael S. Yesley, "The Use of an Advisory Commission," *Southern California Law Review* 51 (1978):1452.

5. For a discussion of the implications of philosophers' participation in these bodies, see "Symposium on the Role of Philosophers in the Development of Public Policy," *Ethics* 97 (July 1987):775-791.

6. Capron, "Looking Back at the President's Commission," p. 8, note 2.

7. Stephen Toulmin, "The Tyranny of Principles, "*Hastings Center Report* 11, no. 6 (December 1981):32.

8. Alan J. Weisbard and John D. Arras, "Commissioning Morality: An Introduction to the Symposium, Commissioning Morality: A Critique of the President's Commission for the Study of Ethical Problems in Medicine and Biomedical and Behavioral Research," *Cardoza Law Review* 6 (1984):226. Ronald Bayer makes the further point that often consensus is illusory, being merely the common view of those who share the same ideology. (See Ronald Bayer, "Ethics, Politics, and Access to Health Care: A Critical Analysis of the President's Commission for the Study of Ethical Problems in Medicine and Biomedical and Behavioral Research," *Cardoza Law Review* 6 [1984]:309.)

9. Morris B. Abram and Susan M. Wolf, "Public Involvement in Medical Ethics," *New England Journal of Medicine* 310, no. 10 (March 8, 1984):629. Alexander Morgan Capron, executive director of the President's Commission, noted the benefits of consensus but was more cautious, observing that "only time will tell whether consensus was ever bought at too great a cost; my sense is that it was not" (Capron, "Looking Back at the President's Commission," p. 8, note 2).

10. This point was made by several commentators on the work of the President's Commission. For example, Jay Katz said: "The morality of commission reports, past and future, requires study of the question of whether societal morality is better served by documenting the complexities inherent in any ethical recommendation for the conduct of human affairs than by making light of the complexities through striving for a consensus report" (Jay Katz, "Limping Is No Sin: Reflections on Making Health Care Decisions," *Cardoza Law Review* 6 [1984]:247).

11. With respect to the issue of human fetal tissue transplantation research, private groups have attempted to fill this void. The efforts of the Center for Biomedical Ethics at the University of Minnesota are particularly noteworthy. See Dorothy E. Vawter et al., *The Use of Human Fetal Tissue: Scientific, Ethical, and Policy Concerns,* A Report of Phase I of an Interdisciplinary Research Project conducted by the Center for Biomedical Ethics (Minneapolis: University of Minnesota, 1990).

12. For a list of questions, see Weisbard and Arras, "Commissioning Morality," p. 226, note 8.

13. The Bioethics Board expired in 1989 (135 Cong. Rec. S15309 [November 9, 1989]). It was charged with examining on a continuing basis "ethical issues arising from the delivery of health care and biomedical and behavioral research."

Commentary

Walter Harrelson

It is good to have a case study outlining the process by which a group of medical and nonmedical specialists arrived at a set of recommendations to a governmental body concerned with health. The case study by James Childress charts the course traversed by the HFTTR panel in reaching the conclusions and recommendations contained in its report to the U.S. Department of Health and Human Services. The work of this panel shows the value and limitations of using panels of medical and nonmedical experts, working together over time, to frame policy for the nation in instances that involve highly controversial and divisive issues. Both the value and the limitations of such groups are related to their process.

Often, the issues can come into clearer focus through such deliberations if panelists are carefully selected and the panel has sufficient time to work together under a leadership that presses for clarity and consensus. Even under optimal circumstances, however, it is difficult to reach a useful consensus about such matters and to agree on language that is publicly comprehensible and aesthetically appealing to general readers.

The list of questions presented to the panel by the assistant secretary for health was quite specific, but the questions invited, and may have been intended to produce, debate over a rather wide front. Some of them were general

Walter Harrelson is Distinguished Professor of Hebrew Bible, emeritus, at Vanderbilt University and former dean of its Divinity School.

public policy questions; some were legal and others medical questions. Some in particular required extended deliberations by moral philosophers, ethicists, and theologians. The members of the panel seem to have been well equipped to deal with most, if not all, of these questions. Some panel members focused almost exclusively on the question of how the use of human fetal tissue might encourage abortion or constitute an action that could involve "complicity" in abortion. As a result, most of the panel's time was devoted to this central question.

The case study indicates that the Department of Health and Human Services received what it desired: a sophisticated set of responses to questions touching on legal, medical, moral, and general public policy aspects of the use of fetal tissue for transplantation, questions that, because of their link to the politically volatile issue of abortion, were under rigorous discussion within U.S. society. The panel composition may not have been ideal, because the responses of some panelists did not allow the discussion to maintain its focus on the use of fetal tissue obtained through induced abortions. But discussions of issues of this sort frequently take the course that the participants demand.

Did, however, Health and Human Services, and the public generally, get what it most needed from the panel's report? I would argue that it did not. What was most needed was not only a cogent, clarifying discussion of the issues by medical and nonmedical experts but also a rhetorically and aesthetically attractive report. When one enters the field of public policy debate on issues that are as strongly controversial as abortion, one must find a language and a set of images that will help a polarized community begin to build elements of consensus. It is important, indeed, that the panel itself was able to arrive at a consensus that included persons with quite different views on abortion. It is equally important that the positions of those panel members who dissented were powerfully and eloquently stated, so that political decisions would not be made without a sharpened awareness of such positions. What was lacking in the case study, and apparently lacking in the report of the panel, was a document of the style that is urgently needed today: an eloquent, appealing, quotable report that can assist the decision maker both in the making and later in the defense of difficult policy decisions.

This report was not primarily a scientific or a fact-finding report but one that described the deliberations of specialists from a number of disciplines who sought to clarify and move to a different level a controversy that urgently required both; that is, clarification and restatement in more useful, usable terms. When the experts themselves fail to provide this second articulation of the fruits of their deliberations, they leave the door open for two particularly unhappy outcomes (plus others, no doubt). One of these outcomes is apparent in this case: the administrator decides to do nothing—to leave standing the moratorium on governmental funding of fetal tissue transplantation research. The other has also appeared, and will appear again and again: administrators and political leaders resort to their own forms of persuasion and demagoguery in dealing with the issue, and the public is neither better informed nor provided with fresh terms and images with which to view and address the issue. In this regard, the panel missed a fine opportunity.

Asilomar and Recombinant DNA:
The End of the Beginning

Donald S. Fredrickson

I remember the Asilomar Conference as an event both exciting and confusing. Exciting because of the scale of the scientific adventure, the great expanses which had opened to research, and because no one could be indifferent to the debate over the powers and responsibilities of scientists. Confusing because some of the basic questions could only be dealt with in great disorder, or not confronted at all. On the frontiers of the unknown the analysis of benefits and hazards were locked up in concentric circles of ignorance . . . how could one determine the reality . . . without experimenting . . . without taking a minimum of risk?[1]

Philippe Kourilsky

At noon on February 27, 1975, the curtain descended on the first act of what is likely to go down in the history of science as the recombinant DNA controversy. The setting was the chapel of a conference center in the peaceful California coastal town of Pacific Grove. The cast included about 150 molecular biologists from some of the world's premier laboratories, and the final scene showed an agreement being struck among

Donald S. Fredrickson was the director of the National Institutes of Health from 1975 to 1981, where he was responsible for the establishment of the NIH Guidelines for Recombinant DNA Research. Presently, he divides his time between consulting and scholarship, including research and writing as a Scholar of the National Library of Medicine.

these scientists regarding the resumption of genetic experimentation, which they had voluntarily stopped six months before. Yet despite this difficult and commendable achievement, the succeeding episodes of this real-life drama rather suddenly took a turn for the worse. Laypersons, scientists, and legislators, on one side or the other, engaged in an angry struggle over the resumption of research. Numerous hearings, forums, and town meetings were held. In townships, states, and Congress, bills governing laboratory research were drafted and debated at length, and injunctions to forbid all such experimentation were sought in the courts. Half a decade of recriminations and anxiety passed before society and biomedical science patched up the largest rents in their mutually beneficial entente. Why did this happen? Could it have been avoided? Can we be sure that such a threat to such a sensitive relationship will not happen again?

The objective of this essay is to reconstruct, from an abundant record,[2] the story of the climactic event of the first act, the Asilomar conference of 1975. The subject should be viewed in the broadest context; therefore, we must zoom in on it from the past, using a wide-angle lens.

THE COMING OF AGE OF MOLECULAR BIOLOGY

In 1944, two noteworthy but unrelated events occurred that precipitated important changes in biomedical research. One was a scientific achievement, the other a political decision. The scientific achievement was the discovery of the chemistry of genes. When the first cautious report was absorbed and accepted, it snapped into focus genetics research of the past 80 years (if one counted the careful notes the monk Gregor Mendel put aside in 1865). Following a much earlier trail of research, especially a clue that different strains of pneumococcus were able to exchange certain characteristics like coat appearance and virulence, Oswald Avery, Colin MacLeod, and Maclyn McCarty at the Rockefeller Institute established that the exchanger was a sticky macromolecule or polymer made up of sugar, bases, and phosphoric acid, known as deoxyribonucleic acid, or DNA. The necessary confirmation that their "transforming principle" was, indeed, the stuff of the gene came eight years later with observations that when viruses (bacteriophages) infected bacteria only, the viral DNA entered the host and there led to expression of the complete virus.[3]

The symbolic political event in 1944 was a directive from President Franklin Delano Roosevelt to his chief of wartime research, Vannevar Bush, to find a way to continue federal financing of medical and other scientific research, which proved so successful after the nation's laboratories had been mobilized for war in what historian Hunter Dupree calls the Great Instauration of 1940.[4] Many members of Congress and the heads of at least one government agency, the Public Health Service, were poised to take full advantage of a positive decision to continue this unprecedented effort. The constitutional silence on a federal mandate to support science for its own sake was forgotten. Academic leaders and scientists were ready to overcome a long-held suspicion that taking government money was bound to mean the sale of academic freedom. The details of how this new policy began with the National Institutes of Health (NIH) in 1945 and how this agency became a magician's wand whose touch gave biomedical research an exponential rate of growth for more than 10 years thereafter are major stories in themselves. The overall result was florid expansion of the capacity of America's academic institutions to carry out research and to train young researchers. The greatest growth occurred in basic research, a high-risk activity dependent on public funds.

This burgeoning scientific community quickly discovered that pre-war fears of government interference with scientific freedoms were groundless. From the first, the new resources were primarily distributed to individual scientists on the basis of judgments on their proposals by scientific peers, managed on a national basis. The briskly expanding network of basic scientists, widely scattered in universities or nonprofit laboratories, was largely self-regulating and united in a worldwide profession with the same objectives and intrinsic ethic. Indeed, this shared belief in the autonomy and right of internal regulation of scientific investigation became the central dramatic theme of the recombinant DNA controversy. By restricting themselves voluntarily the scientists jeopardized the freedom that was absolutely necessary for the vitality and success of their enterprise.

Structure of DNA

In the midst of what became the scientific boom years of the 1950s, another epochal scientific event occurred in England. With dazzling deduction and splendid showmanship, the helical form and base-pairing structure of DNA were unveiled by James Watson and Francis Crick in Cambridge in 1953.[5] The carefully offhand postscript in their report of discovery, noting how this structure might explain the replication of the gene, stimulated resurgence of the crusade to bring back the answers to fundamental questions of living matter and the evolution of the species.

Such a dramatic expansion of the scientific horizon was perfectly timed to the swelling of the ranks of biomedical researchers. A large fraction of the best and the brightest of the decade's graduate students had begun to move into this pool. Being highly competitive, they shared with budding investment bankers and other entrepreneurs the knack for perceiving where the harvest would someday be most bountiful. As a career, experimental research involves a long apprenticeship to acquire specialized techniques that are applicable to one particular subdiscipline. Thus, the young scientist must select his or her special area of interest with care, so that when embarked on a lifetime adventure in independent research, his or her chosen field will be ripe in opportunities for discovery.

By the early 1950s an increasing number of aspirants chose to move to the frontier where the outer edges of genetics, biochemistry, and microbiology were merging, alongside a flood of new technologies such as electron microscopy, crystallography, cell culture, and virology, and in parallel with increased capabilities for information storage and analysis. By mid-century, the center of this fluid, expanding field became known as molecular biology, a term arguably attributed to the English x-ray crystallographer W. T. Astbury, who used it in 1950 to describe studies of "the forms of biological molecules and their ascent to higher and higher levels of organization."[6] Already the most interesting molecular forms were the genes, around which a limitless series of questions were framed. What was the full nature of genes? How were they organized in the chromosomes? Were they conserved in evolution? Were they interchangeable among species? What were the mysterious codes they carried? How were they translated? How was expression regulated with such exquisite timing to produce differentiation throughout the growth and decline of such a complex machine as man? What were the nature and origin of abnormal genes that failed in their assignments or caused disease?

The birth and early growth of the discipline now centering on genetics were hastened and greatly enlivened by the participation of scientists, many of them British or European, who were attracted to biology from such disciplines as mathematics, physics, and chemistry. Their presence among the leaders on the new frontier helped lend élan and eminence to the cadre of young scientists calling themselves molecular biologists.[7]

Fruit Flies, Corn, and Molds

The techniques available to get at the gene, however, were crude and cumbersome, and it took some time for the field to mature. In early studies of gene recombination—which is an important process for reproduction—pioneers like Thomas Hunt Morgan had profitably used the fruit fly (drosophila), creatures that are still invaluable for this purpose today. Others, like Barbara McClintock, turned to corn or other plants to learn about the organization of genes in the chromosomes and their mobility or susceptibility to rearrangement. In their classical work in the 1930s and 1940s, George W. Beadle and Edward L. Tatum used bread molds (neurospora), which are easy to culture and reproduce rapidly by genetic crosses. Simple as they were, the molds taught these pioneer geneticists the fundamental tenet of the central dogma: one gene controls the structure of one protein.[8]

The Need for Germs

Those researchers who were primarily interested in studying growth, differentiation, and genetics in mammalian tissues, including humans, now turned by necessity to the microbiological world for answers. The inhabitants of this ancient kingdom of living things had been the most instructive tutors of biologists since the promulgation of the germ theory of disease by Pasteur and Koch in the nineteenth century. Bacteria were readily available, had short generation times, and were cheap and simple to culture as well as generally predictable and reliable in behavior. Until 1950 a large share of the growth in understanding of biochemistry and nutrition and the great maturation of enzymology was attributable to studies of bacteria.

For genetic studies there are fundamental differences between the bacteria and viruses and most other living things. The former are termed prokaryotes because they have no cellular nucleus and the chromosomes are free in the cell juice, or cytoplasm. In bacteria some of these genes are in circular DNA molecules, or plasmids, which are often exceptionally mobile and can transfer genes to other bacteria. All the other cellular forms are called eukaryotes, and their cell nuclei hold all but a few of their genes arranged in a certain number of pairs of chromosomes. All the genes of either a prokaryote or a eukaryote are known collectively as the genome. In 1950 the major processes of exchange of genetic characters between organisms, so-called transductions or transformations, could only be observed in a few strains of microorganisms, one of which was the intestinal bacterium *Escherichia coli*, a laboratory partner in many invaluable studies. Of particular importance was, and still is, a stable strain of *E. coli* known as K-12, which was cultured from a patient at Stanford Hospital in the 1920s and eventually used in laboratories around the world. It was in this strain that a precocious Joshua Lederberg, while studying with Tatum at Yale, observed a third method of the transfer of genetic characters, called conjugation. In this process—the first intimation of sexuality in bacteria—a "male" and "female" *E. coli* bacteria join together side-by-side, and an end of the male chromosome enters the female. The entering DNA recombines with the host genome, and, after replication and cell division, the new recombinant cell has genetic features of the two parental DNAs.[9]

Viruses also began to make invaluable contributions to molecular biology after techniques for cultivating cells in culture were devised in the 1940s. Viruses are invisible packets of genes and proteins so small they can pass through filters that capture bacteria. In the simplest sense, the virus is a "transportable genome," stealing entry into the host cell where the viral genes replicate and sometimes combine with the host genome but invariably direct the cell machinery to synthesize their products, called virions, which in turn enable the viral genes to be transferred to other cells. Certain viruses are the only organisms in the biosphere that utilize a genome that contains not DNA but RNA (ribonucleic acid). RNA molecules are complementary to DNA in structure and have essential functions in the translation of the DNA code to proteins. The RNA viral genome of one class of RNA viruses, the retroviruses, contains the code for the enzyme reverse transcriptase, which transcribes RNA to DNA.[10] The DNA from such retroviruses may also recombine with DNA in the host genome. By such "natural" recombinations, retroviruses and mammalian cells may exchange and activate cellular genes called oncogenes (the expression of which may underlie cancerous transformation in the host).[11]

Viruses have long been known to cause tumors in animals—indeed, as long ago as 1906, when Peyton Rous found a retrovirus that causes sarcoma in chickens. Since then many other RNA and DNA viruses that are tumorigenic in animals, particularly rodents, have been identified. The Epstein-Barr virus, a DNA virus isolable from a rare tumor called Burkitt's lymphoma, is one of the few viruses suspected of being tumorigenic in man.

The potential hazards of infections from bacteria and viruses did not retard early work in molecular biology. By the second decade after the transforming principle had been enunciated, the laboratories of virologists and microbiologists had been thoroughly infiltrated by biochemists, geneticists, and cell and molecular biologists. The whir of the Sharples centrifuge, surrounded by its misty aerosol of *Escherichiae* in harvest, was commonplace in the most advanced laboratories and a sign that higher science was in progress. Viruses were handled on open laboratory tables, and—there being as yet no better methods—cultures were transferred by mouths separated from the contents of the pipette by a cotton plug. The microbiologists had learned, in their apprenticeships, respectful behavior toward organisms known to cause disease (pathogens) and compulsively washed down the lab tops and their hands if a drop of viral culture was spilled. Outside of the effects of the later extensive use of antibiotics, however, a general belief prevailed that man and microbes had reached a state of equilibrium that was not likely to be easily upset by human manipulation.

The interests of most of the molecular biologists did not lie in classical bacteriology, and many had received only rudimentary instruction in handling pathogens or in the ecology of microorganisms. Any anxieties they harbored were directed more toward maintaining a competitive edge in the hunt for new paradigms, and their laboratory technique with respect to germs often reflected this priority.

The possibility of using the insights and methods of molecular biology to better the lot of mankind was already being discussed by the mid-1960s.[12] It would only be a little longer before the discovery of restriction enzymes, tools capable of cutting DNA selectively and with precision at points along the chain.[13] And just a few years later, a particularly useful enzyme of this type would be the precipitating cause of the recombinant DNA controversy.

An International Frontier

The ever-expanding territory of molecular biology spread across two continents and occupied floors in the top universities and research centers of a number of countries. A half-dozen British laboratories, including ones at Cambridge, London, and Edinburgh, largely supported by the Medical Research Council, were highly productive. Europe was developing a European Molecular Biology Laboratory (EMBO), with a major communal laboratory in Heidelberg. In the 1950s and 1960s France also had its centers, particularly in Paris, at both the university and the Pasteur Institute. At the latter there were many workers, such as André Lwoff and François Gros, whose speciality was bacteriophages, viruses that can live parasitically with bacteria, sometimes fatally turning upon their host. At the Pasteur Institute, the laboratories of François Jacob and Jacques Monod were a particularly popular center of intellectual ferment that attracted many Americans for training and later collaborative work. Here an elegant conception of how the expression of (bacterial) genes is regulated was being shaped. First, bacteria, prominently including E. coli, were exposed to mutagens, including ultraviolet light; then their capacity to adapt to stringent change in growth media was tested. From these experiments gradually emerged the concept of the operon, a cluster of genes controlled by a single promoter. This idea led to an understanding of repression and induction of gene expression.[14]

By far the largest number of molecular biologists were working in the United States in laboratories extending from Boston and Cold Spring Harbor in New York to southern California. NIH was a major source of support, and NIH grants also went to European laboratories, including those of Jacob and Monod. In addition, the NIH intramural laboratories committed substantial resources to molecular biology in the 1960s, with the heaviest concentration being in virology. The National Cancer Institute (NCI) would soon erect one of the very few maximum security laboratories in the world to search for the elusive viruses some thought were at the root of human cancers.

The National Science Foundation (NSF) at this time was also providing important financial support to nonmedical scientists. During the 1960s Herman Lewis, the head of its Section on Cellular Biology, organized an informal Human Cell Biology Steering Committee (HCBSC). Its stated purpose was to offer advice on establishing large-scale cell cultures at different sites to foster a scale-up of studies in molecular biology, but it was also a clearinghouse for ideas of some of the leaders in the field. The HCBSC met fairly regularly, usually in Washington, D.C., and its membership included several faculty members from Stanford University.[15] It was at Stanford in the early 1970s that experimentation in molecular biology would first lead to serious controversy.

SETTING THE STAGE: THE EXPERIMENT AND ITS EFFECTS

In the late 1960s, Paul Berg, professor of biochemistry at Stanford, took sabbatical leave to work in the laboratory of virologist Renato Dulbecco at the Salk Institute. Berg had worked on molecular aspects of protein synthesis and was no stranger to the use of *E. coli* mutants. Like many others, he had become interested in the molecular genetics of viruses. His curiosity about whether a virus might be used to transfer a foreign gene into eukaryotic cell cultures led him to become familiar with simian virus 40 (SV40). Berg considered the relationship between phage and bacteria to be closely analogous to that between SV40 and eukaryotic cells, and he wondered if the virus might work more efficiently as a vector for a bacterial gene. The chosen gene already existed in highly enriched form in the bacterial plasmid. Berg enlisted two co-workers to determine if they could insert a bacterial galactose operon gene held by a modified lambda phage into the SV40 genome. Janet Mertz, a graduate student newly arrived from the Massachusetts Institute of Technology (MIT), was intrigued by the possibility that SV40 chromosomes would be reproduced in bacteria. Krimsky describes the Stanford laboratory activity at that time, including Mertz's growing ambivalence about such an experiment.[16]

SV40 was first isolated from monkeys in 1960 and was carried in cultured monkey kidney cells. Within a short time researchers discovered that the virus-infected cells caused tumors in hamsters.[17] This finding was of exceptional interest to the makers of poliomyelitis vaccine because monkey kidney cells had been indispensable for cultivating the poliovirus for the first vaccine. When investigators began to look for the virus, they soon found that the level of contamination of rhesus monkey kidney cells with SV40 was, indeed, high. It was by then no surprise, yet still a most unpleasant revelation, that some lots of the vaccine also contained the simian virus. A survey in 1961-1962 revealed that many of the recipients of the vaccine had antibodies to both the poliomyelitis and SV40 viruses.

Using the fairly cumbersome techniques then available, Berg and his co-workers were able to delete portions of the circular, helical coils of the SV40 genome in mapping studies. In spring 1971 they began to make preparations to couple SV40 genes to bacterial galactose genes for insertion into eukaryotic cell cultures.

Critique

In June, Mertz attended a workshop at Cold Spring Harbor and while there discussed the proposed experiments at Stanford with other students and her instructor. John Lear opens his book with a full-stop rendition of the outcome of her revelation: "On the afternoon of Monday, June 28, 1971, Robert Pollack, a 31-year-old microbiologist on the research staff of the Cold Spring Harbor Laboratory, Long Island, made a telephone call that would fundamentally change the relationship of American science to the society that sheltered it."[18] Pollack's call was to Paul Berg and it did not catch Berg completely by surprise, for Mertz had already relayed to him some of her instructor's criticisms. Pollack told Berg in effect that he should "put genes into a phage that doesn't grow in a bug that grows in your gut," and reminded him that SV40 is a small-animal tumor virus that transforms human cells in culture and makes them look like tumor cells. Pollack later described the idea as a "pre-Hiroshima condition—it would be a real disaster if one of the agents now being handled in research should in fact be a real human cancer agent."[19] At the end of the course, Pollack is said to have complained in his final lecture that "[n]o one should be permitted to do the first, most messy experiments in secret and present us all with a reprehensible and/or dangerous fait accompli at a press conference."[20]

After Pollack's call Berg undertook further opinion sampling of other peers about the proposed experiment and renewed discussions he had had much earlier about the general nature of such research. In 1970 Berg dined at the home of Maxine Singer, a molecular biologist at NIH, and her husband, a lawyer and trustee of the Hastings Institute.[21] Another guest was Leon Kass, who in 1971 was to publish a widely read article on the social consequences of the new biology.[22] Kass and Berg later exchanged correspondence over the subject of their dinner conversation. On a later trip to Washington in 1971, Berg paid a visit to scientists in the so-called Memorial Laboratories of Building 7 on NIH's Bethesda, Maryland, campus, which was dedicated to several scientists who had contracted fatal diseases during laboratory or field studies. There he talked to virologists working on SV40, one of whom was Andrew Lewis. Lewis still remembers Berg's admission that some of the scientists he had talked to felt that there was some line in the process of manipulating the genome that should not be crossed until more was known.[23]

The Encounter

Shortly before Berg's visit Lewis had been reminded of the rising tensions in the competitive field of molecular biology. In August 1971 he had gone to Cold Spring Harbor to make a presentation of his work on hybrids of adeno-SV40 viruses. (Adenoviruses are large viruses that cause respiratory infections.) Experiments in which these viruses had been grown in monkey kidney cells for purposes of preparing vaccines had led to the discovery of hybrid viruses, in which the genomes of adenoviruses also were contaminated with the genes of SV40. Most of these hybrids were defective, that is, unable to reproduce, and for a decade they had attracted little attention. Lewis's hybrids, however, were nondefective, and therefore capable of independent growth. Because these hybrids were much more likely to lead to information about the tumorigenic property of the virus, interest in them was steadily rising at laboratories like Cold Spring Harbor. Berg's proposed experiment was now well known at this institution and Dan Nathans, who was at the same meeting, described headway in dissecting the circular SV40 genome with one of the first restriction enzymes.

After his presentation Lewis had an unexpected encounter—extraordinary for a young and unknown scientist—with one of the *Wunderkinder* of molecular biology. Lewis had never met and did not recognize Watson, who had recently become director of Cold Spring Harbor Laboratory. Without introduction, Watson expressed his displeasure that Lewis had failed to share samples of the viruses with Cold Spring Harbor and proceeded to enumerate ways by which he could force Lewis to provide them. Lewis responded by relating his concerns about the possible hazards of the recombinant DNA in these nondefective hybrids and his reluctance to share samples without agreement by the recipients to acknowledge the possible hazards and follow certain precautions. The next month he supplied samples of the hybrids to the Cold Spring Harbor labs, and stepped up efforts to convince his NIH superiors that they should endorse a policy requiring a memorandum of understanding to accompany the sharing of nondefective hybrids and other potentially hazardous viruses. Lewis's friends and co-workers at NIH did not all share his serious concerns about the hazards of his experimental material, but NIH eventually undertook such precautions.[24]

When Berg returned to his laboratory in fall 1971 he informed his co-workers that he had concluded that they should postpone the part of their proposed experiment that would transfect the SV40-lambda hybrid into *E. coli*. He called Pollack and told him, and asked him to help organize a conference on the hazards of tumor viruses the next year. The departure of Berg's co-worker David Jackson to start a new laboratory at Ann Arbor, Michigan, in spring 1972 made the postponement of the original experiment indefinite.

The "First" Asilomar Conference

In 1972 the controversy over recombinant DNA was still well contained within the community of molecular biologists, and there had been no organized attempt to deal with the major single source of anxiety—the DNA of cancer viruses. Paul Berg, however, refused to let the matter drop. In August 1972 the HCBSC informed its members that a meeting on containment would be held in Asilomar on January 22-24, 1973. As Herman Lewis remembers it, the idea for the conference had come from Berg. NSF was willing to pay for the conference, but Alfred Hellman of NCI wanted his agency to participate, and NCI therefore shared the costs. Pollack, Hellman, and Michael Oxman of the Children's Medical Center in Boston proposed names of participants to Berg, who selected the final list and handled most or all of the preliminaries. It is certain that he picked the location, for the conference center at Pacific Grove had long been a favorite of campus scientists at Stanford.

Sometimes dubbed Asilomar I, the January 1973 meeting involved about 100 biomedical scientists, all but one or two of whom were Americans. There was no effort to invite the press, but the proceedings were edited by Pollack, Oxman, and Hellman and later published. Up-to-date information on many viruses was summarized by the experts, and there was thorough vetting of the evidence (or lack of it) that the known viruses, either pathogens or those studied in the laboratory, caused human cancer. In the end there was no evidence to support a single case. In the case of the polio vaccine that had been contaminated with SV40 in the late 1950s, the available information about the several million recipients of the vaccine did not suggest any alteration in cancer rate or type. It was obvious, however, that a fuller epidemiological search would someday be required to raise the level of certainty. Finally, safety precautions, especially for those engaged in the search for any virus causing human cancer, were outlined. In closing, Berg stated that "prudence demands caution and some serious efforts to define the limits of whatever potential hazards exist." Recombinant DNA experiments were not mentioned in the proceedings. Asked for his impression of the effect of the exercise, Andy Lewis answered, "After the conference we felt less concerned about the hazards of [laboratory] viruses causing cancer." Some of the recorded comments or exchanges from the conference floor, however, indicated that other anxieties were causing tempers to fray, and there was concern that fear was being spread unnecessarily. It was also evident that many scientists were becoming alarmed that research money would not be adequate to cover potentially escalating costs of new containment facilities, epidemiological studies, or other safety requirements.[25]

EcoRI

In spring 1972, R. N. Yoshimori, working on his doctoral thesis in the University of California, San Francisco, laboratory of Herbert Boyer, isolated from *E. coli* a new restriction enzyme that he designated *Eco*RI. The enzyme was quickly shared with other laboratories, and at Paul Berg's suggestion, John Morrow examined its action on the SV40 genome. He found that the SV40 DNA was cleaved at a unique site, and this finding provided a reference site for mapping the SV40 genome. To her great excitement, Mertz discovered that when *Eco*RI cleaved the circular DNA, it produced a linear segment with "sticky" ends that adhered to other ends that had been similarly cleaved. Electron microscopist Ronald Davis quickly confirmed her impression, and Boyer immediately came to see. Within a short time his associate, Howard Goodman, showed how *Eco*RI cuts left complementarity of the bases in DNA, which allows perfect splicing with other DNA that has been similarly cut.[26]

Scientific Exchange and Scrutiny

At the end of September 1972, about 50 molecular biologists from 12 countries, including nearly a score from the United States, attended an EMBO workshop in Basel on DNA restriction and modification. One evening of the workshop was devoted to "an open discussion of the use of restriction endonuclease to construct genetic hybrids between DNA molecules . . . [and] the implications this may have as a useful tool in genetic engineering and the potential biohazards." A few weeks later Honolulu was the site of a three-day U.S.-Japanese conference devoted to all aspects of plasmids, including recombination and genome transformation.[27] This latter meeting also gave Boyer and Stanford's Stanley Cohen the opportunity to discuss collaboration in experiments to probe *Eco*RI's utility in plasmid manipulation. Within a few months the partnership established that the enzyme uniquely cleaved a local plasmid (named pSC101—for Stanley Cohen) and combined two antibiotic-resistant plasmids, inserting the hybrid genes into *E. coli*.[28]

These international scientific meetings in the autumn of 1972 were but two examples of the constant worldwide information exchange among scientists, interactions that sometimes foster long-range collaborations but that are also vital to maintain parity among scattered workers in fast-moving fields of research. Experimental science is an open process that has an existential quality that is the antithesis of secrecy. A scientist who has made a discovery can usually be counted on to make it known. Proof to support a claim, a full report of the evidence, and its submission to confirmation and validation by others are required to ensure the precious priority of discovery that is still the paramount personal reward of scientific research. The worldwide scientific community, including the corps of peer-reviewed publications that serve the different fields, judges and protects these priorities as international properties.

Key judgments about the worth and priority of a scientist's work as criteria for support are largely national decisions, however. Judgments of the ethics or morality of individual scientists or their experiments likewise remain within national boundaries. The major reason for this insularity is the national or regional character of public support for scientific research. Cultural expectations are a major force in the maintenance of fiscal support of science. The continuing public approval of generous appropriations through agencies like NIH is based on expectations of improved public health and the conquest of particular diseases. Basic research, which laypersons cannot always identify as keyed to their aspirations, is nevertheless tolerated and tacitly understood to be necessary to maintain the tide on which practical benefits eventually arrive. The currency of these transactions is the continued credibility of scientists and the ultimate satisfaction of the consumer public, including the public's pride of sponsorship of a worthwhile, popular enterprise. In the early 1970s, the biomedical community began to experience concern about increasing tension in the vital public-science connection.[29]

THE 1973 GORDON CONFERENCE ON NUCLEIC ACIDS

The most effective, continuous self-monitoring of the scientific tribes derives from regular gatherings of its warriors and elders to examine in depth recent performance and progress. One of the favorites among such meetings is the Gordon research conferences, which have played a formative role in the careers of nearly all biomedical researchers. For a week in the summer, members of a subdiscipline take over a number of New England schools and engage in highly informal, intensive review of their particular field. On June 13, 1973, the Gordon Conference on Nucleic Acids began in New Hampton, New Hampshire. The first three days were dedicated to synthesis of DNA, the structure of RNA, and the interaction of proteins and DNA, themselves topics in which movement was rapid and fascinating. The fourth day was given over to bacterial restriction enzymes in the analysis of DNA. In a session chaired by Daniel Nathans, Herbert Boyer was scheduled to speak. According to John Lear, Stanley Cohen had obtained Boyer's promise to say nothing at the Gordon conference about the current work of their partnership. Krimsky, however, cites chairperson Maxine Singer, who recalled how Boyer had shared with the conferees information about the capabilities of the restriction enzyme *Eco*RI to splice DNAs of different origin and how two plasmids bearing genes specifying resistance to two different antibiotics had been joined.[30] It was after Boyer's comments that someone loudly sounded the excited comment, "Now we can combine any DNA."

Other reactions to this hint that biology was approaching something akin to the nuclear physicists' chilling arrival at "critical mass" were delayed until late afternoon, when two researchers at the Cambridge Molecular Biology Laboratory, Ed Ziff and Paul Sedat, sought out the two conference chairpersons, Maxine Singer of NIH and Dieter Söll of Yale. Ziff and Sedat urged the chairs to schedule a discussion of the potential hazards in the experiments disclosed in the afternoon's session. With only a half day to go in the conference, Singer and Söll nevertheless agreed to take up the matter at the beginning of the Friday morning session. Within about a half hour, the conference participants who were still on hand voted to ask the National Academy of Sciences (NAS) and the Institute of Medicine[31] to establish a committee to consider the problem of recombinant DNA research and recommend specific actions or guidelines.[32] The participants also agreed to publish the letter of request.

As later drafted by Singer and Söll and approved by the conferees, this letter began as follows:

We are writing to you, on behalf of a number of scientists, to communicate a matter of deep concern. Several of the scientific reports at this year's Gordon Research Conference on Nucleic Acids . . . indicated that we presently have the technical ability to join together, covalently, DNA molecules from diverse sources.

. . . This technique could be used, for example, to combine DNA from animal viruses with bacterial DNA, or DNAs of different viral origin might be so joined. In this way new kinds of hybrid plasmids or viruses, with biological activity of unpredictable nature, may eventually be created. . . .

The letter further noted that the experiments might advance fundamental knowledge and alleviate human health problems but that some hybrid DNA molecules might prove hazardous to laboratory workers and the public.

The die was cast. The Gordon conference reaction was unprecedented, and its expression of deep concern could not go unheeded. The train of events thus was set in motion that brings us to the principal subject of this narrative.[33]

THE ACADEMY'S TURN

Receipt of the Singer-Söll letter, dated July 17, 1973, was acknowledged by NAS president Philip Handler a few days later.[34] The conference letter appeared in the September 13 issue of *Science*. (Quite coincidentally, an editorial in the same issue by Amitai Etzioni dealt with a recent poll of public attitudes toward institutions and concluded that friends of science had no grounds for "hysterical alarm.")

Having consulted with the NAS council in late August, Handler informed the executive committee of the new Assembly of Life Sciences (ALS) that he was referring the Singer-Söll letter to it. Paul Marks, chairman of ALS's Division of Medical Sciences, replied that he agreed that ALS should establish a study committee and indicated that he was "as concerned with the potential hazards of certain of the hybrid molecules being studied as I am with the potential of unreasonably gloomy predictions [of] these hazards."[35] The ALS executive committee heard directly from Maxine Singer in September and, when asked for a suggestion as to who might head the study committee, she suggested Paul Berg. Handler requested the latter to take charge, and early in January Berg informed the ALS that he had decided to bring together a small group (fewer than 10 individuals) for a one-day planning meeting to consider mechanisms for reviewing potential dangers (as well as benefits) stemming from the ability to generate hybrid DNA molecules.[36]

Berg convened the meeting he had in mind at MIT on April 17, 1974. The six other participants selected by Berg independently were David Baltimore, James Watson, Dan Nathans, Sherman Weissman, Norton Zinder, and Richard Roblin. Herman Lewis of NSF was also there as an observer; Maxine Singer was unable to attend. Much has been written about this historic one-day meeting—for example, that James Watson had wanted an international meeting, that Berg recalled Norton Zinder saying, "If we had any guts at all, we'd tell people not to do these experiments," and how Roblin came to participate.[37] The details of this historic event were overshadowed, however, by its conclusions, which were contained in the report released three months later in a press conference at NAS on July 18, 1974.[38]

The report began with a summation of recombinant achievements since the July Gordon conference: the creation of new bacterial plasmids carrying antibiotic resistance markers; the insertion of toad ribosomal DNA into *E. coli*, where it synthesized RNA that was complementary to the inserted DNA; and unpublished experiments involving incorporation of drosophila DNA into DNA from plasmids and phage ready to be inserted into *E. coli*.[39] The summation was followed by the planning committee's conclusion that this type of unrestricted activity could create artificial recombinant DNA molecules that might prove biologically hazardous. As an example, the report cited the possibility that *E. coli* might exchange new DNA elements with other intestinal organisms with unpredictable effects.

The committee made four recommendations, which are summarized below:

1. Establish a moratorium on certain experiments. The committee commented that such a moratorium was "most important, that until the potential hazards of such recombinant DNA molecules have been better evaluated or until adequate methods are developed for preventing their spread, scientists throughout the world [should] join with the members of this committee in voluntarily deferring" these experiments. Two types of experiments were to be deferred: (1) those involving the creation of new, autonomously replicating plasmids that could carry antibiotic resistance to strains not now having such genes or that could enable toxin formation in now innocent strains (type I) and (2) experiments linking DNA from oncogenic or other animal viruses to plasmid or other viral DNAs (type II).
2. "Carefully weigh" experiments to link animal DNA to plasmid or phage DNA.
3. Request the director of NIH to establish an advisory committee to evaluate hazards of recombinant DNA, develop procedures to minimize those risks, and devise guidelines for work with recombinant DNA.
4. Hold an international meeting of all involved scientists early in the coming year (1975) to discuss appropriate ways to deal with the potential hazards of recombinant DNA molecules.

The relationship of Berg's committee to the Academy and the endorsement of its recommendations by the ALS-NRC, as well as the stress on the international nature of the proposed conference, were important touches added at the final stages of report preparation and review.[40] They were a credit both to the NAS and to the committee and helped to materially buffer possible inferences that a gang of seven (or perhaps, in the end, eleven) American scientists had impulsively doused the boiler of what arguably would become the most powerful scientific engine of the century.

THE ASILOMAR CONFERENCE

On September 10, 1974, the committee appointed to organize the February 1975 Asilomar meeting gathered in room E17 of the MIT Center for Cancer Research. The committee, which consisted of chairman Paul Berg, David Baltimore, Richard Roblin, Maxine Singer, Sherman Weissman, and Norton Zinder, was joined by several other scientists. Donald Brown, Richard Novick, and Aaron Shatkin had been summoned because they were to play key roles as chairmen of three working groups (on plasmid-cell DNA recombinants, plasmid-phages, and animal viruses, respectively) that would issue formal reports. Herman Lewis attended in his familiar role as patron and rapporteur for the HCBSC (many of whose members were directly involved in the conference). William Gartland was present as an observer for NIH, the conference's principal underwriter.

The first order of business was a discussion of foreign participation, ending with two additions to the organizing committee: Sydney Brenner of the Molecular Biology Laboratory at Cambridge and Nils Jerne, chairman of the EMBO council. (Jerne, however, was unable to participate in the committee or the conference.) Brenner, a highly articulate and gifted molecular biologist, was also a member of the Ashby Working Party in Britain, which had been set up by the Medical Research Council to determine how British science should react to the Berg committee report.[41]

A nearly complete format for the three-and-a-half-day conference was produced by the time the meeting ended.[42] Berg solicited suggestions for possible participants, but the final invitation list was his (see the appendix). The slate was in keeping with the intent expressly stated in the July 1974 report: an international meeting of involved scientists. About 90 of the invitees were American; another 60 came from 12 different countries. All were among molecular biology's elite. No organizations were represented per se. Sixteen members of the press were invited, all accepting the condition that no copy would be filed until the conference ended.[43]

The three discussion panels were asked to present completed draft reports at the conference and thus met in November to begin work. Novick's plasmid panel began an extensive analysis that finally would cover most of the potential areas of hazard. Shatkin's animal virus panel, however, apparently misunderstood the work schedule: when they arrived in Asilomar on the Sunday night preceding the conference, they were unaware that their draft report was to have been completed. Organizing quickly, they gathered after dinner to draw one up.

Monday, February 24—Opening Day

The conference's organizing committee had decided at their September meeting that there would be no publication of the conference (because of the manpower and time required), although audiotape recordings of the sessions would be maintained as an archive. Any conferee could ask that recording be suspended during his or her discourse, but none so requested. When the participants then noticed the small forest of microphones set up by members of the press, the discussion ended by permitting the press to use their recorders for preparation of their stories. Allowing any part of the tapes to be broadcast, however, was declared to be against the rules.

David Baltimore opened the conference on Monday morning. He gave a short history of how the meeting had come about and described its auspices and organizers. He noted that conference participants had been invited to the meeting on the basis of their expertise or involvement in the science. He then explained that the meeting had been convened to lay out the existing technology and what had been done to answer the question of what (experiments) should or should not be done, and to determine what should be done before an experiment is undertaken. Baltimore emphasized that the balance of risks and benefits would be considered but that discussion of the hazards was more important than either the benefits or molecular biology per se. His summary of the program ended with the observation that, on the last morning, the organizing committee expected to present a summary statement, including general guidelines for discussion and consensus. Baltimore reminded the audience that if it could not reach consensus, there was no one else to whom it could turn. Paul Berg next stepped to the podium to review the basics of recombinant DNA technology. This discussion set the tone of much of the first three days of the meeting, the format and content tending toward the highly technical, with presentations in the traditional style of experts talking to experts. It reflected scientists doing what they do best—talking about their own work. There was another requirement to be satisfied by such intercourse, however, and that was the need of the participants to be exposed to the different techniques, personalities, and scientific jargon peculiar to each of the three or four major subcultures assembled: the virologists, the "plasmid engineers," the specialists in phage ("lambda people"), and the eukaryotic cell biologists. The insularity of these narrow subspecialities predictably bred suspicions that one's own area of research could emerge from such a meeting unfavorably restricted by strangers.

The expertise on hand at Asilomar was impressive (see the appendix). Speaking after Berg was Stanley Falkow, who combined a medical background with an encyclopedic knowledge of bacteria. After him came Ephraim Anderson from the Public Health Laboratory Service in Britain, who also had medical training and had dealt with epidemics of intestinal infections before concentrating on plasmids. Anderson had taken umbrage at the type I recommendations in the Berg committee report, partly because, in the version printed in *Nature*, a dropped word led to the interpretation that his long-time research had been banned. As soon as he read it, Anderson shot off a note to the journal, which appeared in the next edition, expressing the wish that the "NAS statement had been presented less pompously." At Asilomar, Anderson and a British colleague, William Smith, were asked to present their experimental evidence that *E. coli* K-12 had a low risk for transferring plasmids to other enteric bacteria. After it was all over, however, Anderson's criticism of the conference remained unmitigated.[44]

Another speaker on the first day, Roy Curtiss from the University of Alabama, had displayed a very different reaction to the Berg report. A month after it appeared he had sent a 16-page memorandum to the signatories and distributed hundreds of copies to the world community of molecular biologists, in which he stated, "I heartily endorse the aims, but not necessarily the scope of your recommendations. . . . I personally pledge to cease Type I experiments (to construct bacterial plasmids that are not now known to exist) that I was currently engaged in . . . and not to initiate Type II experiments. . . ."[45] Curtiss moreover argued for specific heightening of the restrictions and spelled out conditions under which he believed *E. coli* might be hazardous. Berg and many others responded to the Curtiss letter, and the reiteration of prior arguments now enriched the debate. The last speaker in the postdinner session that first evening—after presentations by Boyer and Cohen—was Ken Murray of the team of molecular biologists in Edinburgh, who described phages as cloning vehicles. Murray had published a companion (but more conciliatory) note to accompany Anderson's in the July issue of *Nature*, which he closed with a line from the *Manchester Guardian*'s earlier comment on the Berg report: "While welcoming the NAS initiative : . . if we follow the moderate tone set by the NAS we shall be careful not to oversell the social benefits devolving from the recent experiments."[46]

When Berg began his session on the morning of the first day, he mused aloud that the writers of the original letter had not anticipated how it would affect the scientific community and that the organizing group was not prepared or experienced in how to arrive at a decision. He said therefore that a panel of lawyers arranged by Dan Singer would present views on law and public policy issues on the third day. Harold Green, another Washington lawyer and a trustee of the Hastings Institute, spoke after lunch on the first day, however, and told the scientists that the conference and its unique moratorium on research—for which he gave them high praise—would serve as a moral precedent and a model of how science should deal with such issues. He was asked several questions about how the responsibilities for risk, or the framework for proceeding with experimentation, should be determined, and he offered his opinion that the government ultimately would determine the public policy. To end his presentation, Green held out astringent balm to any injured by this forecast by noting that "all institutions in society are imperfect and of these the government is the most imperfect."[47]

Tuesday, February 25—Getting Down to Guidelines

The second day began with Richard Novick's presentation of the report of his working group "Potential Biohazards Associated with Experimentation Involving Genetically Altered Microorganisms, with Special Reference to Bacterial Plasmids and Phages."[48]

The conclusions of this first of the working group reports were most conservative. The document contained extensive recommendations for classifying, monitoring, and designing many classes of experiments, and it would later serve as a template for the future recommendations of the NIH Recombinant DNA Advisory Committee. The mass of information it contained, however, seemed to overwhelm the absorption capacity of the participants. A day later, the organizing committee found it necessary to amend its construction in order to propose a framework for consensus. Long after Asilomar, the comment would continue to be made that the conference had failed to consider the unlikelihood that E. coli K-12 could be converted to a dangerous enteric pathogen or engage in harmful genetic transmission to other organisms under normal circumstances in vivo. The working group report did not neglect such calculations, but the pace of the Asilomar debate outstripped the time for adequate reflection on them. It would not be until 1977 (the Falmouth conference) that similar deductions led to the dismissal of this conversion as a serious hazard.

The mesh of protection proposed by the plasmid-phage panel grated on some of the listeners. Michael Rogers, the correspondent from *Rolling*

Stone, later reported some sample reactions. Josh Lederberg rose to express grave concern about the danger of the panel's recommendations "crystallizing into legislation"; Ephraim Anderson then demanded that the panel indicate, by a show of hands, which of its members "had experience with the handling and disposal of pathogenetic organisms capable of causing epidemic *disease*." When the panel members rather sheepishly admitted that they had all probably had too little, their tormentor added insult to injury by nipping away at the grammar and syntax of the report. Suddenly James Watson uttered a call for an end to the moratorium—moreover, "without the kind of categorical restrictions called for in the plasmid report." Rogers recalled that Maxine Singer was on her feet immediately to ask what had changed in the last six months to cause Watson to abandon the movement he had helped to launch.[49]

In line with the assessment of a number of subsequent commentators, Rogers admired Sydney Brenner ("the single most forceful presence at Asilomar") and described him as rising shortly thereafter to ask waverers in the crowd, "Does anyone in the audience believe that this work—prokaryotes at least—can be done with absolutely no hazard?" After a dramatic pause, Brenner continued, "This is not a conference to decide what's to be done in America next week; if anyone thinks so, this conference has not served its purpose." During the afternoon, Brenner led a session on the desirability of "biological containment," the designing of plasmids, phages, or other vectors that could not survive in a new ecological niche and thereby do mischief if they escaped the "physical containment" that had been thus far discussed. It was not a completely new idea, but Brenner's enthusiasm stimulated much discussion and encouraged thinking about other ways to open up the blocked channels of research. That night a group of "lambda people," concerned that the plasmid group had overly emphasized crippled plasmids in their proposals for biological containment, worked late and by morning had a design on paper for a potentially safer phage vector.[50]

A heavy barrage of virology was laid down in the late afternoon and evening session of the second day. Undoubtedly, in the minds of some scientists—especially those to whom viruses were unfamiliar territory—any anxieties over *E. coli*-triggered epidemics paled in comparison with concerns about human cancer being caused by some devilish recombination of DNA from tumorigenic viruses. Among the presentations was that of Andrew Lewis, who described his work on the adeno-SV40 hybrids, accompanied by the precautions he considered desirable for the use and sharing of the nondefective forms of these organisms. But after Aaron Shatkin came forward with the recommendations of the virus working group, the panel appeared to disappoint some who considered viruses to be the greater menace. The report consisted of two pages, the first signed by all but one member of the panel, and began with a reaffirmation of the potential benefits of such research, a theme the organizers at Asilomar had requested be muted. The preamble to the report read as follows:

The construction and study of hybrid DNA molecules offer many potential scientific and social benefits. Because the possible biohazards associated with the work are difficult to assess and may be real, it is essential that investigations be re-initiated only under conditions designed to reduce the possible risks. Although the need for the development of new and safer vectors is clear, we believe that the study of these recombinant DNAs can proceed with the application of existing National Cancer Institute guidelines for work involving oncogenic viruses . . . with the exceptions noted below [highly pathogenic viruses] we recommend that self-replicating recombinant DNA molecules be handled according to guidelines for moderate risk oncogenic viruses . . . the vast majority of experiments will fall into the moderate risk category.

The second page of the report was Andrew Lewis's minority report of one, which called for experiments on recombination of DNA from animal viruses to take place in moderate-risk facilities as defined by NCI, and only when theoretically safe vectors had been developed. A day later, an amended report was issued by the viral group that endorsed the desirability of both physical and biological containment for experiments inserting viral or eukaryotic cell DNA into prokaryotic hosts. The number of signatories of this unanimous statement had increased to eight.[51]

Time would prove whether Andrew Lewis was right or wrong. It should be noted, however, that although there were other participants at Asilomar who expressed conservative views (e.g., Curtiss, Falkow, and Robert Sinsheimer), Andrew Lewis was the one "dove" who most clearly and steadfastly maintained his convictions against a popular tide.

Wednesday, February 26—Dissonance and Lessons in the Law

On the morning of the third day copies of several communications were passed out, one of which was an open letter to the conference from Science for the People, a grass-roots science watchdog organization. Its principal message was that "decisions at this crossroad of biological research must not be made without public participation" and that the signers did "not believe that the molecular biology community . . . is capable of wisely regulating this development alone." It called for a continuation of the moratorium until several proposals for widening public input were put into effect. The authors were bacterial geneticists and molecular biologists, among whom was Jonathan Beckwith. (In 1969 a Beckwith team had became the first to isolate a gene, the *lac* operon.) There was no formal discussion of the letter at the conference, however, and scientific presentations filled the morning.[52]

After lunch Donald Brown presented the report of the Working Group on Eukaryotic Recombinant DNA. This group believed recombinant eukaryotic DNA could be hazardous in three ways:

1) a gene could function in the bacteria in which it is cloned and produce a toxic product; 2) a DNA component could in some way enhance the virulence or change the ecological range of the bacterium in which it is cloned; or 3) a DNA component could infect some plant or animal, integrate into its genome, or replicate, or by its expression could produce a modification of the cells of the organism. [53]

As they were painfully aware, however, the scientists here were grappling with questions for which existing knowledge was woefully inadequate, and the very experiments proscribed as potentially hazardous were the ones from which the answers ultimately would have to come. Already there was skepticism that *E. coli* might simply replicate animal genes and never translate them into proteins, but the fundamental difference between translation of DNA by prokaryotes and eukaryotes had yet to be discovered. The frustration engendered by the tireless invention of scenarios invited baroque and temporary constructions. The recommendations of the working group included a classification of three major levels of hazard, with additional subclasses, to which a complicated hierarchy of containment conditions was arbitrarily applied. "Shotgun" experiments, in which a vector might be exposed to pieces of the total genome of a eukaryotic cell, were all consigned to the highest hazard class, with mammalian DNA being particularly suspect because it "more likely contained pathogens for humans." Such rulings caused dismay among researchers who would now be forced to carry out their experiments inside scarce high containment facilities. Disagreements over classification of hazards quickly cropped up and continued until the final hour of the conference.

After dinner, at the evening session, the chair introduced Daniel Singer, who presided over a small panel of lawyers he had selected in hopes of strengthening the framework for the final discussion the following morning. Singer began by complimenting the scientists on the exercise of public responsibility he perceived in their undertaking. He reminded them that the benefits and risks of their research were not only scientific but social issues, and the public, which was paying for the research, would have to have its say. Alexander Capron, professor of law at the University of Pennsylvania, began with his impressions of the conference, likening it to typical scientific meetings (highly technical in content—"like Cold Spring Harbor"). "In other words," Capron snapped, "counter-phobic behavior." He too believed that the public would have to become involved, and "the public" meant government and the law. Capron then coursed across the terrain of regulation, rule making, and legislation, concluding that he hoped he had led the scientists to accept three things: some regulation is necessary, it may lead to restrictions, and public and governmental bodies would insist on having a say.

The third speaker, Roger Dworkin, professor of law at Indiana University, led the scientists into the chilling landscape of legal liability. He described dangerous crevasses with names like proximate cause, negligence, and strict liability, and created courtroom litigation scenes. Dworkin hit a particularly sensitive nerve when he discussed worker's compensation and regulatory agency involvement, including the roles of the Occupational Safety and Health Administration. Here he off-handedly suggested that even the secretary of labor might have final authority over the rules for recombinant DNA research. Like Banquo's ghost, this specter reappeared several times before the discussion ended late that evening. Listening to the lawyers predict what might happen to the decisions to be made on the morrow, the scientists stiffened their resolve to close ranks so that the world would see that the scientific community was able to finish what it had begun. And more than the others, the members of the organizing committee now realized that the product of their long, last-evening's work had to be definitive.

Thursday, February 27—The Final Hours

The final session opened at 8:30 a.m. Keenly conscious that his deadline was noon, Paul Berg began by recapitulating the three responsibilities the organizing committee had accepted: (1) to organize the conference to bring experts together for a discussion of the risks of recombinant DNA research; (2) to determine what consensus existed and to embody this in a statement; and (3) to prepare a statement to the NAS concerning the outcome of these deliberations. Each participant had received a copy of the provisional statement that the organizing committee had spent the night preparing. There were six sections in the statement, and Berg opened discussions on the first. It was a statement of scientific accomplishments and an intimation that the situation was somewhat clearer than it had been the previous July. Several participants, however, immediately raised procedural questions about how to handle inputs to the wording. Others inquired if all chance for modification ended with the close of the session. A member of the organizing committee reminded the conferees that the committee's report was not "written in a vacuum, but reflected the Committee's views of what seemed to have been agreed upon thus far." "Will we get to vote on each paragraph?" someone asked, and the chairman replied that he would prefer a more informal means to arrive at consensus.

Notwithstanding his reluctance to begin a series of time-consuming ballots, Berg quickly found that a vote was being forced by Brenner's suggestion that reaction to the following statement be tested: "Work should proceed, but with appropriate safeguards; the pause is over." Hands went up, and the chairman said he would record an overwhelming consensus on this statement. There was also a palpable sense of relief at this forward movement, and discussion turned to the second point. It too was greeted by suggestions for improvement of grammar and form. After the participants, however, had been encouraged to concentrate on substance, they allowed the chair to decree general agreement with the statement, "with reservations, some form of experiments should proceed; some, however, should not." The discussion began to deteriorate, it moved to issues of actual levels of containment for experiments, but the chair gamely kept order. He patiently listened to great differences of opinion on details and permitted polls whenever it appeared they might be useful. Feelings ran high. There were numerous attempts, for example, to amend some definitions of hazard from the floor. A voice cried out to protest that the carefully prepared statement of his working group had "been prostituted."

As the first lunch bell sounded, the moment for the final question could no longer be delayed. Berg, making himself heard over the commotion that had begun, said, "All those in favor of this as a provisional statement, please raise your hands." Stanley Cohen protested loudly that he could not support something without seeing the wording of it. "All those opposed to the statement," Berg now demanded. Roberts counted "somewhere about four hands." Two of these belonged to Lederberg and Watson. A third was Cohen's. Waclaw Szybalski recalls, "I was strongly opposed, vocally objected, and raised my hand when negatives were requested." Philippe Kourilsky, agreeing with the count of "four or five," says his was also a negative vote. Thus, the statement with which they had begun the morning—although frayed and variously patched along the way—had made it through, still holding to the framework fashioned by the organizing committee in their last night's vigil.[54]

Someone had asked the Russian delegates to remain to the end. A spokesman for the group rose and, in a brief statement, said that a world partitioned politically could nevertheless hold an undivided scientific community.[55]

By 12:15 p.m. on February 27, 1975, Asilomar II had ended.

A press conference was held the following day. The members of the press who had attended throughout (earning honorary degrees in molecular biology) were now freed from their imposed silence and released generally laudatory, respectful commentary. The same day, the new NIH Recombinant DNA Advisory Committee met for the first time and adopted the provisional statement of the conference as interim rules for federally supported laboratories in the United States.

CONCLUSION

The conference organizing committee—Berg, Baltimore, Brenner, Roblin, and Singer—submitted the final report of the Asilomar Conference on Recombinant DNA Molecules to the NAS Assembly of Life Sciences under a cover letter from Berg, dated April 29, 1975. In keeping with Academy policy, the report was reviewed on this occasion by members of the ALS executive committee, who also received some comments from Academy president Handler. It was approved on May 20 and appeared in the June 6, 1975, edition of *Science* and the Academy *Proceedings* as a "Summary Statement."[56]

Read today, this statement still stands as a lucid, fair description of the conference consensus. It does not seek to go beyond the facts as they were considered by the participants, neither in predicting benefits nor in dismissing any of the biohazards considered possible at the time. As Handler commented in passing the report to the ALS, it was written "only to the cognoscenti in the field" and was not concerned with ensuring that other audiences understood the conclusions.[57]

Fifteen years have now passed since the participants in the Asilomar conference went home to explain to anxious co-workers and laboratory staff what the new restrictions meant. Many also went to university leaders and institute administrators to argue for the new security facilities now required for their work. A few soon found themselves "on the barricades" in their own communities like Ann Arbor, Cambridge, and the Pasteur Institute, where tensions were rising. As fears diffused among the general population, not only laypersons but dissident scientists as well turned militant, and—as the lawyers had predicted—representatives of government in the United States and several other countries rose to play their different roles.

The Asilomar agreements were not substantively relaxed until the end of 1978. Indeed, elements of the original final consensus remain in the NIH guidelines that still govern the public and private use of recombinant DNA technology in the United States. In February 1990, the NIH Recombinant DNA Advisory Committee held its forty-second meeting, the first in this sixteenth year of its existence. The principal items on the agenda were possible revision of the definition of recombinant DNA molecules (unchanged since 1976) and the consideration of extension of an experiment to insert a recombinant gene into patients as a marker for new therapeutic approaches to cancer. One member (the Environmental Protection Agency) of the quintet of federal agencies forming the Biotechnology Science Coordinating Committee, which was established in 1986 to coordinate the regulation of recombinant DNA biotechnology in the United States, has declared it will no longer attend meetings until the committee is reformed. In England, the Advisory Committee on Genetic Modification advises the Health and Safety Executive and Ministry of Environment, the statutory authority for regulation of use of recombinant DNA technology in Her Majesty's government. In Brussels, proposed council directives dealing with "contained use of genetically modified organisms" and "deliberate release to the environment of genetically modified organisms" have been sent to a commission. On the basis of these directives, as amended, all member states are expected to enact statutes that provide for harmonization of the rules for recombinant DNA technology throughout the European Economic Community.

Long before the outcomes of the Asilomar conference could be properly assessed, lists of its putative deficiencies or limitations as a policymaking model for the recombinant DNA debate were being compiled.[58] Yet hindsight, though a powerful weapon, can easily be warped by time. Judgments of the Asilomar conference must be conducted using tight rules of what is admissible as evidence. Certainly, there should be no mention of the lack of appearance over the 15 or so years since the conference was held of any of the hypothetical hazards that were so earnestly debated there. Likewise, evidence of the bottomless cornucopia of invaluable new knowledge that these same techniques have already provided and will continue to supply to humankind must also be scrupulously barred. The scales that weigh Asilomar have to be calibrated using the context of all that contributed at that time to give the event its significance as the climactic end of the beginning of recombinant DNA research.

NOTES

1. Philippe Kourilsky, *Les Artisans de L'Hérédité* (Paris: Editions Odile Jacob, 1987), pp. 143-144. One of six French participants at Asilomar, Kourilsky provides a foreign scientist's view of this American conference, including his concern that missing among the participants were "ecologists with a global point of view." See also Philippe Kourilsky, "Manipulations génétiques in vitro: compte-rendu de la conférence de Pacific Grove," *Biochimie* 57, No. 2 (1975): vii; and the transcript of an interview with Philippe Kourilsky, March 20, 1976, contained in the Massachusetts Institute of Technology (MIT) Archives, MIT Recombinant Historical Collection, Box 9, Folder 113.

2. At least four books on the early history of the recombinant DNA controversy contain detailed descriptions of the 1975 Asilomar conference: Michael Rogers, *Biohazard* (New York: Knopf, 1977); John Lear, *Recombinant DNA: The Untold Story* (New York: Crown, 1978); Nicholas Wade, *The Ultimate Experiment: Man-made Evolution* (New York: Walker, 1979); and Sheldon Krimsky, *Genetic Alchemy* (Cambridge, Mass.: MIT Press, 1982). In the preparation of this essay the author also made extensive use of other sources: the MIT Recombinant DNA Historical Collection at the MIT Archives; the Archives of the National Academy of Sciences, including the original tape recordings of the conference; the National Institutes of Health (NIH) Central Files; and the collections of the National Library of Medicine. Between November 1989 and June 1990, the following conference participants were interviewed in person or by telephone: William Gartland, Leon Jacobs, Philippe Kourilsky, Arthur Levine, Andrew Lewis, Herman Lewis, Malcolm Martin, Robert Martin, Anna Marie Skalka, Waclaw Szybalski, and Pierre Toillais.

3. The clue came from F. Griffith, "The significance of pneumococcal types," *J. Hygiene* 27 (1928):113-159. The key discovery is described in Oswald Avery, C. M. MacLeod, and M. McCarty, "Studies on the chemical nature of the substance inducing transformation of pneumococcal types," *J. Exp. Med.* 79 (1944):137-158. The confirmation appears in A. D. Hershey and M. Chase, "Independent functions of viral protein and nucleic acid in growth of bacteriophage," *J. Gen. Physiol.* 36 (1952):39-56.

4. A. Hunter Dupree, "The great instauration of 1940: the organization of scientific research for war," in *The Twentieth Century Sciences*, Gerald Holten, editor (New York: Norton, 1970).

5. J. D. Watson and F. H. C. Crick, "A structure for deoxyribonucleic acid," *Nature* 171 (1953):737-738.

6. W. T. Astbury, "Molecular biology or ultrastructural biology?" *Nature* 190 (June 17, 1961):1124-1125.

7. Horace Freeland Judson has composed an unparalleled romance on early molecular biology (*The Eighth Day of Creation* [New York: Simon and Schuster, 1979]) in which he introduces us to a galaxy of performers, including, among many others, John Kendrew and Max Perutz, crystallographers who worked out the structures of myoglobin and hemoglobin; Erwin Schrödinger, the mathematician considering the adaptation of quantum mechanics to living organisms (*What Is Life? The Physical Aspect of the Living Cell* [Cambridge: University Press, 1944]); Max Delbrück, the phage expert whose early training was with the atomic physicist Niels Bohr; Leo Szilard, who was with Fermi at the Manhattan Project before he took up the study of phage and became an ardent pilgrim among the biologists; and Francis Crick, who first read physics but fortunately turned to the study of living things and was the perfect complement to James D. Watson, a very young biologist who came to Cambridge after obtaining his doctorate under Salvatore Luria at Indiana University. Among many others who coursed in and out of room 103 in the Austin Wing of the Cavendish Laboratory—where the helical model of Crick and Watson was rising—were Linus Pauling, the Nobel Prize-winning chemist, who was in hot pursuit of the crucial structure of DNA, and Sydney Brenner, the South African scientist destined to play a catalytic role at Asilomar.

8. These three classical geneticists eventually would receive Nobel prizes in physiology or medicine: Morgan in 1933, McClintock 50 years later in 1983, and Beadle and Tatum (with Lederberg) in 1958. The increasingly rapid succession of Nobel honors thereafter show the surging importance of molecular genetics up to the time of the Asilomar conference: Arthur Kornberg in 1959; Crick, Watson, and Wilkins in 1962; Jacob, Lwoof, and Monod in 1965; Holley, Khirana, and Nirenberg in 1968; and Delbrück, Hershey, and Luria in 1969. Four of the molecular biologists who participated in the Asilomar meeting subsequently received Nobel awards: Baltimore, 1975; Nathans, 1978; Berg, 1980; and Bishop, 1989.

9. Joshua Lederberg, "Gene recombination and linked segregations in *Escherichia coli*," *Genetics* 32 (September 1947):505.

10. David Baltimore, "The strategy of RNA viruses," *Harvey Lect*. Series 70 (1974-1975):57-74; Howard Temin, "On the origin of the genes for neoplasia: the G. H. A. Clowes Memorial Lecture," *Cancer Res*. 34 (November, 1974):5842-5846.

11. R. C. Parker, H. E. Varmus, and J. M. Bishop, "Cellular homologue (c-src) of the transforming gene of Rous sarcoma virus: isolation, mapping, and transcriptional analysis of c-src and flanking viruses," *Proc. Natl. Acad. Sci. USA* 78 (September, 1981):5842-5846.

12. See the description of a meeting at Rockefeller University, October 2, 1966, reported in the MIT Archives, MIT Recombinant DNA History Collection, Box 16, Folder 204.

13. M. Meselson and R. Yuan, "DNA restriction enzyme from E. coli," *Nature* 217 (March 23, 1968):1110-1114.

14. The international traffic to and from the Pasteur Institute and the charisma of the late Jacques Monod is poignantly revived in the recollections of his colleagues edited by André Lwoff and Agnès Ullmann, *Un Hommage à Jacques Monod: Les Origines de la Biologie Moléculaire* (Paris-Montreal: Etudes Vivantes, 1980).

15. Among the members of the HCBSC were Paul Berg, James Darnell, Gerald Edelman, Phillip Robbins, Harry Eagle, William Sly, Matthew Scharf, James Watson, Herbert Weissbach, Charles Yanofsky, and Norton Zinder.

16. Krimsky, *Genetic Alchemy*, pp. 26-29.

17. B. H. Sweet and M. R. Hilleman, "The vacuolating virus SV40," *Proc. Soc. Exper. Biol. Med*. 105 (1960):420; R. J. Huebner, R. M. Chanock, B. A. Rubin, and M. J. Casey, "Induction by adenovirus type 7 of tumors in hamsters having the antigenic characteristics of SV40 viruses," *Proc. Natl. Acad. Sci. USA* 52 (1964):1333-1340.

18. Lear, *Recombinant DNA—The Untold Story*, p. 1.

19. Wade, *The Ultimate Experiment: Man-made Evolution*, p. 33; Nicholas Wade, "Microbiology: hazardous profession faces new uncertainties," *Science* 182 (November 9, 1973):566.

20. Lear, *Recombinant DNA: The Untold Story*, p. 28.

21. Krimsky, *Genetic Alchemy*, p. 33.

22. Leon R. Kass, "The new biology: what price relieving man's estate?" *Science* 174 (November 19, 1971):779-788.

23. Interview with Andrew M. Lewis, NIH, Bethesda, Maryland, November 17, 1989.

24. The NIH Biohazards Committee was established in 1972, with Robert Martin as the first chairman. The committee's jurisdiction was restricted to intramural operations. It approved Andrew Lewis's concept that viral cultures should be shared with those outside investigators who signed and returned a memorandum of understanding, but a number of the researchers failed to live up to the agreement.

25. These tensions are evident in the published record of the meeting, edited by A. Hellman, M. N. Oxman, and R. Pollack, *Biohazards in Biological Research: Proceedings of a Conference at Asilomar, January 22-24, 1973* (New York: Cold Spring Harbor Laboratory, 1973). Several excerpts appear below:

M. N. Oxman: "Almost any form of biological research involves some potential biohazards. [This has] only recently become of concern to many people outside of those few laboratories that are directly involved with agents of known pathogenicity for man and other animals. This sudden expansion of concern in the absence of adequate information has resulted in a good deal of fear and confusion. . . ."

Francis Black (Yale): "We have come to realize that the cost will inevitably reduce the number of grants available and increase the time available to reach our ultimate goal. If we do believe in our mission of trying to control cancer, it behooves us to accept some risks . . . if five or ten people were to lose their lives, this might be a small price for the number of lives that might be saved."

James Watson (Cold Spring Harbor): "I'm afraid I can't accept the five to ten deaths as easily as my colleague across the aisle. They could easily involve people in no sense connected with the experimental work and most certainly not with the recognition and fame (for discovery of) the cause of human cancer . . . NCI has to face up to paying for the costs of safety or declaring all the viruses we work with as not dangerous. . . ."

26. Janet E. Mertz and Ronald W. Davis, "Cleavage of DNA by RI restriction endonuclease generates cohesive ends," *Proc. Natl. Acad. Sci. USA* 69 (November 1972):3370-3374; A. Dugaiczyk, H. W. Boyer, and H. M. Goodman, "Ligation of EcoRI endonuclease-generated DNA fragments into linear and circular structures," *J. Mol. Biol.* 96 (July 25, 1975):171-184.

The volume of recombinant DNA research at Stanford at that time is indicated by the fact that, as the paper by Mertz and Evans was sent to the *Proceedings of the National Academy of Sciences* by sponsor Paul Berg, a report of similar findings from another department was on its way to the same journal (Vittorio Sgaramella, "Enzymatic oligomerization of bacteriophage p22 DNA and of linear simian virus 40 DNA," *Proc. Natl. Acad. Sci. USA* 69 [November 1972]:3389-3393).

27. EMBO workshop on DNA restriction and modification, Basel, Switzerland, September 26-30, 1972, reported in the MIT Archives, MIT Recombinant DNA History Collection, Box 16, Folder 205. U.S.-Japan conference on bacterial plasmids, Honolulu, 1972, reported in the MIT Archives, MIT Recombinant DNA History Collection, Box 16, Folder 206.

28. Lear, *Recombinant DNA: The Untold Story*, pp. 64-65. See also Stanley N. Cohen, Annie C. Y. Chang, Herbert W. Boyer, and Robert B. Helling, "Construction of biologically functional bacterial plasmids in vitro," *Proc. Natl. Acad. Sci. USA* 70 (November 1973):3241-3244.

29. From the onset of its extramural grants program, NIH protected to the utmost the autonomy and freedom of basic researchers. The clinical investigators—who many molecular biologists considered a foreign culture—were meanwhile feeling governmental restraints. Beginning in 1966, all institutions receiving NIH, and later any federal, support had to have a local institutional review board (IRB) approve their clinical experiments. Soon at least one member of the IRB had to come from outside the institution. (After Asilomar, a similar requirement would be imposed on recombinant DNA experimentation.) Potentially far more serious was the appearance in the early 1970s of the first proscriptions of federally funded research. First, studies of abortifacients were forbidden; then in 1974 all fetal research was proscribed. These prohibitions remain in force today.

30. Lear, *Recombinant DNA: The Untold Story*, p. 69; Krimsky, *Genetic Alchemy*, pp. 72-73, citing the transcript of an interview with Maxine Singer, July 31, 1975, contained in the MIT Archives, MIT Recombinant DNA Historical Collection, Box 13, Folder 151.

31. The Institute of Medicine (IOM) was in the third year of its existence as a new partner of NAS and the National Academy of Engineering. The president of IOM responded to the letter of Singer and Söll with the suggestion that their request should be handled by the National Research Council (NRC). (See the letter from John Hogness to Maxine Singer and Dieter Söll, August 1973, contained in the NAS Archives, Folder ALS [Assembly of Life Sciences], Committee on Synthetic Nucleic Acids: Ad Hoc, Proposed, 1973.) Rather than IOM, a new organization within the academies had that year been created to oversee NRC activities in biology and health. This Assembly of Life Sciences had yet to have its first meeting when the communications from the Gordon conference arrived.

32. Maxine Singer and Dieter Söll, "Guidelines for hybrid DNA molecules," *Science* 181 (September 21, 1973):1114.

33. Both Lear (*Recombinant DNA: The Untold Story*, pp. 69-74), and Krimsky (*Genetic Alchemy*, pp. 73-80) describe the origins and depth of concern for the ethics of science held by the Gordon conference chairperson, Maxine Singer. (For his sources, Krimsky makes particular use of a transcript of an interview with Maxine Singer on July 31, 1975 [MIT Archives, MIT Recombinant DNA Historical Collection, Box 13, Folder 151] and a transcript of an interview with Daniel Singer, July 28, 1975 [MIT Archives, MIT Recombinant DNA History Collection, Box 13, Folder 150].) Singer recollected that when she and Söll had been confronted by the two scientists, she had no doubt that the conference should seriously consider the concerns they had raised.

34. Letter from Philip Handler to Maxine Singer and Dieter Söll, July 20, 1973, contained in the NAS Archives, Folder ALS, Committee on Synthetic Nucleic Acids: Ad Hoc, Proposed, 1973.

35. Letter from Paul Marks to Philip Handler, August 30, 1973, contained in the NAS Archives, Folder ALS, Committee on Synthetic Nucleic Acids: Ad Hoc, Proposed, 1973.

36. Letter from Paul Berg to Leonard Laster, January 2, 1974, contained in the NAS Archives, Folder ALS, Committee on Recombinant DNA Molecules: Ad Hoc, 1974.

37. See Wade, *The Ultimate Experiment: Man-made Evolution*, and Rogers, *Biohazard*, p. 44. Richard Roblin had met Berg at Dulbecco's laboratory in the 1960s. In the course of preparing a lecture on bioethics, he remembered the letter from the Gordon conference and wrote to the Academy inquiring what had happened to the issue (letter from Richard Roblin to Leonard Laster, March 20, 1974, contained in the NAS Archives, Folder ALS, Committee on Recombinant DNA Molecules, Ad Hoc, 1974). Roblin was referred to Berg, who suggested that he attend the planning committee meeting. Thereafter Roblin served as scribe, one of his tasks being the reworking of the several drafts of the committee's report before it was released by the Academy.

38. P. Berg, D. Baltimore, H. W. Boyer, S. N. Cohen, R. W. Davis, D. S. Hogness, D. Nathans, R. Roblin, J. D. Watson, S. Weissman, and N. D. Zinder, "Potential biohazards of recombinant DNA molecules," *Science* 185 (July 26, 1974):3034. See also *Proc. Natl. Acad. Sci. USA* 71 (July 1974):2593-2594. The "Berg letter," as it is often called, was signed by more scientists than the seven who met at MIT as the planning committee. Lear says that when Stanley Cohen learned Berg had been invited by the Academy to form a committee, he asked to be a member. Reportedly, Berg declined his offer, saying that the committee would consist of cancer workers. Cohen appeared at MIT one day after the planning committee meeting and learned from David Baltimore that no plasmid experts had been in attendance. Concerned that the committee's actions might selectively harm research in his area of interest, Cohen threatened to write his own letter and asked Boyer to join him. Berg then called Cohen and asked him to join in endorsing the report of his committee. A number of other scientists at Stanford thereafter asked to be included, and Berg eventually invited Hogness, Davis, and Boyer to sign the report as well (Lear, *Recombinant DNA: The Untold Story*, pp. 83-84).

39. Annie C. Y. Chang and Stanley N. Cohen, "Genome construction between bacterial species in vitro: Replication and expression of staphylococcus plasmid genes in Escherichia coli," *Proc. Natl. Acad. Sci. USA* 71 (April 1974):1030-1034; John F. Morrow, Stanley N. Cohen, Annie C. Y. Chang, Herbert W. Boyer, and Howard Helling, "Replication and transcription of eukaryotic DNA in Escherichia coli," *Proc. Natl. Acad. Sci. USA* 71 (1974):1743-1747; and unpublished data of David R. Hogness, Ronald W. Davis, and Herbert W. Boyer cited in Berg et al., "Potential biohazards of recombinant DNA molecules."

40. Documents in the NAS archives (especially Folder ALS, Committee on Recombinant DNA Molecules, Ad Hoc, 1974) record interesting efforts in late May 1974 to adjust to concerns on the part of NAS president Philip Handler, who was determined that the report of the planning committee not appear to be a private letter from the scientists to their colleagues. As one part of such efforts, the committee agreed to be constituted immediately as an ad hoc committee of the ALS. In addition, a comparison of Richard Roblin's drafts of the report suggests that the ALS reviewers helped stress the international importance of follow-up to the document and improved the stance of the report, re-

placing an impression of self-sacrifice on the part of the signers with a call to all scientists to join in the moratorium.

41. The French government also reacted quickly to the publication of the Berg letter. The Délégation Générale de Recherche Scientifique et Technique (DGRST) set up an organization for some form of control over "research which nobody denies can be dangerous." Two committees were formed. One was to consider ethical problems arising from the research; it was chaired by Jean Bernard and included Monod, Jacob, Gros, Monier, Ebel, Chabbert, and Slonimsky. The second committee of 15 experts, researchers, physicians, and biologists later defined the safety limits of recombinant research using the Asilomar guidelines. DGRST reviews of research grants in the summer of 1974 imposed a moratorium along the lines proposed by the Americans ("Asilomar and the Pasteur Institute [from La Recherche]," *Nature* 256 [July 3, 1975]:5; P. Kourilsky, personal communication).

42. See R. Roblin's notes on the planning meeting for the Asilomar conference, and Herman Lewis's notes on the biohazard conference organizing committee meeting, MIT, September 10, 1974, contained in the MIT Archives, MIT Recombinant DNA History Collection, Box 16, Folder 207.

43. Lear, *Recombinant DNA: The Untold Story*, pp. 115-118, describes how the press coverage was arranged.

44. "NAS ban on plasmid engineering," *Nature* 250 (July 19, 1974):175; Ephraim S. Anderson, "Indiscriminate use of antibiotics has exerted more pressure on the bacterial population than could be wielded by all research workers in the world put together," *Nature* 250 (July 26, 1974):279-280, and "Viability of, and transfer of a plasmid from, E. coli K12 in the human intestine," *Nature* 255 (June 5, 1975):502-506; William H. Smith, "Survival of orally administered E. coli K12 in alimentary tract of man," *Nature* 255 (June 5, 1975):500-502. A few months after the Asilomar conference Anderson presented his impression of the proceedings in an interview with Charles Weiner. (The transcript of the interview on May 31, 1975, is contained in the MIT Archives, MIT Recombinant DNA History Collection, Box 1, Folder 2.) Anderson notes:

> In some ways, the Asilomar meeting reminds me of Bernard Shaw's definition of the English gentleman hunting the fox: the unspeakable in pursuit of the uneatable. When I say that, I'm not actually decrying the people who were considering the problem. But here was a bunch of people, with no experience in the handling of pathogens, virtually, with the sole exception of a mere handful, considering hazards that were not even known to exist. There's a certain comic atmosphere about it. It's true that this is the first occasion on which such hazards have been considered possible. But, in fact they were a bunch of innocents abroad.

When interviewed by telephone at his home in London on February 6, 1990, Anderson emphasized that he did not intend his remarks to be unkind but that he still felt strongly that the conference was seriously hampered by an insufficient number of participants with experience in handling pathogens and infectious disease. Asked how he had voted on the final show of hands on the provisional statement, Anderson answered, "Aye, because I hadn't had time to consider all the issues, and therefore couldn't be completely negative. One had to leave the matter open at that moment."

45. Roy Curtiss III memorandum to Paul Berg et seq., August 6, 1974, "On potential biohazards of recombinant DNA molecules," contained in the NIH Central Files, Box Comm-4-4-7-1A.

46. K. Murray, "Alternative experiments?" *Nature* 250 (July 26, 1974):279.

47. H. Green, transcribed from the tape recording of the Asilomar conference, February 1975, NAS Archives.

48. The members of the Plasmid-Phage Working Group were R. C. Clowes, S. N. Cohen, R. Curtiss III, S. Falkow, and R. Novick (chairman). I am indebted to Andrew Lewis for copies of the original reports of the working groups.

49. Rogers, *Biohazard*, pp. 62-65.

50. Among the "lambda people" at Asilomar were D. Botstein, A. Campbell, P. Kourilsky, A. Skalka, and W. Szybalski.

51. The members of the Animal Virus Working Group were M. Bishop, D. Jackson, A. Lewis, D. Nathans, B. Roizman, J. Sambrook, and A. Shatkin (chairman).

52. Open letter to the Asilomar conference on hazards of recombinant DNA from Science for the People, contained in the MIT Archives, MIT Recombinant DNA History Collection, Box 17, Folder 219. The signers of this letter from the Genetic Engineering Group of Science for the People were Fred Ausubel, Jon Beckwith, and Luigi Gorini (Harvard); Kostia Bergmann, Kaaren Janssen, Jonathan King, Ethan Signer, and Annamaria Torriani (MIT); and Paulo Strigini (Boston University). Although there are differences in their reports, Krimsky (*Genetic Alchemy*, pp. 110-111) and Lear (*Recombinant DNA: The Untold Story*, p. 124) agree that Berg extended an invitation to Jonathan Beckwith to attend the conference, although the latter did not attend. The record is not clear whether Jonathan King was invited. He was not present.

53. The members of the Plasmid-Cell DNA Recombinant Working Group were S. Brenner, D. D. Brown (chairman), R. H. Burris, D. Carroll, R. W. Davis, D. Hogness, K. Murray, and R. C. Valentine.

54. Sources of the voting tallies are Lear, *Recombinant DNA: The Untold Story*, p. 145; Rogers, *Biohazard*, p. 100; P. Kourilsky, personal communication; W. Szybalski, personal communication.

55. Five Soviet scientists attended the Asilomar conference (see the appendix). A. A. Bayev, a well-known nucleic acid chemist, spoke for the delegation. He and his colleagues were in accord with the consensus, he said. His remarks also gave the wistful impression, however, that molecular biology was lagging in the Soviet Union. As all the participants knew, research in genetics had been gravely damaged during the Stalin era, a stark reminder of the vulnerability of science in a totalitarian milieu. In 1978, I visited Bayev at the U.S.S.R. Academy of Sciences' Institute of Molecular Biology in Moscow and delivered a copy of proposed revisions of the NIH recombinant DNA guidelines.

56. Paul Berg, David Baltimore, Sydney Brenner, Richard O. Roblin III, and Maxine F. Singer, "Summary statement of the Asilomar conference on recombinant DNA molecules," *Science* 188 (June 6, 1975):991; also *Proc. Natl. Acad. Sci. USA* 72 (June 1975):1981-1984.

57. Letter from Philip Handler to James Ebert, May 20, 1975, contained in the NAS Archives, Folder ADM, International Relations, International Conferences, Recombinant DNA Molecules, Organizing Committee, Report.

58. A summary of Krimsky's list of the severe limitations of Asilomar as a policymaking model for the recombinant DNA debate covers the selection of participants, clarity of the decision-making process, boundaries of discourse, public participation, and control of dissent. He suggests some alternatives that could have been employed: nominations from health organizations in the relevant areas (infectious diseases, immunology, and medical microbiology); open requests for papers; contacting environmental organizations for expertise; and soliciting participation from organizations concerned about occupational health. He admits, however, that opening up the process in this way posed the risk of losing control of the issues (*Genetic Alchemy*, p. 151).

APPENDIX

Participants in the International Conference on Recombinant DNA Molecules
Asilomar Conference Center, February 24–27, 1975

Organizing Committee

Paul Berg *(Chair)*, Professor, Department of Biochemistry, Stanford University Medical Center

David Baltimore, American Cancer Society Professor of Microbiology, Center for Cancer Research, Massachusetts Institute of Technology

Sydney Brenner, Scientific Staff of the Medical Research Council, United Kingdom, Cambridge, England

Richard O. Roblin III, Professor of Microbiology and Molecular Genetics, Harvard Medical School, and Assistant Bacteriologist, Infectious Disease Unit, Massachusetts General Hospital

Maxine F. Singer, Biochemist, National Institutes of Health

Domestic Participants

Edward A. Adelberg, Department of Microbiology, Yale University

W. Emmett Barkeley, Head, Environmental Control Section, National Cancer Institute

Louis S. Baron, Chief, Department of Bacterial Immunology, Walter Reed Army Institute of Research

Michael Beer, Department of Biophysics, The Johns Hopkins University

Jerome Birnbaum, Basic Microbiology, Merck Institute

J. Michael Bishop, Professor of Microbiology, University of California Medical Center, San Francisco

David Botstein, Cold Spring Harbor Laboratory

Herbert Boyer, Department of Microbiology, University of California Medical Center, San Francisco

Donald D. Brown, Staff Member, Department of Embryology, Carnegie Institution of Washington

Robert H. Burris, Professor of Biochemistry, University of Wisconsin, Madison

Allan M. Campbell, Department of Biology, Stanford University

Alexander Capron, University of Pennsylvania School of Law

John A. Carbon, Professor of Biochemistry, Department of Biological Science, University of California, Santa Barbara

Dana Carroll, Department of Embryology, Carnegie Institution of Washington

A. M. Chakrabarty, Physical Chemistry Laboratory, General Electric Company

Ernest Chu, Department of Human Genetics, University of Michigan Medical School

Alfred J. Clark, Department of Molecular Biology, University of California, Berkeley

Eloise E. Clark, Division Director, Division of Biological and Medical Sciences, National Science Foundation

Royston C. Clowes, Professor of Biology, Institute for Molecular Biology, The University of Texas at Dallas

Stanley Cohen, Associate Professor, Department of Medicine, Stanford University Medical School

Roy Curtiss III, Department of Microbiology, University of Alabama Medical Center

Eric H. Davidson, Department of Developmental Biology, California Institute of Technology

Ronald W. Davis, Assistant Professor, Department of Biochemistry, Stanford University Medical Center

Peter Day, Connecticut Agricultural Experiment Station, New Haven

Vittorio Defendi, Chairman, Department of Pathology, New York University Medical Center

Roger Dworkin, Department of Biomedical History, University of Washington Medical School

Marshall Edgell, Department of Bacteriology, University of North Carolina, Chapel Hill

Stanley Falkow, Department of Microbiology, University of Washington School of Medicine, Seattle

W. Edmund Farrar, Jr., Department of Medicine, South Carolina Medical University

Maurice S. Fox, Department of Biology, Massachusetts Institute of Technology

Theodore Friedman, Department of Medicine, University of California, San Diego

William Gartland, National Institute of General Medical Sciences

Harold Green, Fried, Frank, Harris, Schriver, and Kampelman, Washington, D.C.

Irwin C. Gunsalus, Professor of Biochemistry, University of Illinois, Urbana

Donald R. Helinski, Professor, Department of Biology, University of California, San Diego

Robert B. Helling, Department of Botany, University of Michigan

Alfred Hellman, Head, Biohazards and Environmental Control, National Cancer Institute

David S. Hogness, Professor, Department of Biochemistry, Stanford University Medical Center

David A. Jackson, Department of Microbiology, University of Michigan Medical School

Leon Jacobs, Associate Director for Collaborative Research, National Institutes of Health

Henry Kaplan, Department of Radiology, Stanford University Medical Center

Joshua Lederberg, Professor, Department of Genetics, Stanford University Medical Center

Arthur S. Levine, Head, Section on Infectious Diseases, National Cancer Institute

Andrew M. Lewis, Laboratory of Viral Diseases, National Institute of Allergy and Infectious Diseases

Herman Lewis, Head, Cellular Biology Section, Division of Biological and Medical Sciences, National Science Foundation

Paul Lovett, Department of Biological Sciences, University of Maryland, Baltimore

Morton Mandel, Department of Biochemistry and Biophysics, University of Hawaii School of Medicine

Paul Marks, Vice President, Medical Affairs, College of Physicians and Surgeons, Columbia University

Malcolm A. Martin, Head, Physical Biochemistry Section, National Institute of Allergy and Infectious Diseases

Robert G. Martin, Biochemist, National Institute of Arthritis, Metabolism, and Digestive Diseases

Carl R. Merril, Laboratory of General and Comparative Biochemistry, National Institute of Mental Health

John Morrow, Department of Embryology, Carnegie Institution of Washington

Daniel Nathans, Boury Professor and Director, Department of Microbiology, Johns Hopkins University School of Medicine

Elena O. Nightingale, National Academy of Sciences Resident Fellow, Division of Medical Sciences

Richard P. Novick, Department of Microbiology, Public Health Research Institute, New York

Ronald Olsen, Department of Microbiology, University of Michigan

Richard J. Roberts, Cold Spring Harbor Laboratory

William Robinson, Department of Infectious Diseases, Stanford University Medical Center

Stanfield Rogers, Department of Biochemistry, University of Tennessee Medical Units

Bernard Roizman, Professor of Microbiology and Biophysics, University of Chicago

Joe Sambrook, Cold Spring Harbor Laboratory

Jane Setlow, Brookhaven National Laboratory

Philip Sharp, Center for Cancer Research, Massachusetts Institute of Technology

Aaron J. Shatkin, Roche Institute of Molecular Biology

George R. Shepherd, Los Alamos Scientific Laboratory

Artemis P. Simopoulous, Staff Officer, Division of Medical Sciences, National Research Council

Daniel Singer, Vice President, Hastings Institute of Society, Ethics, and Life Sciences

Robert L. Sinsheimer, Chairman, Division of Biology, California Institute of Technology

Anna Marie Skalka, Associate Member, Department of Cell Biology, Roche Institute of Molecular Biology

Mortimer P. Starr, Department of Bacteriology, University of California, Davis

Dewitt Stetten, Jr., Deputy Director for Sciences, National Institutes of Health

Waclaw Szybalski, McArdle Laboratory, University of Wisconsin, Madison

Charles A. Thomas, Jr., Department of Biological Chemistry, Harvard Medical School

Gordon M. Tompkins, Professor of Biochemistry, Department of Biochemistry and Biophysics, University of California, San Francisco

Jonathan W. Uhr, Professor and Chairman, Department of Microbiology, University of Texas Southwestern Medical School

Raymond C. Valentine, Assistant Professor in Residence, Department of Chemistry, University of California, San Diego

Jerome Vinograd, Professor of Chemistry and Biology, California Institute of Technology

Duard Walker, Department of Medical Microbiology, University of Wisconsin, Madison

Rudolf G. Wanner, Associate Director for Environmental Health and Safety, Division of Research Services, National Institutes of Health

James Watson, Professor, Department of Biology, Harvard University

Peter Weglinski, Department of Biology, Massachusetts Institute of Technology

Bernard Weisblum, Professor, Department of Pharmacology, University of Wisconsin Medical School, Madison

Sherman Weissman, Professor, Department of Medicine, Biology, and Molecular Biophysics, Yale University

Pieter Wensink, Brandeis University

Frank Young, Department of Microbiology, University of Rochester

Norton D. Zinder, Professor, The Rockefeller University

Foreign Participants

Ephraim S. Anderson, Director, Enteric Reference Laboratory, Public Health Laboratory Service, London, England

Toshihiko Arai, Department of Microbiology, Keio University, Shinjuku, Tokyo, Japan

Werner Arber, Department of Microbiology, University of Basel

A. A. Bayev, Academician, Institute of Molecular Biology, Moscow, U.S.S.R.

Douglas Berg, Département de la Biologie Moléculaire, Université de Genève, Geneva, Switzerland

Yuriy A. Berlin, Professor, M. M. Shemyakin Institute of Bioorganic Chemistry, Academy of Sciences of the U.S.S.R., Moscow, U.S.S.R.

G. Bernardi, Institut de la Biologie Moléculaire, Faculté des Sciences, Paris, France

Max Birnstiel, Institute of Molecular Biology II, University of Zurich, Switzerland

Walter F. Bodmer, Genetics Laboratory, Department of Biochemistry, Oxford, England

N. H. Carey, G.D. Searle and Company, Ltd., Research Division, England

Y. A. Chabbert, Professor, Bacteriology Department, Institut Pasteur de Paris, France

François Cuzin, Institut Pasteur de Paris, France

Julian E. Davies, Professor, Département de la Biologie Moléculaire, Université de Genève, Switzerland

Ray Dixon, ARC Unit of Nitrogen Fixation, University of Sussex, Brighton, England

W. A. Englehardt, Professor, Institute of Molecular Biology, Academy of Sciences of the U.S.S.R., Moscow, U.S.S.R.

Walter Fiers, Laboratorium voor Moleculaire Biologie, Ghent, Belgium

Murray J. Fraser, Professor, Department of Biochemistry, McGill University, Montreal, Quebec, Canada

W. Gayewski, Professor, Department of Genetics, Warsaw University, Ujazdowskie, Poland

Stuart W. Glover, Department of Psychology, University of Newcastle-upon-Tyne, England

Walter Goebel, Professor Gesellschaft für Molekularbiologische Forschung, Braunschweig, West Germany

Carleton Gyles, Department of Veterinary Microbiology and Immunology, The Ontario Veterinary College, University of Guelph, Ontario, Canada

Gerd Hobom, Institut für Biologie II der Universität Freiburg, West Germany

Peter H. Hofschneider, Professor, Max-Planck-Institut für Biochemie, München, West Germany

Bruce W. Holloway, Department of Genetics, Monash University, Victoria, Australia

H. S. Jansz, Professor, Nederlandse Dereniging voor Biochemie, Amsterdam, The Netherlands

Mikhail N. Kolosov, Academician, M. M. Shemyakin Institute of Bioorganic Chemistry, Academy of Sciences of the U.S.S.R., Moscow, U.S.S.R.

Philippe Kourilsky, Institut Pasteur de Paris, France

Ole Maaloe, Professor, Department of Microbiology, University of Copenhagen, Denmark

Alastair T. Matheson, Senior Research Officer, Division of Biological Sciences, National Research Council, Ottawa, Ontario, Canada

Kenichi Matsubara, Department of Biochemistry, Kyushu University, Fukuoka, Japan

Andrey D. Mirzabekov, Professor, Institute of Molecular Biology, Academy of Sciences of the U.S.S.R., Moscow, U.S.S.R.

Kenneth Murray, Senior Lecturer, Department of Molecular Biology, University of Edinburgh, Scotland

Haruo Ozeki, Department of Biophysics, Faculty of Sciences, University of Kyoto, Japan

James Peacock, Division of Plant Industries, CSIRO, Canberra City, Australia

Lennart Philipson, Department of Microbiology, The Wallenberg Laboratory, Uppsala University, Sweden

James Pitard, Department of Microbiology, University of Melbourne, Parkville, Victoria, Australia

Mark H. Richmond, Head, Department of Bacteriology, University of Bristol, England

A. Rorsch, Department of Biochemistry, Leiden State University, The Netherlands

Vittorio Sgaramella, Instituto di Genetica, Pavia, Italy

Luigi G. Silvestri, Gruppo Lepetit, Milan, Italy

Lou Siminovitch, Department of Medical Genetics, University of Toronto, Toronto, Ontario, Canada

H. Williams Smith, Houghton Poultry Research Station, Huntingdon, England

Peter Starlinger, Institut für Genetik der Universität Köln, Germany

Pierre Tiollais, Institut Pasteur de Paris, France

Alfred Tissières, Professor, Département de la Biologie Moléculaire, Geneva, Switzerland

John Tooze, EMBO, Heidelberg, West Germany

Alex J. van der Eb, Laboratory of Physiological Chemistry, Leiden, The Netherlands

Robin Weiss, Imperial Cancer Research Fund Laboratories, London, England

Charles Weissmann, Professor, Institut für Molekularbiologie, Universität Zurich, Switzerland

Robert Williamson, Beatson Hospital, Glasgow, Scotland

Ernest Winocour, Professor, Department of Genetics, Weizmann Institute of Science, Rehovot, Israel

E. L. Wollman, Institut Pasteur de Paris, France

Hans G. Zachau, Professor, Institut für Physiologische Chemie und Physikalische Biochemie, Universität München, West Germany

Press Participants

George Alexander, *Los Angeles Times*
Stuart Auerbach, *Washington Post*
Jerry Bishop, *Wall Street Journal*
Graham Chedd, *New Scientist* and *Nova*
Robert Cooke, *Boston Globe*
Rainer Flohl, *Frankfurter Allgemeine*
Angela Fritz, Canadian Broadcasting Corporation
Gail McBride, *Journal of the American Medical Association*
Victor McElheny, *New York Times*
Colin Norman, *Nature*
Dave Perlman, *San Francisco Chronicle*
Judy Randal, *Washington Star-News*
Michael Rogers, *Rolling Stone*
Cristine Russell, *Bioscience*
Nicholas Wade, *Science*
Janet Weinberg, *Science News*

Commentary

Dorothy Nelkin

The Asilomar conference of February 1975 was a pivotal event in the controversy over the potential hazards of recombinant DNA research. In a commendable and responsible act, several scientists had called attention to possible risks. The subsequent conference at Asilomar was organized to develop a scientific consensus on interim guidelines to assure standards of safety. Scientists were stunned and dismayed at the public response and the widespread indications of mistrust. What then was the social meaning of Asilomar? Was the conference and the subsequent struggle over the safety of this research an isolated "threat" to the relationship between biomedical science and society? Or did these events simply express existing tensions between science and society? Have biomedical science and society restored "their mutually beneficial entente," as Fredrickson says? Or was the incident the beginning of an even more strained relationship?

Asilomar was about the autonomy of science. Stanley Cohen expressed the intent of the scientists who organized the conference: "If the collective wisdom of this group doesn't result in recommendations, the recommendations may come from other groups less well qualified." It was, in many ways, a symbolic event. It symbolized the sense of social responsibility among scientists concerned about the potential hazards of their research. It demon-

Dorothy Nelkin is a University Professor at New York University, affiliated with the department of sociology and the School of Law.

strated that scientists were able to mobilize an enormous international effort to shape research decisions—or, as Fredrickson puts it, to "march in ranks" in the face of external threats to their autonomy. But above all, Asilomar, and the highly publicized events in its wake, crystallized growing public concerns about the wisdom of allowing scientists to regulate themselves. Scientific autonomy was the issue at stake.

The Asilomar conference was neither the beginning nor the end of public efforts to constrain the autonomy of science. During the 1970s biomedical scientists conducting experiments on the effect of antibiotics on the human fetus were indicted for "grave-robbing." Public pressure forced the termination of a Harvard Medical School project to test the association between certain chromosomal abnormalities and predisposition to antisocial behavior, and protest groups obstructed research on the effect of psychotropic drugs on behavioral disorders. Even the teaching of evolution in public schools came under persistent attack. In the 1980s, public pressure persisted—recall the public hearings that challenged science-based programs such as genetic screening of workers in chemical plants, and the critical questions, aired in the media, about the appropriate methods of research to detect carcinogens in food additives. In recent years, the remarkable growth of the animal rights movement and its significant influence on research practices hardly suggest a "mutually beneficial entente." Indeed, many issues, long perceived as internal to science—methods of research, control of fraud, sharing of research data—are now aired in the public arena. For better or worse, the public is entering decisions about the practices as well as priorities of science.

These public pressures on science reflect several types of concerns. The Asilomar decisions dealt rather narrowly with one issue, the containment of potentially pathogenic organisms. Such fears about risks to human health remain at the center of many disputes. But public concerns about science also extend well beyond the fear of risk. Some disputes reflect a growing uneasiness about the social implications of scientific knowledge—the fear that research findings may be put to harmful use. Other disputes occur when people consider scientific research to be morally dubious—a threat to traditional values or religious beliefs. Still others crop up when science appears to infringe on the rights of individuals, threatening, for example, the right to privacy. Whatever the concern, disputes over research decisions are challenging the autonomy of scientists, as activists call for greater regulation and public involvement in decisions concerning research priorities and practices.

The relationship between science and society has been one in which the public provided research support but made limited demands for accountability and control. This relationship rested on a set of assumptions about science as a source of objective, disinterested knowledge. Science has been considered an agent of the general public, removed from political biases and economic interests. Whether myth or reality, this was the image that sustained the acceptance of scientific autonomy. But recent changes in the way the public perceives science have increasingly involved scientists in economic and political liaisons with special interest groups. As these liaisons develop, issues of patenting and property, of ownership and control, are inevitable. In this changing context, scientists will find it more and more difficult to project the image of objectivity and neutrality that in the past has served them so well. Current controversies reveal a growing cynicism about science as critics talk of the "commodification" and the "inhumanity" of science, its "corporate culture," and the erosion of its moral authority.

The economic and policy implications of scientific research, the dominance of costly projects in the research infrastructure, and the increased involvement of commercial interests evident in industry-university relationships and the involvement of scientists in biotechnology firms will exacerbate changes in the autonomy of science. Ironically, the more directly science is called upon to contribute to specific economic and policy goals, the less it can effectively retain its image of moral authority as a source of disinterested, unbiased information. The more science is valued as a political and economic resource, the less scientists can expect to avoid increasing public control.

In this context, the Asilomar conference and the events it subsequently provoked were more a beginning than an end. For they were events that called very wide attention to the public character of science, its potential implications, and the need to set priorities that reflect the public will.

Commentary

Paul Slovic

Donald Fredrickson's chronicle of the Asilomar conference brings us to the end of the beginning of the debate about the acceptability of risks from recombinant DNA technology. As the conference faded into history and safety guidelines for research were being prepared, a new and even more turbulent era began. News of the scientists' concerns about the possibility of serious, unpredictable consequences of crossing natural genetic barriers triggered strong opposition to DNA research in many communities and led legislators to begin drafting strict regulation to control the specter of risk raised at Asilomar.

Despite an exemplary record of safety, public perceptions of risk have had a continuing impact on recombinant DNA research and development. Early battles in what have been labeled the "gene-splicing wars" (Zilinskas and Zimmerman, 1986) focused on containment of genetically altered organisms in the laboratory. Subsequent confrontations have focused on the perceived risks from deliberate release of such organisms into the environment. For example, a field test of frost-retarding bacteria was declared safe by an NIH expert committee in 1983 but was prevented from taking place until 1987 by lawsuits and public hearings. This delay prompted one observer to comment: "Perhaps the most ironic aspect of this long-running . . . controversy is that the

Paul Slovic is president of Decision Research in Eugene, Oregon and professor of psychology at the University of Oregon.

brilliant minds that figured out this world-transforming technology in the first place have yet to figure out a way to ease public fears about it" (Hall, 1987).

Recombinant DNA technology is not unique in its problems with perceived risks. After smooth sailing in its first two decades of development, nuclear power became embroiled in risk-based opposition, triggered by its association with weapons of destruction and by scientists' worst-case accident scenarios. The opposition was subsequently maintained by the cumulative impacts of numerous small and few and not so small accidents. Alvin Weinberg (1976) has observed: "As I compare the issues we perceived during the infancy of nuclear energy with those that have emerged during its maturity, . . . public perception and acceptance . . . appears to be the question that we missed rather badly. . . . This issue has emerged as the most critical question concerning the future of nuclear energy." During the past decade, public concern and dissatisfaction have also become increasingly associated with the production, use, transport, and disposal of many types of chemicals.

At present, nuclear power and chemical technologies are under siege in the United States and many other countries, whereas biotechnology, despite past controversies, is flourishing. What accounts for the differences in public perception and acceptance of these technologies? What does the future hold for biotechnology? I do not pretend to have complete answers to these questions, but I shall speculate about them from the perspective of research on risk perception.

THE NATURE OF PERCEPTION

Serious studies of risk perception began in the mid-1970s, about the same time as the Asilomar conference. These studies have sought to determine why the public is anxious about some technologies (e.g., nuclear power) but not others (e.g., dams, motor vehicles) and why people's concerns are often unrelated to what experts believe they should worry about. Early research demonstrated that people's judgments of probability and risk are strongly determined by the ease with which adverse consequences can be imagined (Tversky and Kahneman, 1973; Lichtentenstein et al., 1978). Both nuclear power and biotechnology prove vulnerable in this regard because of associations with improbable but highly imaginable scenarios such as nuclear explosions and viral epidemics.

Other studies have found that the public has a different, and in some sense richer, conception of risk than do the experts (Slovic, 1987). Public perceptions and acceptance of risk are intimately connected to the qualities or nature of the hazard—that is, whether exposure is voluntary, whether the risks are familiar, controllable, catastrophic, dread, known to science and to those exposed, fair (in the sense of risks being borne equitably by those who benefit from the hazardous activity), and so on. Experts' assessments of risk, in contrast, are driven by probability and magnitude of adverse consequences and tend not to be related to the qualities of risk that concern the public.

Although one can draw many parallels between nuclear power and recombinant DNA technologies (both transform matter in powerful ways that can be used for good or evil), nuclear power is perceived somewhat more negatively on the qualities that most strongly determine perceptions of risk. Nuclear power's risks are judged to be less controllable, more dread, more catastrophic, and less equitably distributed among those who benefit from the technology. However, biotechnology risks are judged less well known and less understood.

Close examination of specific hazards within a particular domain such as radiation or chemicals shows that perceptions of risk are not homogeneous. Within the domain of radiation hazards, nuclear power and nuclear waste are perceived much more negatively than medical x-rays and radon gas. Similarly, industrial and agricultural uses of chemicals are perceived far more negatively than prescription drugs and vaccines. The favorable view of x-rays and medical uses of chemicals indicates that acceptance of risks is conditioned by familiarity, by perceptions of direct benefits, and by trust in the managers of the technology—in this case the medical and pharmaceutical professions. Those in charge of managing nuclear power and nonmedical chemical technologies are clearly less trusted. In addition, the benefits of these technologies are not highly appreciated; hence, their risks are less acceptable. The public's apathetic response to the risk from radon appears to result from the fact that it is of natural origin, occurring in a comfortable, familiar setting with no one to blame.

Biotechnology, of course, encompasses an enormous range of activities ranging from familiar fermentation technologies to deliberate release of genetically altered microorganisms into the environment. Based on the above findings, one would expect that perceptions of risk and benefit would vary considerably across these various activities, with application in medicine being perceived most favorably. One would also expect that the benefits of many nonmedical applications would not be apparent to the public, no matter how obvious they appear to scientists and industrialists. When benefits are not perceived as significant, the public is intolerant of any risk, even a small one.

THE EFFECTS OF PERCEPTIONS

Whether or not one agrees with public risk perceptions, they form a reality that cannot be ignored. During the past decade, research has shown that individual risk perceptions and cognitions, interacting with social and institutional forces, can trigger massive social, political, and economic impacts. Risk analyses typically assess the impacts or seriousness of an unfortunate risk event (e.g., an accident, a discovery of pollution, an adverse drug reaction) in terms of direct harm to victims or property. Yet the adverse impacts of a risk event sometimes extend far beyond these direct harmful effects and may include indirect costs to the responsible government agency or private company that far exceed direct costs. In some cases, all companies in an industry are affected, regardless of which company was responsible for the mishap. In extreme cases, the indirect costs of a mishap may even affect companies, industries, and agencies whose business is minimally related to the initial event. Thus, an unfortunate event can be thought of as a stone dropped in a pond. The ripples spread outward, encompassing first the directly affected victims, then the responsible company or agency, and, in the extreme, extending beyond industry boundaries.

Some events make only small ripples; others make big ones. The challenge is to discover characteristics associated with an event and the way it is managed that can predict the breadth and seriousness of these effects. Early theories equated the magnitude of impact to the number of people killed or injured, or to the amount of property damaged. The accident at the Three Mile Island (TMI) nuclear reactor in 1979, however, provided a dramatic demonstration that factors besides injury, death, and property damage impose serious costs. Despite the fact that not a single person died at TMI, and few if any latent cancer fatalities are expected, no other accident in our history has produced such costly societal impacts. The accident at TMI devastated the utility that owned and operated the plant. It also imposed enormous costs on the nuclear industry and on society through stricter regulation, reduced operation of reactors worldwide, greater opposition to nuclear power, and increased costs of subsequent reactor construction and operation.

The proliferation and spread of ripple effects is a phenomenon that has been termed "the social amplification of risk" (Kasperson et al., 1988). It appears that multiple mechanisms contribute to social amplification, causing even "small" events to have significant effects on industries and society. One such mechanism is the finding that the perceived seriousness of an accident or other unfortunate event, the media coverage it gets, and the long-range costs and other high-order impacts on the responsible company, industry, or agency appear to be determined, in part, by what the event signals or portends. *Signal value* reflects the perception that the event provides new information about the likelihood of similar or more destructive future mishaps.

The informativeness or signal value of an event, and thus its potential social impact, appears to be systematically related to the characteristics of the hazard. An accident that takes many lives may produce relatively little social disturbance (beyond that caused to the victims, families and friends) if it occurs as part of a familiar, well-understood system (e.g., a train wreck). However, a small accident in an unfamiliar system (or one perceived as poorly understood), such as a nuclear reactor or a recombinant DNA laboratory, may have immense social consequences if it is perceived as a harbinger of further and possibly catastrophic mishaps.

In a recent survey of college students, "DNA research" was rated highest among 97 activities with respect to "risks unknown to science." It was also highest in terms of a direct judgment of signal value (the degree to which an accident would increase one's perception of the likelihood of similar or more destructive future mishaps). This survey implies that the first evidence that recombinant DNA activities pose *real* physical risks is likely to result in strong, restrictive sociopolitical responses. Francis Black's position (i.e., his willingness to risk losing five or ten lives in recombinant DNA research as a small price for the number of lives that might eventually be saved) was thus unwise (see Fredrickson, footnote 25). "Small" fatal accidents in the early stages of this activity could have stymied its development for many years. In this light, the cautious approaches recommended at Asilomar and thereafter were indeed justified.

A second important mechanism of social amplification is the action of special interest groups, which bring risk issues to public attention and then try to keep them there. Fredrickson notes the involvement of one such group, Science for the People, which urged the Asilomar contingent to allow the public to participate in the regulation of biological research. Many activists and groups subsequently played a role in the "recombinant-DNA wars" of 1976-1978 (Zinder, 1986). Now there are many more such groups, and they are increasingly well funded and more sophisticated in getting their message across to the public, legislators, and regulators.

Many believe that the gene-splicing wars are over. I disagree. For better or for worse, our society manages risk through public controversy and adversarial confrontation (recall the "chilling landscape of legal liability" described by the lawyers at Asilomar). Members of the public, acting individually or through powerful special interest groups, increasingly demand control over the risks to which they may be exposed. Technical assessments of risk carry little weight, unless those who construct them and those who present them are deemed trustworthy. In fact, trust is in short supply, hard won (by actions such as those of Asilomar), and quickly lost in the adversarial arena. Technologies that alter genetic material will be watched carefully for ominous signs of imperfection and danger and will be treated roughly when such signs appear. On the positive side, people will tolerate what they perceive to be significant risks if the benefits appear to be commensurate—and biotechnology certainly promises great benefits in medicine and other domains.

Although many have labeled public perceptions of risk uninformed or irrational, research on this topic paints a different picture. Whereas experts define risk in a narrow, quantitative way, the public has a broader view, incorporating legitimate value-laden considerations such as uncertainty, controllability, catastrophic potential, and equity into the risk-benefit equation. The impacts of public perceptions of risk cannot be lessened without drastic, politically unacceptable changes in the structure of our society. Thus, we must learn to treat perceptions as legitimate. We must attempt to understand them and to incorporate public concerns and wisdom into decision making, along with the wisdom gleaned from scientific assessments of risk.

REFERENCES

Hall, S. 1987. One potato patch that is making genetic history. Smithsonian 18(5):125-136.

Kasperson, R. E., O. Renn, P. Slovic, H. S. Brown, J. Emel, R. Goble, J. X. Kasperson, and S. Ratick. 1988. The social amplification of risk: A conceptual framework. Risk Analysis 8:177-187.

Lichentenstein, S., P. Slovic, B. Fischoff, M. Layman, and B. Combs. 1978. Judged frequency of lethal events. Journal of Experimental Psychology: Human Learning and Memory 4:551-578.

Slovic, P. 1987. Perception of risk. Science 236:280-285.

Tversky, A., and D. Kahneman. 1973. Availability: A heuristic for judging frequency and probability. Cognitive Psychology 5:207-232.

Weinberg, A. M. 1976. The maturity and future of nuclear energy. American Scientist 64:16-21.

Zilinskas, R. A., and B. K. Zimmerman, eds. 1986. The Gene-Splicing Wars: Reflections on the Recombinant DNA Controversy. New York: MacMillan.

Zinder, N. D. 1986. A personal view of the media's role in the recombinant DNA war. In The Gene-Splicing Wars: Reflections on the Recombinant DNA Controversy, R. A. Zilinskas and B. K. Zimmerman, eds. New York: MacMillan.

Conclusions

. . . Extend the sphere, and you take in a greater variety of parties and interests; you make it less probable that a majority of the whole will have a common motive to invade the rights of other citizens; or if such a common motive exists, it will be more difficult for all who feel it to discover their own strength, and to act in unison with each other.

Federalist Papers 10

Conflict and controversy about values occur in any society. Controversy over science and technology, however, entails unique clashes between expertise and ignorance, encompassing ideals about rationality and progress and challenging our traditional notions of legitimacy and authority.

There are several significant messages delivered by the preceding case studies. They tell us that pluralism and democracy are not very efficient but are robust in the conduct of American science and medicine. They illustrate that advances in science not only are complex but have a multiplier effect in U.S. society, giving birth to complexity upon complexity, that makes rational decision making as to the best way to proceed exceedingly difficult. Yet somehow we muddle through, adjusting the system in incremental ways through a variety of processes. The process we use to make decisions might give us clues as to whether the decision will succeed, even if it is impossible to predict what the decision will be.

For those who believe in rationality, there is the disappointing message that chance, fate, and just plain politics lurk behind every decision. Only historians will know at what point they play a significant role. The cases also illustrate the fact that putting a "human face" on a problem means it will probably be solved sooner, if not better. Several cases reveal that precedent setting makes people uncomfortable because they are reluctant to be held responsible for future decisions in which they have no part. Other cases demonstrate that, for some decision makers, making history is important—the positive side to setting precedents. Finally, and fortunately, the selected cases show us that, in general, people want to do the right thing.

Each case is a unique constellation of occurrences. They address issues of equity; strongly held ethical values; trustworthiness of actors, numbers, and techniques; authenticity of experiences; the influence of competition; the dilemma of setting precedents; and the challenge of effectiveness. They are about the search for legitimation and empowerment of the lay public. They illustrate our concern as a society for sufficiency of information and authority. Together the cases illustrate a spectrum of problem solving, ranging from coexistence to conflict to cooperation.

THEMES OF DECISION MAKING

Although there are structural similarities among the six cases in this book, a reliable taxonomy of biomedical decision making failed to emerge from this exercise. This is not to say that one could not be developed. Rather, the case study method militates against a normative approach. A different approach to the study of decision making would be needed to develop a solid theoretical framework. While a rational approach to decision making was not the expected finding of this exercise, themes were anticipated to emerge. And they did. Across the six cases were the complexities of pluralism and democracy, the frustrations of incrementalism, the surprises of chance and fate, the danger of precedents, and the tension between politics and expertise.

Pluralism and Democracy

A significant social trend in this country over the past few decades has been an increase in direct participation by the public in social and organizational decisions. Simultaneously, the problems facing our nation seem to have grown in complexity and volatility. History and the development of social events such as the civil rights and women's movements have sensitized different groups and forever moved certain issues such as reproductive rights, environmental standards, and re-

search missions into the public domain. As groups became more sensitized, they also became more assertive (Nelkin, 1984).

The trend toward more citizen involvement in decision making follows from the evolution of authority, which was first held by religious
groups, slowly moved to scientific and technical experts, and most recently has been held by the law. Recent years have seen more authority being held by the public, and this change has required increased
negotiation. As a result, decisions are made in broad daylight and the
public can now choose whether to participate. Such freedom of choice
on the public's part, however, does not exist when moral authority is
held by any single body within society.

The philosopher Tristram Engelhardt asks, "How do we resolve policy disputes in a society where there is no longer a moral authority,
and absence of shared faith?" He answers that, somehow, we must
accommodate a plurality of viewpoints (Engelhardt, 1990), but accommodation can be a painful and prolonged process. In the RU-486 and
fetal tissue cases, the nation's polarization on the abortion issue created paralysis. The degree of opposition appears to make a compromise
or rational adjudication of differences impossible. Even open discourse is inhibited. The fetal tissue case is about socially acceptable
public policy with respect to a new procedure. Like the RU-486 case, it
is about moral politics and its influence in decisions.

When Alexis de Tocqueville first warned of the "tyranny of the majority," he could never have foreseen the impact of mass media and public
opinion polls, which have forever altered our perceptions of the majority and minority in America. Today, more than ever, all views claim
legitimacy, and the views that are able to mobilize votes have power.
The Bill of Rights has always protected the voices of those in the minority, but it has been only in recent history that those on the fringe have
been able to use the media to penetrate the mainstream.

This new capability is the lesson of the ddI and RU-486 cases, in
which groups not in the majority were already organized. When the issue of nonsurgical abortion through RU-486 arose, antiabortion groups
were there to react and slow the testing and distribution of the drug.
When AIDs therapeutics proved too slow in coming and often a failure,
the gay community, already organized to fight discrimination, was there
to demand change. The ddI case illustrates the unprecedented involvement of persons affected by the disease in decision making at the
drug development level. The gay community was predisposed to question and distrust the health and scientific establishments. Those making
decisions about new drug development were obliged to involve the activists in their decisions. Although there was some confrontation, there
was also a great deal of dialogue.

The lesson to be learned from these examples is that decisions made in modern pluralistic society require that all those with a vested interest in the outcome be brought to the discussion at some point. One might argue that knowing whether a decision is right generally requires time; thus, only time will clarify whether the early use of ddI or RU-486 will have the positive effects some anticipate. One test that can be applied is asking whether the decision will hold up over time, and the answer may have to do with who sits around the table. Of course, this was not the case in the fetal tissue example, in which the "right" people were brought to the table to debate the issue only to have political forces negate their efforts.

The end-stage renal disease case shows us that even the best intentions and bringing together collective wisdom can still result in a decision that has proven over time to be very expensive for society. Crafted as a mechanism to provide financial equity, it has become an inequitable decision in that it favors those with one disease and not another.

Not inviting the right people to the table can prove troublesome later. Critics of the Asilomar process have argued that the public was not adequately involved in the initial discussions, and it was only good judgment and proper restraints on the part of the scientists that prevented disaster. Had a moratorium not been in place, and had a biohazard occurred, science would have been set back severely once the public realized what had happened.

In an ideal decision-making situation, involving people from the start invests them in the process and possibly in the outcome as well. There is a caveat, however. Involving people in the process of deciding, without giving them the authority to decide, may result in decisions that are impractical. The fetal tissue case reminds us that advisory panels rarely have authority. Lack of authority may sometimes embolden panels to make recommendations that are intellectually and even spiritually sound, but politically untenable.

Is there a problem in the way we try to involve multiple actors in the decision-making process, or do these cases merely describe unusually complex issues? Certainly, there will always be tensions. Religion is no longer a particularly useful mechanism for resolving disputes. Some people resort to the law, but laws can be wrong or ambiguous. Others turn to procedural approaches—if we follow a process that everyone agrees is correct, then we should come up with an answer that we can agree on or accept. The questions, however, then become, was the process ethically defensible? Did we stimulate dialogue instead of confrontation? Did we recognize new constituencies and try to determine who stands to get hurt? Answering yes to these questions may be as close as we can get to the truth. We may have to settle for the politics of the second best because there may not be a best. And what is best by scientific or medical standards may not be the best political option.

Incrementalism

Policymaking is the totality of the decisional processes by which a group decides to act or not to act. Traditionally, there have been two views of this process, the rational approach (Lasswell, 1963) and the incremental approach (Lindblom, 1968). The incremental theory, popularly known as the science of muddling through, claims that the rational approach is unrealistic. The rational approach, which begins with information gathering and ends with appraisal and determination of a policy, allows for a scholarly dissection of the policy process in retrospect but is difficult to follow prospectively.

Incrementalist accounts of decision making stress the impossibility of making the correct choice and the need to limit the costs of the errors that will inevitably occur (Collingridge, 1989). These principles are illustrated in Rettig's account of the decision to provide reimbursement for ESRD, when the decision makers believed that national health insurance would soon be in place. Obviously, the problem with incrementalist approaches is that their result is public laws that are disjointed, incomplete, and sometimes contradictory.

Science and technology challenge the incrementalists because they often cause revolutions both in technical possibilities and in thinking. In the cases described here, scientific and technological uncertainty is complicated by the presence of multiple stakeholders with conflicting values and beliefs about the most desirable direction and magnitude of progress. The cases illustrate how biomedical public policies are made by actors in a political system. They inform us that decision making, even in science, has becomes less an analytic endeavor than a process of mediating among parties with differing levels and types of knowledge —a kind of "knowledge management" (Hart, 1986).

Decision making is not merely the process of choosing among competing alternatives. The cases show us that decisions, even on the grandest of scales, are made on an interpersonal level through haggling, pressing, and persuading. In some of the cases, such as those involving ESRD and the human genome, timing and chance seem to play as much of a role as any other more rational or controllable factor.

All six cases show that decision making involves the bringing together of facts and values. It is relatively easy to separate the facts from the values retrospectively. The problem in complex decision making is to bring all the relevant information together at points where certain choices are made (different roles in decision making) and recognize at the time where facts or values reign. Because advances in science and technology come in two very different forms—revolutions, or the slow accumulation of knowledge leading to breakthroughs—there is no easy way to align facts and values.

Chance, Fate, and Politics

Frequently in decision making, one or two people can really make a difference, such as Charles DeLisi and David Smith of the Department of Energy in the human genome project, Anthony Fauci in the ddI case, and Paul Berg in the Asilomar example. With excellent judgment and good luck, they can make the right choices.

Sometimes timing is the controlling factor. The ESRD case shows us that the time was right for the Senate to pass the legislation providing funds for treatment of kidney disease. A year sooner or later might have produced a different result. It was also chance, or fate, that led to two critical events: the alleged miscommunication about the actual costs of treatment and the good luck that Shep Glazer did not die during dialysis before the House Ways and Means Committee. No one could have calculated these two events into any a priori evaluation of possible outcomes.

Chance was also a critical factor in the ddI case. The fact that the Reagan administration was actively promoting deregulation of all industries was a convenient coincidence that helped facilitate the parallel track. In the genome case we see that, by chance, construction of the Keck telescope inadvertently but directly set in motion discussions that would lead to the human genome project, proving that momentous ideas can be born in unlikely places.

Depending on one's view of the value of cost estimates, luck might also play a role in their accuracy. The ESRD and genome cases illustrate the hazards of trying to assign costs to events that will continue far into the future. It is not that these estimates should not be made, but rather that they should be made on various scales, with plausible scenarios assigned to each figure. In such cases preparedness appears to be more important (and more possible) than correctness.

Precedents and the Slippery Slope

In several of the cases, key actors expressed concern about the possible impact of current decisions on future choices. The ddI case is a good example: Levi describes the worry at FDA about modifying the regulatory process in such a way that the changes would complicate the approval of new non-AIDS drugs. The AIDS activists felt they were already sliding and initially had little concern about the effect of their lobbying efforts on future drugs and future disease groups. It was only later in the debate that they recognized that their requests for use of an experimental drug in a dying population might affect other groups of patients. In the fetal tissue case, Childress documents the concern, on the part of some panelists and key administration officials, that condoning the use of fetal tissue would set a precedent resulting in an increased demand for surgical abortions. At Asilomar, some scientists expressed concern about imposing a moratorium because of the lasting effect it might have on future decisions. The ESRD case is about entitlement, access, and equity, and the slippery slope of precedents.

Why this concern about precedent? It seems that although individuals are usually willing to take responsibility for their own actions and decisions, they do not want to be held responsible for future decisions that may be much more troubling. The fear of the slippery slope can be put into very concrete terms: once we head down this path, can we turn back? Some writers have argued that if rationales are given for why a decision was made, the slippery slope argument can be addressed (Mendeloff, 1985). If a group can agree on a decision, even though they disagree on principles, then rationales should be provided for why they chose to agree—even if those rationales are as simple as accommodation to the realities of limited time, information, and reasoning ability.

Sometimes if the problem has a clear human aspect, such as it did in the ddI and ESRD examples, concerns about precedent take a back seat. In both of these cases the present and the future placed uneven demands on those making the decision. A decision made today could literally save lives, and it seemed immoral or indecent not to provide funds where they could have such an immediate impact. The value in the present thus overshadowed the cost to the future. The decision makers were not unaware of this dilemma, but perhaps did not perceive the place their decision might assume in history.

Politics, Expertise, and Process

There is a continuing tension over the degree to which politics should be modulated by scientific expertise (Levine and Benda, 1986). Many scientists feel that to make decisions about science, one must know science. But the centrality of science and scientific knowledge to American life implies that science is too important to be left to the scientists (Hill, 1989). The ddI case highlights the public dimensions of science and medicine and shows that science cannot always dictate the terms of engagement.

Congress now has the help of such agencies as the Office of Technology Assessment and the Congressional Research Service to help it understand scientific and technological issues. Executive agencies routinely seek the advice and presumably the principled guidance of scientific experts. Recently, the boards advising the U.S. government comprise not just scientists but theologians, ethicists, lawyers, and laypersons.

Boards and panels were convened to discuss the human genome project; a committee was formed to advise the Bureau of the Budget on treatment for ESRD; and an advisory panel debated the use of fetal tissue for therapeutic transplantation. What were the roles of these groups? How well did they succeed? Did they inform the debate, reassure the public, or build consensus? To some extent they might have accomplished all of these objectives, had their deliberations been more widely publicized. They each draw attention to the issue of how scientific panels and reports are used in the political process. The Gottschalk report was never seen by the members of Congress and their key staff in making the landmark ESRD decision. The deliberations of the fetal tissue panel were never widely distributed but instead summarized in single-column press coverage. For political reasons, the sponsors of such expert bodies might not always want their recommendations publicized. Nevertheless, if the sponsors are public agencies, then there seems to be a duty to make the results known.

In the Asilomar case, scientific experts submerged themselves in an emerging policy problem and attempted to extrapolate beyond what was known scientifically. In doing so, they resorted to cognitive processes that are not significantly different from those of the layperson. Yet the cutting-edge nature of the research could only be assessed by its practitioners. If the audience at Asilomar could not reach consensus, there was no one else to turn to.

Consensus building in science is traditionally aided by three conditions: autonomy, disciplinarity, and a low level of critical public scrutiny (Collingridge, 1989). These break down as soon as the science is thought to be relevant to policy. Autonomy becomes limited and disciplinary barriers become confused because policy problems are by nature interdisciplinary. In addition, public problems are more critically scrutinized. If one accepts these notions of consensus building inside and outside of science, the Asilomar case represents a remarkable example of how scientists overcame their amateur standing in policymaking. They were neither prepared nor experienced in how a group should arrive at the kind of decision they were attempting to make, yet they did so with remarkable expediency and, in retrospect, with admirable responsibility. Some feel that the Asilomar case sends a positive message to the nonscientific community: their mistrust of the professional elite can be laid to rest because such individuals can and will adopt moral precedents in the realm of science and technology. Even so, there is no mechanism in place for dealing with this type of issue again.

In contrast, the human genome case is about the decision to fund a very costly program in the face of dissent within the scientific community. The case describes the ad hoc process by which it was conceived, formulated, and ratified at several levels in the federal science agencies. It involves visionary scientists, skilled bureaucrats, timing, and pure politics. The budget process was the mechanism by which the policy was made. In many ways, this was an invisible decision, made in Washington, about Washington, by a small number of people. If the public knew what was being planned, would they have stopped it? Perhaps it was the informal, ad hoc nature of the process that helped the project get funded. There was no focal point; the issue was a moving target. It was easy for those in the scientific community who were opposed to the project to get lost in the process. Some have charged that the project was steamrollered through Congress without adequate debate. Politically, the project left the arena of scientific debate and took on a life of its own because it had to do with power and "turf." Again, as in the case of Asilomar, there was a vacuum in place of an adjudicating body.

Nowhere is the lack of adequate process more visible than in the RU-486 case, where political events rather than informed discussion led the debate. In the controversy over abortion in this country the lines are so sharply drawn that any deliberative body would probably be viewed as too political to have any legitimacy. Because of this, the RU-486 case is likely to unfold in as diffuse and decentralized a process as one could conceive. It is the case of not making a decision that in effect is a decision in favor of one side of the controversy.

In defense of the bureaucracy, however, one might point to ddI. In an age when bureaucracy seems to be unresponsive and at times unacceptably slow, the ddI case reminds us that we are all capable of remarkable shifts of attitudes. This was certainly true of the scientists and regulators involved in the decision about ddI who were able to forgo a strongly held position in favor of one they had bitterly opposed. The case also reminds us that hard choices often bring together strange partners. Levi illustrates an unusual confluence of interests—among AIDS activists, regulators, drug companies, and scientists. Each group had different reasons for seeking parallel track and early release of ddI, and ordinarily the missions of these groups would conflict. The unexpected coalition that did, indeed, result remind us of the importance of carefully assessing the "whos" and "whys" of any decision's dynamic.

The case of ddI is also about seeking change through traditional formats. No new regulations were needed—just a new way to use an accepted process, which is perhaps why the ddI effort succeeded. The United States is a pragmatic society, and Americans often seek the path of least resistance.

QUESTIONS FOR RESEARCH

Each of the cases in this volume raises its own set of issues and areas of uncertainty, but questions common to most, if not all, of the cases became apparent as the committee read through and discussed them. Some of these questions reflect a lack of understanding of the interactions of science and policy; others are raised because of lack of good data; and still others come from concerted introspection into how scientists as experts can operate in a society where authority is sometimes viewed as insufficient for action. One goal of this effort was to develop a set of questions that might be pursued through future research. Nine overarching issues were identified and are described below.

How and Why Does an Issue Become Public, and What Is the Proper Response?

People who make policy in areas of biomedical research would benefit from a greater understanding of why some issues trigger immediate, intense public reaction and others do not. For example, the RU-486 case demonstrates the power of the antiabortion lobby in influencing the decisions of pharmaceutical executives. On the other hand, the human genome project, which is likely to lead to improved capabilities for prenatal diagnosis of genetic defects, was never targeted by groups concerned about termination of unwanted pregnancies. What roles do immediacy, magnitude, and cost play in the public's reaction to an issue? Is there any way to predict with any certainty that an emerging technology or application is going to receive more public scrutiny than others?

What Are the Roles of Science Versus the Public in Risk Recognition, Perception, Assessment, and Management?

In the Asilomar case study, the scientific community took the risk of raising the issue of potential biohazards from recombinant DNA research. Since Asilomar, numerous grassroots and national efforts have been directed toward monitoring and, in some cases, delaying the conduct and siting of research on recombined organisms. Would the public outcry have been as strong or as swift if the scientific community had not come forward with their concerns? Some scientists say they regret this experience, that it discouraged them from being forthright in future situations. Yet the willingness of the scientific community to be the first to warn also allowed them to play a primary role in the development of guidelines and regulations—a sort of preemptive strike. Similarly, in the human genome case, Watson recognized that issues related to acceptable risk, ethics, and legality would follow the project and thus set aside a portion of the project budget to address those questions.

The issue of risk perception is integral to formulating biomedical policy. In the case of ddI and AIDS treatment, the gay community asked that individuals be allowed to determine their own acceptable risk and that scientific judgment take a back seat to personal choice. Decision makers could benefit from a greater understanding of how people perceive risk, which might also allow for more autonomy in decision making. In addition, it would benefit the assessment and management of risk, two critical areas of underfunded research.

What Are the Role and Impact of the Media in Publicizing and Defining the Debate?

The media are often the first line of communication to the public on issues of science and technology (Nelkin, 1988). Keeping in mind the old saying that it is easier to form public opinion than to change it, the manner in which the press defines the issue, presents its dimensions, and follows up on it may be more important than any other factor in a biomedical debate. How the media collect information deserves more study, as do media attitudes toward science. Impediments to effective communication between scientists and the media should be explored, including such topics as how to present complex information, how to convey uncertainty, how to overcome lack of public interest, and how to deal with the reluctance of scientists to step beyond the facts into values and opinion.

How Can We Evaluate and Predict the Impact of Single-Issue Politics?

The cases on RU-486, fetal tissue, and to some extent ddI illustrate the remarkable emergence of single-issue politics in America. Very often, biomedical disputes arise over moral differences—whether to terminate a pregnancy, refuse to resuscitate or prolong life, or risk a life through experimental therapies. Because single issue voters tend to tie their vote to moral issues, it seems that biomedicine is bound to become enmeshed in the politics of single issues as public involvement overwhelms the debate, driving the experts out of the dialogue. More needs to be known about how these influences affect decision makers and whether there is any way to bring all viewpoints into the process.

How Have the Ground Rules and Institutions Changed in Biomedical Decision Making?

The six cases, because they span the years 1969 to the present, reveal that the environments in which decisions are made change rapidly. In addition, decision making is continuous. To understand policies, therefore, one must look at the context in which they were made, recognizing that decisions do not have an internal autonomy. Policy analysts as well as decision makers might be more effective if they understood that precedents might not always apply to a new situation and that rules made in another time may no longer be relevant.

For example, the Congress described in the ESRD case study was a different body than the one found in the human genome story. It was organized differently, and its expertise was more centralized. Furthermore, it operated under a very different set of assumptions about the future. Although both cases illustrate spending decisions, and appear to be quite diverse when the nature of that spending is considered, greater differences are apparent in the way that costs were developed and negotiated. History is instructive in highlighting similarities and differences; its uses for decision making deserve more attention (Neustadt and May, 1986).

How Can Costs of Research and Treatment Be Estimated to Diminish Future Conflicts?

Cost estimates can be used to promote or discourage a new initiative, and seriously erroneous estimates can literally cost lives. Yet we often let the numbers carry us away. We need not only better methodologies for estimating costs but also greater understanding of how much weight cost estimates carry in the minds of those making decisions. At what point do decision makers allow costs to counterbalance effectiveness?

The cases on ESRD and the human genome project demonstrate the role costs can play in a decision. In both cases, uncertainties were not adequately factored in. For ESRD, the unanticipated and widespread use of dialysis in elderly and terminally ill populations was not considered. In the human genome case, the decision makers did not seem to calculate the relative costs of such a large-scale project in times of budgetary constraint. Where there is overconfidence, it must be identified. Where there is uncertainty, wider bands must be drawn around costs. In sum, more research is needed on the methodology of cost estimates, specifically on the assumptions underlying them.

When Is Consensual Decision Making the Most Desirable Approach?

To answer this question, we need a better understanding of the behavioral and social aspects of consensus seeking and building. Consensus can be obtained in many ways. In the case of fetal tissue transplantation, an advisory panel was asked to deliberate on 10 issues and reach a consensus that could be communicated to the assistant secretary for health. In the case of ddI, consensus was arrived at slowly and informally, and to some was hard won. What are the assumptions behind the consensus type of decision making, and what do decision makers feel they gain from following that route?

In consensual decision making, panel composition is crucial. How panels are selected will influence outcome. The selection process and its effect on outcome deserve further study.

What Are the Domains of Politics and Science? Where Do They Overlap? What Is the Role of Expertise?

There is general agreement that science should be accountable and communicative, given its public nature (as a result of both its funding and its application). Very often, scientists' knowledge is a result of society's investment in them. In addition, scientists are valuable and sometimes exclusive sources of important information. That information can be powerful, and it is the duty of the scientist to share that power. Increasingly, the public is a partner in determining the adoption of new technology and is likely to become more litigious as it becomes more informed. The role of science is not to prevent litigation but to provide accurate information so that debates will be more informed.

As science and politics mix more frequently, as was illustrated in every case in this book, exploring the domains of the two cultures and understanding where they can conspire or clash become more compelling.

Who Represents the Public?

Although the public increasingly intervenes in biomedical decision making, it is often through proxies. For example, citizens may call or write their elected officials (as well as vote for those who represent their interests) or donate money to advocacy groups. In some cases, the media take on the responsibility of proxy by investigating and reporting on stories deemed to be in the public interest. On the side of decision makers, public officials and elected representatives may feel that they are acting in the public interest. Scientists can also act in what they perceive to be a civic role. Who represents the public and when do they have legitimacy?

QUESTIONS FOR POLICY MAKERS

Is it possible to plan better and to make more rational decisions in an irrational world where there are no absolute standards and where people hold diverse views? Or must we forever bear the social costs of learning by trial and error? One way to reduce the costs and the level of error is to involve the public in the decision, thereby enhancing social learning (Nelkin, 1984; Rip, 1986). By nature, however, the process will be ongoing, pluralistic, and fragmented. Policymakers are accustomed to that kind of discomfort; scientists are not. Decisions made by following democratic procedures need not be better than those made autocratically, but they will be more acceptable and carry more weight in a society that values democracy.

Problems can be dealt with on the organizational level, where the goal is to satisfy and reduce uncertainty, or on the personal level, by evaluating stakeholders and their interest, and estimating power struggles. The six cases suggest that decisions must be made on both levels. To achieve this balance, decision making must allow for interaction among the issue's key stakeholders in order to minimize serious cognitive or judgmental bias.

Yet the democratic process requires rules for interaction, the basis for which is due process guarantees, hearings, and administrative law. What makes the rules hard to follow is the use of moral discourse in policy determination. When the nation cannot agree on values, it finds it hard to agree on solutions to difficult problems. What then can be done? We can ask the following questions before taking any action.

Do we understand the problem?
Can we formulate the issue?
Do we understand the scientific facts or the technology?
Have we identified the uncertainty and recognized its implications?
How explicit are the values involved?
Have we identified and involved the constituencies?
Have we articulated all of the options?
Do we know how to extrapolate beyond our present knowledge?
Have we tried to stimulate dialogue, not confrontation?
What is our personal stake in the decision?
Where can we find advice and authority, and what role will they play?
What is the best social forum for resolving the conflict so that polarization will not prove paralytic?

Answering some of these questions can provide decision makers not with the right decision, but with a more enlightened framework within which to make a decision. Because most of the decisions described in this book are still being played out, one can only speculate whether they were correct. One way of viewing the biomedical decision-making process is through a sort of existential paradigm, whereby no decision is exhaustively describable or understandable in scientific terms. The irreducible uniqueness of each situation deserves special consideration in analysis. The paradigm of science as it relates to utility is set within the existential paradigm. Science is so much a part of our society that it is no longer useful, or helpful, to consider it in isolation. A decision maker who does not recognize the tensions within the paradigm is more likely to make a decision that will gain little support and may eventually have to be abandoned.

REFERENCES

Collingridge, D. 1989. Incremental decision making in technological innovation: What role for science. Science, Technology, & Human Values 14(2):141-162, spring 1989.

Engelhardt, H. T. 1990. Integrity, humaneness, and institutions in secular pluralistic societies. In Integrity in Health Care Institutions: Humane Environments for Teaching, Inquiry, and Healing, R. E. Bulger and S. J. Reiser, eds. Iowa City, Iowa: University of Iowa Press.

Hart, S. L. 1986. Managing knowledge in policy making and decision making. Knowledge: Creation, Diffusion, Utilization 8(1):94-109, September 1986.

Hill, C. 1989. How science policies are determined in the United States. The Evaluation of Scientific Research. New York: John Wiley & Sons.

Lasswell, H. 1963. The Future of Political Science. New York: Atherton.

Levine, C. H., and P. M. Benda. 1986. Expertise and democratic decisionmaking: A reader. Science Policy Background Report No. 7, Committee on Science and Technology, U.S. House of Representatives. Washington, D.C.: U.S. Government Printing Office.

Lindblom, C. 1968. The Policymaking Process. Englewood Cliffs, N.J.: Prentice-Hall.

Mendeloff, J. 1985. Politics and bioethical commissions: 'Muddling through' and the 'slippery slope.' Journal of Health Politics, Policy, and Law 10(1):81-92, Spring 1985.

Nelkin, D. 1984. Controversy: The Politics of Technical Decisions, 2nd edition. Beverly Hills, Calif.: Sage.

Nelkin, D. 1988. Selling Science: How the Press Covers Science and Technology. San Francisco: W. H. Freeman.

Neustadt, R. E., and E. R. May. 1986. Thinking in Time: The Uses of History for Decision Making. New York: The Free Press.

Rip, A., 1986. Controversies as informal technology assessment. Knowledge: Creation, Diffusion, Utilization 8(2):349-371, December 1986.

Appendixes

A

The Public and the Expert in Biomedical Policy Controversies

Stanley Joel Reiser

The landmark health policy cases of the last two decades have seen the American public and experts from the scientific and medical communities linked in dialogue (and sometimes controversy) to resolve issues of far-reaching social as well as scientific import. Before such a dialogue could occur, however, a set of events in the field of medicine brought both parties together and facilitated these exchanges. With World War II as a backdrop, the public and the community of experts sparred over the authority to enter each other's private domain and influence the actions that took place there. This essay examines the developments that brought these two groups to their current positions as partners in the public policymaking process.

QUESTIONING THE EXPERTS: THE CHALLENGE FROM LAYMEN

By the end of the Second World War, science and technology had come to be seen as fundamental forces impelling social growth, whose prominence caused rising exhilaration and deepening apprehension. Some saw such advances as the harbingers of a new age in which the drudgery and dangers of life would be lifted from the shoulders of humanity through, for instance, increased automation and the discovery of cures for many dread diseases. Others, no less intrigued with these benefits, nevertheless perceived a darker side. Their concern had sev-

Stanley Joel Reiser is the Griff T. Ross Professor and Director of the Program on Humanities and Technology in Health Care at the University of Texas Health Science Center, Houston.

eral dimensions. Would seeking technological solutions to the problems of life cause human activities to be reduced to expressions of technique (Ellul, 1967)? Would the weapons made possible by technology, already powerful and with greater destructive capacity certain to follow, ultimately destroy humanity (Brown, 1963)? Would planning and change based on technological transformations of basic social institutions, such as cities, damage essential human values and relationships (Mumford, 1934)? These questions were all being raised, but in the context of the subject of the report to which this appendix is attached, a major concern dealt with the functioning of democracy (Aron, 1962).

As all fields of human endeavor were enhanced by scientific and technological knowledge, experts appeared who claimed mastery over this learning, which had now grown too voluminous and complicated for the average person to grasp. These experts ("technocrats," as some called them) were increasingly recruited to provide advice about and manage social enterprises and policies, and their very expertise became a source of concern. If knowledge was now so vast that only specialized experts could penetrate the intricacies of a particular subject, what would be the fate of democracy? How could the ordinary citizen with a general education, the legislator, for example, be expected to understand the different sides of a complex issue? How could legislators or citizens retain firm control of the reins of social enterprises like government when experts held sway over society's most essential knowledge—the reach and limits of its technology? What would happen to democratic institutions if technological authority became subtly transposed into political power, with the expert piper increasingly calling the policy tune?

A response to the question of whether citizens as individuals and collectively as the public could meet the challenge of experts came in the 1960s, from the sphere of medicine. The physician had long been an archetype of authority, able to wield an expanding array of technology of much complexity and variety. The public had a level of personal and intimate contact with this technology, and with those who wielded authority over it, that was greater than its contact with perhaps any other area of learning. In addition, post-World War II developments in medical science had brought the technological side of medicine to high public visibility by the 1960s, both through personal experiences with therapy and through the media.

The physician's expert authority had a long history. Early records, such as those from the Hippocratic literature of ancient Greece, recognize this power and seek to ensure that it not be abused. The Hippocratic oath, for example, is quite emphatic that physicians must not take advantage of the person who, to regain health, entrusts them with access to his or her physical self and the secrets of personal experience. The doctor is bound by this oath to respect the person of the patient and to keep information received from the patient confidential.

Yet the doctor through history has also believed strongly in the duty to shield a patient from harm. The exercise of this duty required, as physicians viewed it, authority over the therapy they were providing subject to their expert learning and large experience. For instance, the conviction that knowledge of a threat to life or limb would wound a patient by causing despair and depression has led doctors from Hippocratic times until the present to systematically withhold such information from patients. A Hippocratic statement on this issue in the essay *Decorum* explains this dominant medical view about wielding benevolent authority: "Give necessary orders with cheerfulness and serenity, turning his [the patient's] attention away from what is being done to him; sometimes reprove sharply and emphatically, and sometimes comfort with solicitude and attention, revealing nothing of the patient's future or present condition. For many patients have taken a turn for the worse, I mean by the declaration I have mentioned of what is present or by a forecast of what is to come" (Jones, 1923a). In the 1960s this ancient authority, bolstered by a new technological capability that gave physicians a therapeutic power rivaling long-held diagnostic and prognostic ones, was challenged successfully by individual patients and the public alike (Jones, 1923b).

The challenge was strengthened by two of the most prominent right movements in the twentieth century—the civil rights and women's rights movements. The 1960s were filled with calls for American society to take heed of these groups, which had been deprived of human dignity and of access to political freedoms and social position. They called for recognition of an inherent self-worth shared by all, with "everybody a somebody," as Martin Luther King, Jr., put it. Along with the notion of worthiness, the ideal of autonomy was advanced particularly by women's rights advocates, who were concerned, among other things, about being deprived of the power to direct their reproductive lives.

These movements dovetailed with events in medicine, particularly in the field of research, that were refocusing attention on the ethical aspects of its landscape. Heinous experiments on prisoners during World War II by Nazi scientists and physicians had led to the formulation of a code to guide research on humans, which was presented at the Nuremberg war crimes trials. The 10 principles were the pillars of a protective wall of rights designed to secure the well-being of future research subjects. The code's central protection was announced in its first principle: "The voluntary consent of the human subject is absolutely essential" (Nuremberg Code, 1949). The requirement of voluntariness meant subjects must be located in a noncoercive environment that allowed, in the code's words, "free power of choice." They were also to be fully informed about the research to make enlightened consent possible.

This code and the events that brought it into existence significantly heightened recognition of ethical responsibilities within the scientific community, but by themselves were not enough to produce sustained action. Thus, several decades passed before the rights-concerned environment of the 1960s produced the U.S. surgeon general's 1966 directive on research. It required all health care institutions that were receiving federal funds to empanel human studies committees to oversee the ethical dimensions of a research project. A key feature of the directive was to ensure that a process of informed consent for subjects was integrated into each research proposal. This requirement subsequently stimulated similar actions in clinical medicine.

Rapidly, physicians began to shed millennia-old views that justified, through the "do-no-harm" principle, their determining the best interests of patients. Measures that had been adopted under this view, such as concealing threatening diagnoses, in general were shown to be unwise. In the new ethos, harm was also generated by the disregarding of patients' views in deciding among the benefits and risks of therapeutic alternatives. Respect for the person of the patient came to mean respecting his or her autonomy and right to know about and help choose the risks he or she would face. Formal recognition of this new situation, that the medical relationship was a partnership, was expressed in the 1973 "Statement on a Patient's Bill of Rights" adopted by the American Hospital Association: "The patient has the right to obtain from his physician complete current information concerning his diagnosis, treatment, and prognosis in terms the patient can be reasonably expected to understand" (American Hospital Association, 1973).

These events were major steps forward for the subjects of scientific research and the patient community. The daunting authority of the scientist and especially the physician—certainly the most accessible expert of the twentieth century—had been successfully challenged. These experts now acknowledge that it is possible to share detailed scientific and technical knowledge—and the resulting decisions that vitally concern a patient's health and life—with laypeople who are in uniquely vulnerable situations with respect to this knowledge and decision process. Thus, the authority of laypeople to help determine how science and technology would be developed and used was purchased initially with the coin of ethical assertion and political persuasion. That clinicians and scientists acquiesced in sharing their authority was due to an ability to draw on internalized traditions of ethical reflection to sanction the arguments that became the engines of change. Disciplines lacking such traditions would have been at a disadvantage. Neither ethical nor political pressures, however, would have maintained satisfactory adherence to these changes if experience and formal studies had not demonstrated that they were an improvement. For example, physicians recognized that their expertise was in how particular classes of patients, rather than particular individuals, fared under different regimens. The doctor reigned as expert on general population reactions; the well-informed patient came out best in determining personal preference. Merging both views produced the best choice. In the end, clinicians and medical scientists saw as part of their professional responsibility respect for the views of and provision of knowledge to their public of patients and subjects who, in turn, learned to act on their new understanding.

QUESTIONING THE EXPERTS: THE CHALLENGE FROM OFFICIALDOM

The challenge of the ordinary citizen to the authority of the expert was paralleled in the 1960s by a similar engagement between medical experts and political officialdom. Until that time, power in medicine generally had been exercised within the private professional enclosures, and encounters of professional authorities with public officials were sporadic. For instance, in 1960, basic decisions about how medical care was to be provided were made by doctor, patient, and family acting privately. The level or extent of care was not influenced by social agencies through payment or treatment guidelines, which by 1990 had become routine.

Passage of the Medicare and Medicaid acts in the mid-1960s began to alter permanently the private character of medicine. For the first time, the federal government assumed a major role in delivering medical services. Medicine now became a public enterprise: as its benefits and costs increasingly caused public authorities and society to take notice, an array of new values, disciplines, and social institutions joined existing professional ones in shaping future actions.

The debate that emerged concerned the relative balance to be struck in the governance of medicine between medical institutions such as professional societies and governmental agencies such as legislatures. How beneficial but expensive medical resources should be shared and paid for earned a place on the political stage of the nation in the 1960s, and the question has retained a leading role ever since. The experiences of experts and laypeople in their private encounters, however, established the possibility for more productive exchange as this discourse moved to public forums.

THE EXPERT'S JOURNEY INTO PUBLIC DOMAIN

The changes in the role of the layman, as patient or official, in decisions involving research and therapy were paralleled by discussions among experts in medicine and science on the implications of entering the public domain and participating in the resolution of controversial public problems. The social power that could be wielded by experts in science and technology derived from their ability to direct natural forces and understand alternative uses to which such forces could be put. Holders of this knowledge could exert great influence on national decisions and goals by entering the political scene and becoming deeply involved in public debate; in fact, however, most did not. By the 1960s some had come forth to write articles in popular publications or submit testimony to congressional committees; fewer still devoted large portions of time to policy matters.

A number of factors accounted for this behavior. In the first place, the role of the scientist and physician in public discourse remained controversial within their own professions. Could scientists or physicians remain current with the very knowledge that made them expert if they spent too much time and remained too far from their professional workplaces? Would such distancing endanger their productivity as clinicians or researchers and thus their standing with colleagues? If they lacked training in the social science disciplines that explained the policy process, how could they participate meaningfully in it? Given these kinds of questions, before and during the 1960s physicians and scientists resisted leaving the secure environment of clinics and laboratories to join officials in developing policy alternatives. Thus, fears that these experts would exert excessive control over policy and democracy were exaggerated. Instead, society grappled with the difficulties of gaining their aid in the political marketplace.

By the end of the 1960s, first in clinical medicine and later in medical science, expert participation in public discourse had begun to grow. This participation stemmed in part from the recognition during the 1960s that medicine and science were losing their identity as private professions and were gradually becoming social enterprises. This transformation of viewpoint was not merely the result of growing social support. Rather, it represented an emerging public recognition that the activities of clinical medicine and medical science bore heavily on significant national goals, which justified public dialogue about the character, costs, and directions of those activities. Only by recognizing and addressing these public interests—which meant periodically leaving laboratory and clinic and educating the next generation of students about these issues—could physicians and scientists maintain their own standing as leaders, protect the integrity of their professions, and affect a public agenda that increasingly shaped their own professional lives.

CONCLUSION

Such social and medical developments, from the 1940s to the 1960s, set the stage for the relation between public and expert in later cases from the Asilomar controversy to the human genome debate. Firmly entrenched as participants, the public now plays a key role in deciding the uses of science and technology, just as the expert has formed a clearer view of appropriate action in matters of policy. Both groups have yet to sort out questions that repeatedly appear in contemporary biomedical policy debates such as those discussed in this volume. For the public, what kind of justification is necessary for a given interest group to place a particular subject on the public agenda? How do they justify their own claim, as opposed to the claims of other groups, to sit at the policy table and help formulate solutions? For the expert, how is the appropriate level of knowledge for policymaking to be determined? When do we know enough to act? And for both, having developed policies acceptable to contemporary constituencies, what burdens are appropriate to pass on to our successors, particularly when we create policies that may either set important precedents or encumber later generations?

The ability to address these issues will grow to the extent that we continue to introduce factors into our new methods of policy development—such as better handling of the uncertainty factor and recognizing and explicating the ethical dimensions of policy issues. Participants in policy debates will also be aided by an awareness of tradition and the methods of their predecessors. Particular cases are unique, but the approaches to basic decisions that they demonstrate reflect previous events. Although the past cannot predict the present, like gravity, it exerts on us an inescapable pull.

REFERENCES

American Hospital Association. 1973. Statement on a patient's bill of rights. Hospitals 47(February):41.

Aron, R. 1962. The education of the citizen in industrial society. Daedalus (Spring):253.

Brown, H. 1963. The dangers we face. Pp. 170-177 in The Atomic Age: Scientists in National and World Affairs, M. Grodzins, and E. Rabinovitch, eds. New York: Basic Books.

Ellul, J. 1967. The Technological Society. New York: Alfred A. Knopf, Inc.

Jones, W. H. S., ed. 1923a. Decorum. Pp. 293-301 in Hippocrates, Vol. 2. Cambridge: Harvard University Press.

Jones, W. H. S., ed. 1923b. The Hippocratic Oath. Pp. 164-165 in Hippocrates, Vol. 1. Cambridge: Harvard University Press.

Mumford, L. 1934. Technics and Civilization. New York: Harcourt, Brace and Co.

The Nuremberg Code. 1949. Pp. 181-182 in Trials of War Criminals Before the Nuremberg Military Tribunals Under Control Council Law, No. 10, Vol. 2. Washington, D.C.: U.S. Government Printing Office.

B
Biographical Notes on Authors and Commentators

PAUL BERG earned a Ph.D. in biochemistry from Western Reserve University in 1952. After serving on the faculty at Washington University, Dr. Berg moved to Stanford, where he is presently Willson Professor of Biochemistry and director of the Medical School's Beckman Center for Molecular and Genetic Medicine. His research uses biochemical molecular genetic approaches for the analysis of eukaryotic gene expression and recombination, basic knowledge for understanding, preventing, managing, and curing genetic diseases. He is a member of the National Academy of Sciences, the Institute of Medicine, the American Academy of Arts and Sciences, and the American Philosophical Society. He is also a foreign member of the French Academy and the Japanese Biomedical Society. In 1980, Dr. Berg received the Albert Lasker Medical Award and the Nobel Prize in Chemistry for his studies of the biochemistry of nucleic acids, particularly recombinant DNA. He was awarded the National Medal of Science in 1985.

PETER F. CARPENTER is a visiting scholar at the Center for Biomedical Ethics at Stanford. He is the retired president of the ALZA Development Corporation, former executive director of the Stanford University Medical Center, and deputy executive director of the U.S. Price Commission. He serves on a number of nonprofit foundation boards and is an advisor on institutional missions, values, and ethics.

R. ALTA CHARO is assistant professor of law and medical ethics at the University of Wisconsin Law and Medical Schools. She has also served as a legal analyst for the Biological Applications Program of the congressional Office of Technology Assessment, and as an American Association for the Advancement of Science Fellow in Science, Technology, and Diplomacy at the U.S. Agency for International Development. Prior to her joint appointment at the University of Wisconsin, Ms. Charo lectured in law at Columbia University in New York and at the Sorbonne in Paris.

JAMES F. CHILDRESS is the Edwin B. Kyle Professor of Religious Studies and professor of medical education at the University of Virginia, where he is also chairman of the Department of Religious Studies and principal of the Monroe Hill Residential College. He is the author of numerous articles and several books on biomedical ethics, including *Principles of Biomedical Ethics* (with Tom L. Beauchamp), *Priorities in Biomedical Ethics*, and *Who Should Decide? Paternalism in Health Care*. Formerly vice chairman of the national Task Force on Organ Transplantation, he serves on the Board of Directors of the United Network for Organ Sharing (UNOS) and is a member of the Recombinant DNA Advisory Committee, the Human Gene Therapy Subcommittee, and the Biomedical Ethics Advisory Committee. He is a fellow of the American Academy of Arts and Sciences and of the Hastings Center, and he has been the Joseph P. Kennedy, Sr., Professor of Christian Ethics at Georgetown University and a visiting professor at the University of Chicago Divinity School and Princeton University. He received his B.A. from Guilford College, his B.D. from Yale Divinity School, and his M.A. and Ph.D. from Yale University.

ROBERT MULLAN COOK-DEEGAN, is the director of the Division of Biobehavioral Sciences and Mental Disorders at the Institute of Medicine (IOM), National Academy of Sciences. Prior to his appointment at the IOM, he was a senior research fellow at the Kennedy Institute of Ethics at Georgetown University and an associate in the Department of Health Policy and Management at Johns Hopkins University. He was previously an outside consultant to the National Center for Human Genome Research at the National Institutes of Health. Dr. Cook-Deegan served as the acting executive director of the Biomedical Ethics Advisory Committee of the U.S. Congress from December 1988 until October 1989. Before that, he was a senior associate at the Office of Technology Assessment (OTA) of the U.S. Congress, where he worked for six years. While at OTA, he directed the project "Mapping our Genes—Genome Projects: How Big? How Fast?" and subsequently obtained an award from the Alfred P. Sloan Foundation to write a book on the science and politics of the human genome. He is currently at work on that book and on establishing a public archive of the material gathered for it, under a grant from the National Science Foundation.

LEON EISENBERG received his M.D. from the University of Pennsylvania and did his internship at Mount Sinai Hospital in New York City. After a year as an instructor in physiology at the University of Pennsylvania and two years in the Army Medical Corps at Walter Reed Medical Center, he served as a resident in psychiatry at the Sheppard and Enoch Pratt Hospital and then as a fellow in child psychiatry at the Johns Hopkins Hospital under Professor Leo Kanner, whom he succeeded as chief of child psychiatry in 1961. His research interests include early infantile autism, the influence of the social environment on cognitive development, and the relationship between culture and mental disorder. He moved to Harvard in 1967 as chief of psychiatry at Massachusetts General Hospital, later becoming chairman of the Executive Committee of the Harvard Department of Psychiatry and Presley Professor of Psychiatry. In 1980, he assumed the chair of the newly created Department of Social Medicine, which brings the disciplines of anthropology, history, sociology, economics, political science, and law to bear on research and teaching in medicine.

DONALD S. FREDRICKSON, a graduate of the University of Michigan, began a career in biomedical research at Harvard Medical School before he moved to the National Institutes of Health (NIH) in 1953. After many years in both clinical and laboratory research and several leadership posts in the National Heart Institute, he became president of the Institute of Medicine in 1974. A year later, however, he returned to NIH to become its director ("just in time to reap the whirlwind from Asilomar") and to accept responsibility for the establishment of the NIH Guidelines for Recombinant DNA Research as the rules for conduct of genetic engineering in the United States. Resigning the directorship of NIH in 1981, Dr. Fredrickson later became president and chief executive officer of the Howard Hughes Medical Institute. At present, he divides his time between consulting and scholarship, including historical research and writing as a Scholar of the National Library of Medicine.

CARL W. GOTTSCHALK is a career investigator of the American Heart Association and Kenan Professor of Medicine and Physiology at the University of North Carolina, Chapel Hill. He is a renal physiologist and has made extensive use of micropuncture techniques in his research. He has been interested in public policy issues involving care of patients with renal disease and chaired the Bureau of the Budget's Committee on Chronic Kidney Disease. He is a member of the National Academy of Sciences, the Institute of Medicine, and the American Academy of Arts and Sciences.

KATHI E. HANNA is a senior analyst and project director at the congressional Office of Technology Assessment (OTA). She came to the

Institute of Medicine in March 1989 to direct this project and then returned to OTA in late 1990 to participate in assessments of biotechnology in a global economy, basic research for the 1990s, and the implications of population screening for cystic fibrosis. Dr. Hanna is also directing an assessment of the effects of estrogen deficiency on the health of women. Her previous work at OTA consists of science policy studies on such topics as demographics and the scientific work force, the regulatory environment for science, and research funding as an investment. Prior to her work at OTA, she was a science associate at the American Psychological Association, where she was responsible for oversight of policies related to the protection of human participants in research and policies on animal research, and the genetics coordinator at Children's Memorial Hospital in Chicago. Dr. Hanna received her A.B. in biology from Lafayette College, an M.S. in human genetics from Sarah Lawrence College, and a doctorate from the School of Business and Public Management, George Washington University. Her thesis focused on the use of analytical information by policymakers.

WALTER HARRELSON is Distinguished Professor of Hebrew Bible, emeritus, at Vanderbilt University and former dean of its Divinity School. He has written extensively on contemporary ethical questions, on interreligious dialogue, and on the relationship of religion and political life. He lectures widely on these questions as well as on the import of biblical religion for contemporary life. His books include *The Ten Commandments and Human Rights* (1980) and *Jews and Christians: A Troubled Family* (1990, with Rabbi Randall M. Falk).

WILLIAM HUBBARD, JR., received his baccalaureate degree from Columbia University after having completed the first two years of medical school at the University of North Carolina. From 1944 to 1959 he was a house officer and faculty member at New York University-Bellevue Medical Center. From 1959 to 1970 he was dean of the medical school of the University of Michigan. From 1970 through 1984 Dr. Hubbard was president of the Upjohn Company; he is now retired. Previously, he was a trustee of Columbia University, a member and chairman of the Board of Regents of the National Library of Medicine, a member of the National Science Board of the National Science Foundation, and president of the Association of American Medical Colleges. Dr. Hubbard is a member of the Institute of Medicine and a trustee of the W. K. Kellogg Foundation.

PATRICIA A. KING is professor of law at Georgetown University Law Center. She is a graduate of Wheaton College (1963) and Harvard Law School (1969). She specializes in family law and the relationship between biomedical ethics, law, and public policy, particularly reproduction. Professor King has served on numerous public bodies concerning biomedicine and public policy. They include the National Commission for Protection of Human Subjects of Biomedical and Behavioral Research, the President's Commission for the Study of Ethical Problems in Medicine and Biomedical and Behavioral Research, and the Human Fetal Tissue Transplantation Research Panel.

JEFFREY LEVI is a Washington-based health policy consultant. With degrees in government from Oberlin College and Cornell University, he has worked on AIDS policy issues for organizations such as the Institute of Medicine, Gay Men's Health Crisis, and AIDS Action Council. From 1983 to 1989, he served as political director and executive director of the National Gay and Lesbian Task Force, where he was chief lobbyist and spokesperson on AIDS and gay/lesbian civil rights issues. He has testified on AIDS policy issues before numerous congressional committees and served on various government advisory bodies.

ERNEST R. MAY is an authority on American diplomatic history and he has been a professor of history since 1963. He was dean of Harvard College from 1969 to 1971 and acting associate dean of the Faculty of Arts and Sciences at Harvard during the academic year 1971-1972. He was director of the Institute of Politics from 1971 to 1974 and chairman of the Department of History from 1976 to 1979. In 1981, he was named Charles Warren Professor of History. Professor May received his A.B. and Ph.D. from the University of California at Los Angeles. He is a member of the Council on Foreign Relations and a fellow of the American Academy of Arts and Sciences. He has been a consultant at various times to the Office of the Secretary of Defense, the National Security Council, the Lawrence Livermore National Laboratory, the National Endowment for the Humanities, the Smithsonian Institution, and various committees of the Congress. He is currently chairman of the Board of Visitors of the Defense Intelligence College. His publications in the areas of history and diplomacy are numerous.

DOROTHY NELKIN holds a university professorship at New York University, where she is also professor of sociology and affiliated professor in the School of Law. Her research focuses on controversial areas of science, technology, and medicine as a means of understanding their social and political implications and the relationship of science to the public. This work includes studies of antiscience movements, the social impact of new technologies, public policies concerning science and medicine, and media communication of science and risk. Most recently she has examined the social and ethical implications of the diagnostic tests that are emerging from research in genetics and the neurosciences. She has served on the Board of Directors of the American Association for the Advancement of Science and on the National Academy of Sciences Committee on a National Strategy for AIDS. She is currently a member of the Board of Medicine in the Public Interest and of the Council for the Advancement of Science Writing. She has been a Guggenheim fellow, a visiting scholar at the Russell Sage Foundation, and the Clare Boothe Luce Visiting Professor at New York University. Her books include *Controversy: The Politics of Technical Decisions*; *Science as Intellectual Property*; *The Creations Controversy*; *Workers at Risk*; *Selling Science: How the Press Covers Science and Technology*; *A Disease of Society: The Cultural Impact of AIDS* (with D. Willis), and *Dangerous Diagnostics: The Social Power of Biological Information* (with L. Tancredi).

STANLEY JOEL REISER is the Griff T. Ross Professor of Humanities and Technology in Health Care at the University of Texas Health Science Center, Houston. He received his education at Columbia University (A.B.), the State University of New York Downstate Medical Center (M.D.), and Kennedy School of Government, Harvard University (Ph.D.). His first academic post was on the faculty of Harvard University, holding appointments in the Medical School and the College, and also at Massachusetts General Hospital. His teaching and research centered on the humanistic and technological dimensions of health care. In 1982 he moved to Houston to become professor and director of the Program on Humanities and Technology in Health Care. His publications include *Medicine and the Reign of Technology*, *Ethics in Medicine*, and *The Machine at the Bedside*. He is currently co-editor of the *International Journal of Technology Assessment in Health Care*.

RICHARD A. RETTIG joined the professional staff of the Institute of Medicine (IOM), National Academy of Sciences, in 1987, first as director of the Council on Health Care Technology and more recently as director of the IOM study of the end-stage renal disease program of Medicare. Dr. Rettig received his bachelor's degree from the University of Washington in 1958 and his Ph.D. in political science from Massachusetts Institute of Technology in 1967. He has worked for the federal government and for the state of New Jersey, and he has held academic appointments at Cornell University, Ohio State University, and the Illinois Institute of Technology. Dr. Rettig was a senior social scientist with the RAND Corporation from 1975 through 1981 and has written extensively about the Medicare end-stage renal disease program and medical technology. He is the author of *Cancer Crusade: The Story of the National Cancer Act of 1971*.

PAUL SLOVIC is president of Decision Research of Eugene, Oregon, and a professor of psychology at the University of Oregon. During the past 15 years, Dr. Slovic and his associates have developed methods for describing risk perceptions and measuring their impacts on individuals, industry, and society. Their work has included creation of a taxonomic system to understand and predict perceived risk, attitudes toward regulation, and impacts resulting from accidents or failures. Dr. Slovic has been a consultant to numerous companies and government agencies. He is a member of the National Council on Radiation Protection and Measurements and a past president of the Society for Risk Analysis.

Index

Biomedical science is a double-edged sword. While providing advances in the treatment and quality of life for victims of disease, it also raises agonizing and thorny questions: Should scientists be allowed to pursue research on treatment of disease using fetal tissue from induced abortions? Should terminally ill patients be allowed to choose their own treatment, even if the safety and effectiveness of those treatments are unknown? Should American women be denied access to a nonsurgical abortifacient because some groups feel its use is immoral?

Such questions used to be the province of science and medicine. Today, biomedical research is the focus of public scrutiny and debate. Scientific consensus sometimes is forced to concede to political powers or to the organized activities of public interest groups. Decisions regarding the application of biomedical advances often have no precedent, making choices about how to proceed exceedingly difficult. As a result, decisions about biomedical research are often shaped by politics—personal and institutional—and by confusion and uncertainty on the part of the public. As researchers make more advances in life-saving technology and genetic manipulation, the questions society must face are likely to become even more complex.

We do have some important guidance, however, in the form of several recent decisions, arrived at through arduous give-and-take. In this book from the Institute of Medicine, six landmark cases offer insight into how we might confront future decisions more productively.

These highly readable case studies focus not on the particular outcomes but on the *process* of decision making, how the parties involved exchanged information and arrived at a course of action.

In the case of RU-486, the "French abortion pill," the influence of special interest groups exerted enormous influence. On the other hand,